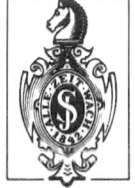

Investigational Techniques in Oncology

Edited by
Norman M. Bleehen

With 103 Figures

Springer-Verlag
London Berlin Heidelberg New York
Paris Tokyo

Professor Norman M. Bleehen, FRCP, FRCR, Honorary FACR,
Cancer Research Campaign Professor of Clinical Oncology;
Honorary Director MRC Clinical Oncology and
Radiotherapeutics Unit, University of Cambridge School of
Clinical Medicine, Department of Clinical Oncology and
Radiotherapeutics, Addenbrooke's Hospital, Hills Road,
Cambridge CB2 2QQ, UK.

Library of Congress Cataloging-in-Publication Data.
Investigational techniques in oncology.
Edited papers from a symposium held in London in February 1986, sponsored by
the Royal College of Radiologists.
Includes bibliographies and index.
1. Cancer – Diagnosis – Congresses. 2. Cancer – Research – Techniques –
Congresses. 3. Diagnostic imaging – Congresses. 4. Radiology, Medical –
Congresses. I. Bleehen, Norman M., 1930–   . II. Royal College of
Radiologists (Great Britain) [DNLM: 1. Neoplasms – diagnosis –
congresses. 2. Neoplasms – radiography – congresses. QA 241 I62
1986] RC270.I53 1987 616.99′4075 86–31429

ISBN-13: 978-1-4471-1436-9   e-ISBN-13: 978-1-4471-1434-5
DOI: 10.1007/978-1-4471-1434-5

© Springer-Verlag Berlin Heidelberg 1987

Softcover reprint of the hardcover 1st edition 1987

Typeset by Wilmaset, Birkenhead, Wirral
Printed by Henry Ling, The Dorset Press, Dorchester

2128/3916-543210

Preface

The eighth annual multidisciplinary symposium on clinical oncology organised by the Royal College of Radiologists discussed the subject of investigational techniques in oncology. It was held in London in February 1986. This volume collects together the edited texts of the papers which were presented at the meeting, together with the George Edelstyn memorial lecture given by Professor J. Einhorn.

Clinicians rely very heavily on pathologists and radiologists to help with the diagnosis and staging of patients who present with malignant tumours. The conventional techniques to which we have become accustomed are fast being supplemented by exciting new approaches. These have moved very rapidly from being purely experimental techniques to being a part of routine clinical practice. Some of these new approaches have been highlighted in this symposium.

Recent advances in molecular biology have produced various specific techniques for looking at phenotypic changes in cells as detected by immunohistochemical probes. Visualisation of genes and their transcripts in human biopsies has become a real possibility using a wide and increasing range of molecular probes. Some of the advantages of these techniques and their potential for the future are presented here.

The radiological techniques of conventional X-rays, nuclear medicine techniques and ultrasound are being complemented, and indeed in some cases overtaken, by the newer techniques of magnetic resonance imaging, computerised tomography and positron emission tomography. Techniques such as digital subtraction angiography are aiding the expanding horizons of interventional radiology. This volume highlights some of these areas of interest to the oncologist.

The problems of assessing image comparisons from a statistical point of view are also discussed. This is an area often ignored in clinical investigations but has been quite rightly emphasised as essential for the comparison of the various techniques discussed.

The George Edelstyn memorial lecture with which this volume concludes considers some of the problems facing the oncologist and the impact that new diagnostic techniques have on those problems. It is hoped that all the papers presented here will stimulate further interest and activity in clinical oncology. This is a rapidly moving field, but the message of these presentations should be of considerable value for some time.

I wish to express my thanks to all the speakers for making the symposium a success and agreeing to provide manuscripts for publication. Mr Michael Jackson of Springer-Verlag has continued to give advice and support in the production of this volume. I should also like to thank my secretaries, Miss Gillian Pickering and Mrs Fiona Brown, and my research associate, Mrs Anne Anderson, for help with the organisation of the meeting and the editing of the manuscripts. Finally my thanks are due to Mr A. J. Cowles, General Secretary of the Royal College of Radiologists, and to his staff, who contributed to the organisation and management of the symposium.

Royal College of Radiologists   Norman M. Bleehen
38 Portland Place, London, W1N 3DG

April 1986

Contents

List of Senior Authors

K. Dewbury
Department of Radiology, Southampton General Hospital,
Shirley, Southampton SO9 4XY, UK

A.K. Dixon
Department of Radiology, University of Cambridge,
Addenbrooke's Hospital, Cambridge CB2 2QQ, UK

J. Einhorn
Director, Radiumhemmet, Karolinska Hospital, S104 01,
Stockholm, Sweden

L.S. Freedman
MRC Clinical Oncology and Radiotherapuetics Unit, Medical
Research Council Centre, Hills Road, Cambridge CB2 2QH, UK

D. Irving
Department of Radiology, Lewisham Hospital, High Street,
Lewisham, London SE13 6LH, UK

R.J. Johnson
Department of Diagnostic Radiology, Christie Hospital & Holt
Radium Institute, Wilmslow Road, Withington, Manchester M20
9BX, UK

T. Jones
Medical Research Council Cyclotron Unit, Hammersmith
Hospital, Du Cane Road, London W12 0HS, UK

J.O'D. McGee
Nuffield Department of Pathology, John Radcliffe Hospital,
Headington, Oxford OX3 9DU, UK

J. McIvor
Department of Radiology, Charing Cross Hospital, Fulham Palace
Road, London W6 8RF, UK

M.V. Merrick
Medical Radioisotope Department, Western General Hospital,
Crewe Road, Edinburgh EH4 2XU, UK

J.M. Polak
Department of Histochemistry, Royal Postgraduate Medical
School, Hammersmith Hospital, Du Cane Road, London W12
0HS, UK

1 Techniques for the Determination of Tumour Neuroendocrine Differentiation and for the Localisation of Intracellular Organelles Involved in Peptide Synthesis, Storage and Release

J. M. Polak and S. R. Bloom

Introduction

The discovery that peptide hormones are produced by specialised endocrine cells diffusely dispersed throughout the body and intermingled within non-endocrine elements (Ballesta et al. 1985) (e.g. the endocrine system of the gut or of the lung) revolutionised previous concepts of glandular (e.g. thyroid, parathyroid and adrenal cortex) endocrinology. It is now generally accepted that the endocrine system is a component of a larger, diffuse neuroendocrine system which consists of peptide-producing endocrine cells and nerves distributed throughout the body. Peptides released from endocrine cells act in the main as circulating or local hormones and peptides present in nerves are regarded as putative neurotransmitters.

Advances in the clinical and biochemical understanding of hormone-producing tumours have led recently to the earlier and more frequent recognition of this class of neoplasms (Polak and Bloom 1985). The terminology proposed for their derivative tumours is varied and confusing (Polak and Bloom 1985). These tumours have been variously termed APUDomas (peptide-producing endocrine cells are synonymous with Pearse's APUD, i.e. Amine Precursor Uptake and Decarboxylation, cells); islet cell tumours, as a good proportion of these tumours originate in the pancreatic islets; and carcinoids, a term originally proposed by Oberndorfer to indicate the carcinoma-like appearance of this special group of tumours. Finally, the comprehensive term of peptide-producing neuroendocrine tumours has lately been adopted. Alternatively, neuroendocrine neoplasms have been named, particularly by clinicians, after the peptide identified to be the main product of a given tumour, as for example insulinomas and glucagonomas. Some tumours are also designated by individual names, such as small cell carcinoma of the lung and medullary carcinoma of the thyroid.

Modern morphological methods have to be adapted for the detailed investigation of neuroendocrine tumours. It is nowadays possible to assess accurately their degree of differentiation and also to visualise intracellular events leading to normal or abnormal patterns of peptide synthesis and release. Moreover, many so-called silent tumours remain clinically and biochemically undiagnosed and it is the duty of the pathologist to provide accurate information about this neuroendocrine differentiation of the tumour.

We will therefore first give an account of the techniques available for the determination of neuroendocrine differentiation and for the analysis of the intracellular apparatus involved in peptide synthesis and storage. We will then describe the main morphological features revealed after using the techniques detailed. The final section deals with the pathology of one of the most common neuroendocrine tumours, the small cell carcinoma of the lung.

Techniques for Assessing Neuroendocrine Differentiation

Conventional histological stains provide useful information, even though these slow-growing, potentially malignant, tumours show few of the cellular features of malignancy as mitoses and atypias are rare. However, it is important to assess the degree of local, blood vessel and lymphatic invasion. Most neuroendocrine tumours present classical carcinoid features, with fairly regular tumour cells (Fig. 1.1) arranged in ribbons, as irregular masses or glandular structures, separated by connective tissue bands where amyloid deposits are found frequently.

Accurate determination of neuroendocrine differentiation is routinely achieved by the application of specialised methods, including silver impregnation procedures and conventional electron microscopy. Immunocytochemistry may be applied at both light and electron microscopical levels directed at specific markers (e.g. peptide/amine) and more general ones (e.g. neuron specific enolase, chromogranin).

Silver Impregnation Procedures

Numerous histological and histochemical methods have been proposed and are still being used for the demonstration of peptide-producing endocrine cells and their derivative tumours. For many of these empirical stains the chemical or physicochemical background is still unknown. The procedures most frequently used can be subdivided broadly into argyrophil and argentaffin reactions.

Cells displaying argyrophilia retain silver ions from the impregnation solution, but visible metallic silver only appears after a subsequent reducing process brought about by an external agent or agents. Cells showing argentaffinity

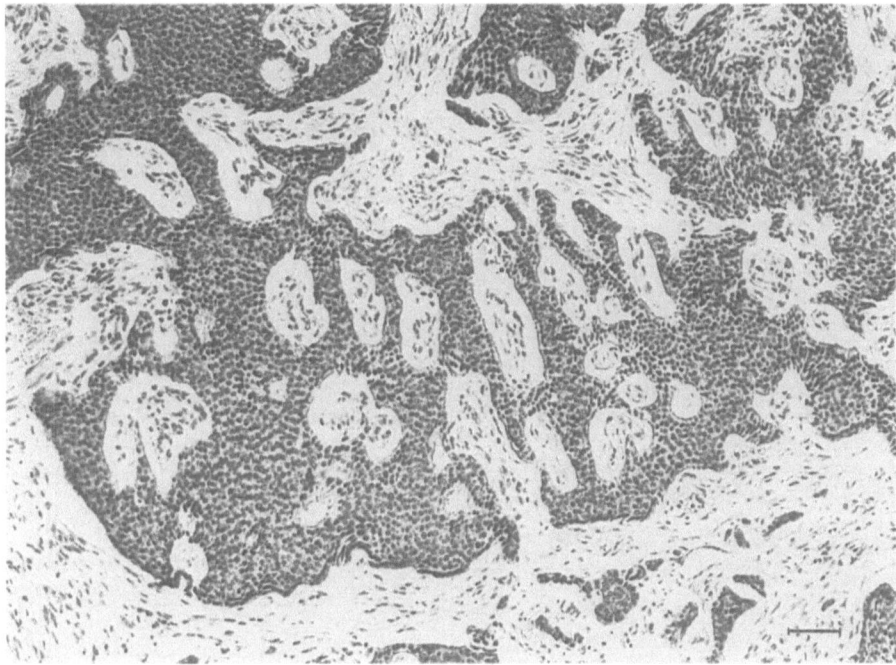

Fig. 1.1. Formalin fixed, wax-embedded 5 μm section of an ileal carcinoid stained with haematoxylin and eosin. The uniform, polygonal cells, with round central nuclei, are arranged mainly in sheets separated by fibrovascular stroma. Scale bar represents 100 μm.

contain one or more chemical substances which retain silver ions from an ammoniacal silver solution, and reduce them to metallic silver. In contrast to the argyrophil reaction, the chemistry of argentaffin staining is better understood. It would appear that serotonin (5-hydroxytryptamine; 5HT) reacts with paraformaldehyde to cause a silver reaction.

Some variants of the original Masson argentaffin reaction are frequently used. Numerous argyrophil stains have been proposed. Of these the most reliable and commonly used is that introduced by Lars Grimelius (Grimelius et al. 1985), which stains most endocrine cell types and tumours (Fig. 1.2). The staining is characteristically granular and occurs in most granule-containing endocrine cells or tumours. Poorly granulated tumours are rarely argyrophilic.

Conventional Electron Microscopy

Peptide-producing tumour cells contain a variable number of intracellular electron-dense secretory granules (Fig. 1.3), which are characteristic of neuroendocrine differentiation. These are spherical or polymorphic (average size ranging from 100 to 350 nm) and are surrounded by a limiting membrane that is either closely apposed, or loosely attached leaving a clear halo between the dense core and the membrane.

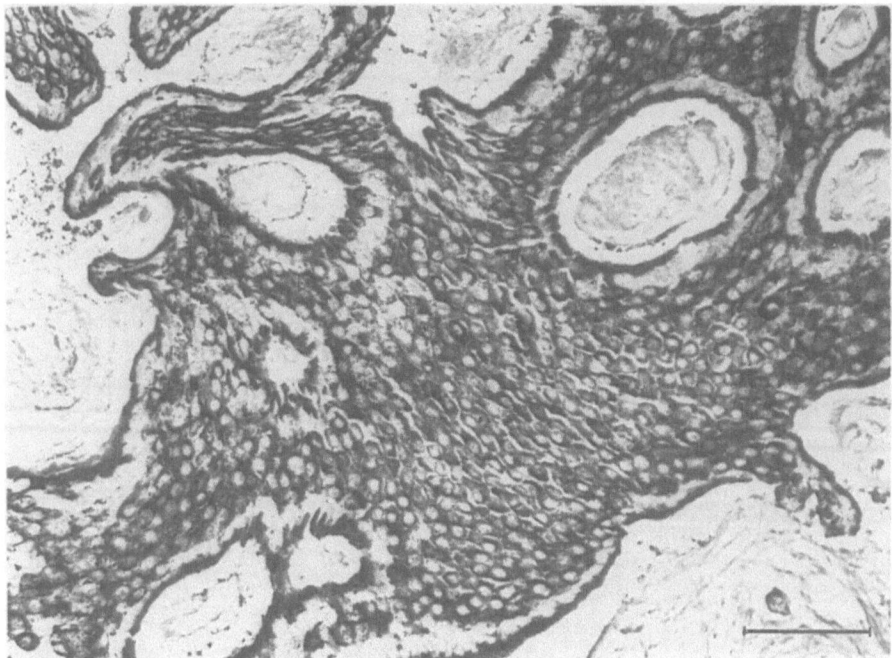

Fig. 1.2. Formalin fixed, wax-embedded 5 μm section of an ileal carcinoid tumour showing argyrophilia. Grimelius silver impregnation method. Scale bar represents 100 μm.

Immunocytochemistry

Immunocytochemistry has revolutionised the study of neuroendocrine tumours. Polyclonal sera and monoclonal antibodies are now widely available, and the staining can mostly be performed using conventional fixation and embedding procedures, both for light and for electron microscopy (Fig. 1.4). A number of enhancement methods have recently been proposed (Van Noorden and Polak 1985). These include the repeat application of the primary or labelled antibody layers, as well as the intensification of the peroxidase–antiperoxidase (PAP)–diaminobenzidine (DAB)/H_2O_2 reaction by gold chloride, and the novel immunogold–silver procedure. All these methods allow the visualisation of antigens present in low concentrations.

General Neuroendocrine Markers

The last 5 years has witnessed an increasing interest in the search for, and use of, general neuroendocrine markers. Neuron specific enolase was one of the first general neuroendocrine markers to be studied. Antibodies to neuron specific enolase revealed the simultaneous presence of this enzyme in peptide-containing

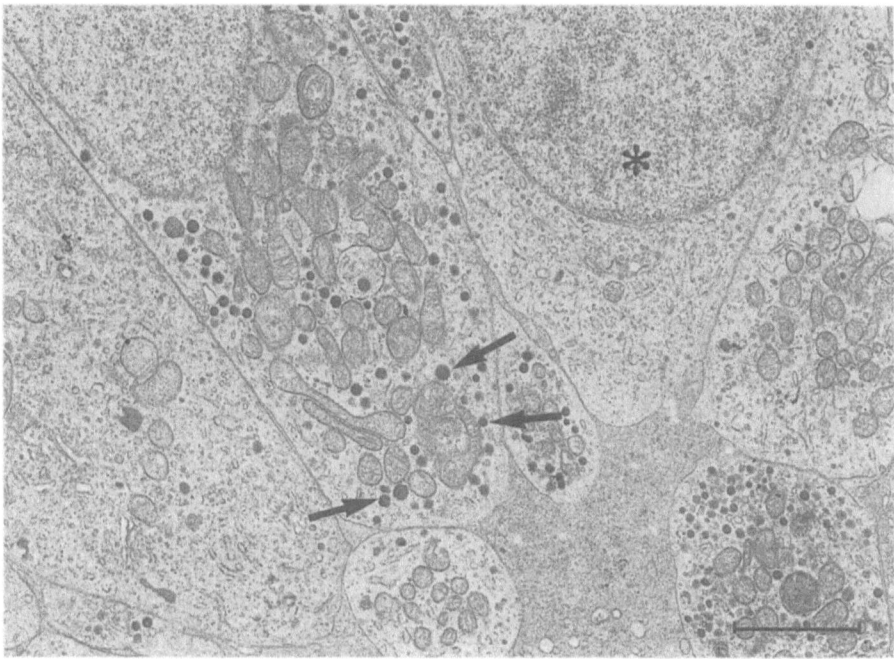

Fig. 1.3. Electron micrograph of a liver metastasis from a human gastrin-producing tumour with the primary in the head of the pancreas. Some cells are heavily granulated (*arrows*) with many mitochondria, whereas others (*asterisk*) have few, if any, granules and a low mitochondrial index. Glutaraldehyde/osmium fixation. Scale bar represents 1.2 µm.

endocrine cells and nerves. Antisera to other markers were subsequently introduced and are similarly capable of staining nerves and/or endocrine cells. The main characteristics of the most widely used neuroendocrine markers are summarised in Table 1.1.

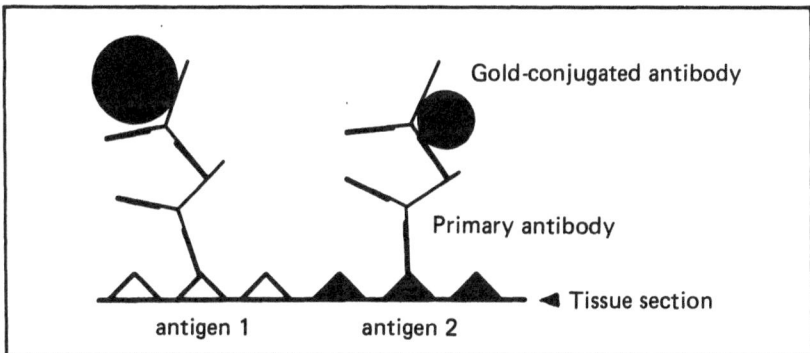

Fig. 1.4. Double immunogold staining procedure. Two primary antisera raised in different species are applied simultaneously to a tissue section. Sites of antigen–antibody complex formation are localised using second layer anti-species IgG adsorbed to two populations of colloidal gold particles.

Table 1.1. Characteristics of general neuroendocrine markers

Marker	Characteristics					
	Endocrine	Neural	Glial	Granular	Cytoplasmic	Cytoskeletal
Chromogranin	+	±	−	+	−	−
7B2	+	NK	−	NK	NK	NK
NSE	+	+	−	−	+	−
PGP 9.5	+	+	−	NK	NK	NK
Neurofilaments	−	+	−	−	−	+
S100	−	−	+	−	−	+
GFAP	−	−	+	−	−	+

Key
+, established.
−, disproved.
±, certain antibodies react.
NK, not known.

Neuron specific enolase (NSE)

Neuron specific enolase is an isozyme of the glycolytic enzyme enolase originally extracted from rat brain and subsequently found by immunocytochemistry to be localised to neurons (Polak and Marangos 1984). Antibodies to NSE were later found to immunostain all components of the diffuse neuroendocrine system.

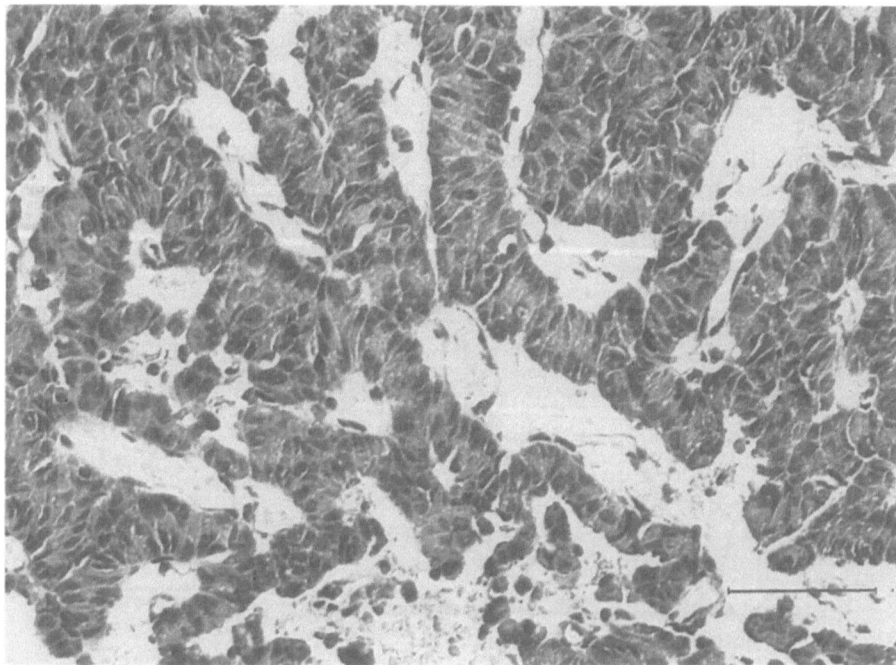

Fig. 1.5. Neuron specific enolase immunostaining of a pancreatic endocrine tumour which secreted vasoactive intestinal polypeptide. Bouin's solution fixed, wax-embedded 5 µm section. Immunoperoxidase (PAP) technique, haematoxylin counterstain. Scale bar represents 100 µm.

NSE is an enzyme apparently unrelated to the presence of secretory granules. Because of its putative involvement in metabolism and its non-granular, cytoplasmic localisation its presence may indicate the functional state of an endocrine cell or a tumour. The staining is often rather diffuse in the cytoplasm, with poorly demarcated areas (Fig. 1.5). It is a particularly useful stain for poorly granulated tumours, such as the small cell carcinoma of the lung. It is very important to be selective when choosing antibodies to NSE. It is a large protein of molecular weight 78 000 and therefore populations of antibodies are likely to react to many separate epitopes of these molecules. The protein, which is not yet synthetically produced, is currently extracted from animal or human brain. Therefore, it is likely that the antigen will be contaminated with material other than pure NSE, and thus spurious staining to non-neuronal elements could be expected. Monoclonal antibodies to NSE are now becoming available and it is predicted that a good mixture of high-quality monoclonal antibodies which would recognise several epitopes of the molecule will be of excellent value for morphologists.

Chromogranin

Chromogranin is one of a family of proteins first shown to be present in adrenal medullary cells and later characterised as a protein of molecular weight 68 000. Chromogranin coexists with catecholamines in the storage granules of adrenal medullary cells and in sympathetic nerves. It has been reported that it is released from catecholamine-containing tissue and its concentration in cells has been used as a means of monitoring sympatho-adrenal function. Although the function of chromogranin has yet to be fully established, it is thought to stabilise the intragranular protein complexes. Polyclonal antisera, staining both sympathetic nerves, adrenal medullary cells and other peptide-producing endocrine cells, as well as monoclonal antibodies staining primarily peptide-producing endocrine cells, have been raised to purified chromogranin. Lloyd's group has carried out extensive studies in order to assess the potential of chromogranin monoclonal antibodies as a marker for peptide-producing endocrine cells (Wilson and Lloyd 1984). Studies carried out so far indicate that chromogranin antibodies stain all endocrine cell types, including those of the gastrointestinal tract (Facer et al. 1985) (Fig. 1.6), the thyroid and adrenal medulla. Ultrastructurally, chromogranin is present in dense-cored secretory granules (Varndell et al. 1985) and thus chromogranin immunostaining is related to the presence of secretory granules within the cells of the diffuse neuroendocrine system.

PGP 9.5

PGP 9.5 is a recently extracted soluble brain protein of molecular weight 27 000. It would appear to be a reasonably good marker for the immunocytochemical identification of neuroendocrine tumours, although possibly less reliable than the demonstration of chromogranin or NSE (Rode et al. 1985). PGP 9.5 is newly discovered and thus further assessment remains to be carried out.

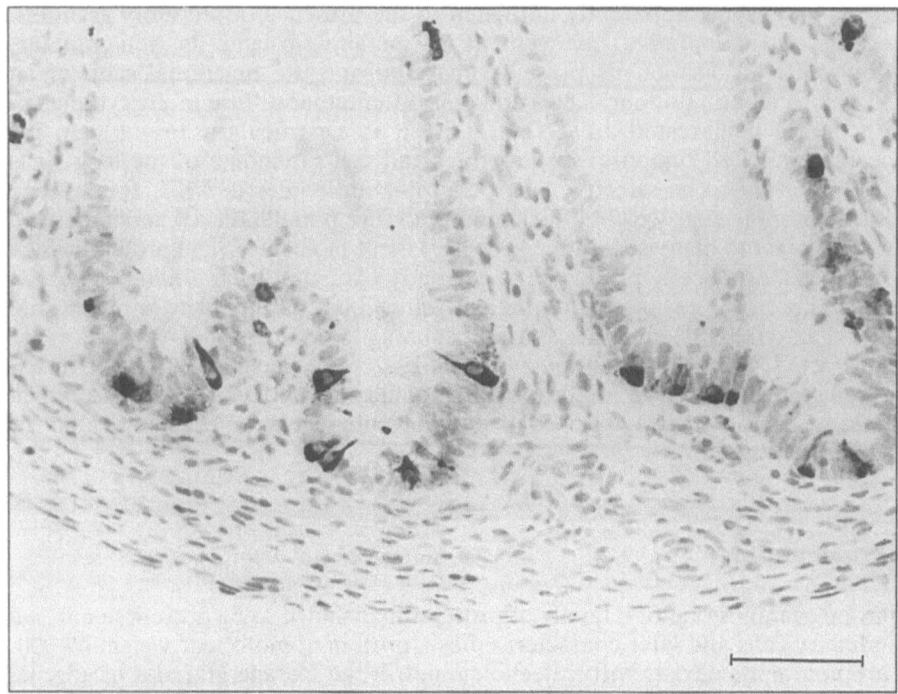

Fig. 1.6. Chromogranin-immunoreactive endocrine cells in human small intestine. Bouin's solution fixed, wax-embedded 5 μm section. Immunoperoxidase (PAP) technique, haematoxylin counterstain. Scale bar represents 100 μm.

7B2 (APPG)

7B2 is a large protein originally discovered by Chrétien's group from the anterior pituitary of the pig (Iguchi et al. 1984), hence its alternative name APPG. Its name derives from the initial chromatographic peak obtained during analysis of extractable pituitary material. Antibodies to a segment of this protein (see Fig. 1.7) have now been raised and have been found to be excellent markers for insulin-producing cells and their derivative tumours (Facer et al. 1986) (Fig. 1.8a,b).

Markers for Nerves and Supporting Elements

The variety of nerves containing not only classical neurotransmitters such as acetylcholine and noradrenaline, 5-hydroxytryptamine and gamma-aminobutyric acid, but also putative peptide neurotransmitters, can now be fully and extensively visualised by the use of polyclonal sera and monoclonal antibodies to neurofilaments (Bishop et al. 1985, Hacker et al. 1985). Neurofilaments belong to the group of cytoskeletal proteins known as intermediate filaments (Dahl and Bignami 1986, Trojanowski 1986) and have been shown to exist in different forms of approximate molecular weights 68 000, 150 000 and 200 000. These

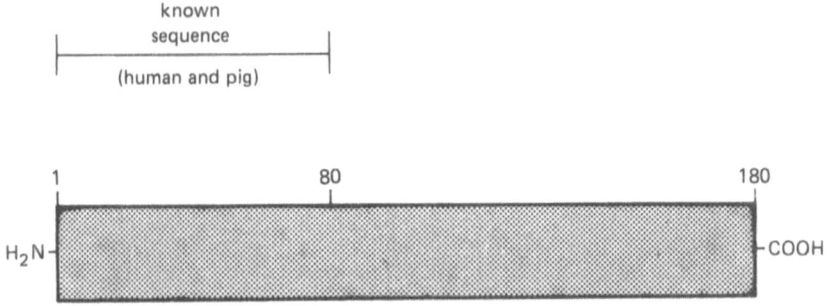

Fig. 1.7. The structure of 7B2.

antibodies have been extensively used in immunocytochemistry to visualise the entire innervation and its derivative tumours. Antibodies to proteins in the supporting elements, such as glial and Schwann cells, are also available. These detect glial fibrillary acidic protein (GFAP) and S100. GFAP is known to be present in astrocytes and well-differentiated neural tumours, while S100 is a good marker for both Schwann and glial cells of peripheral tissue and sheath tumours. S100 antibodies are also good reagents for identifying melanomas.

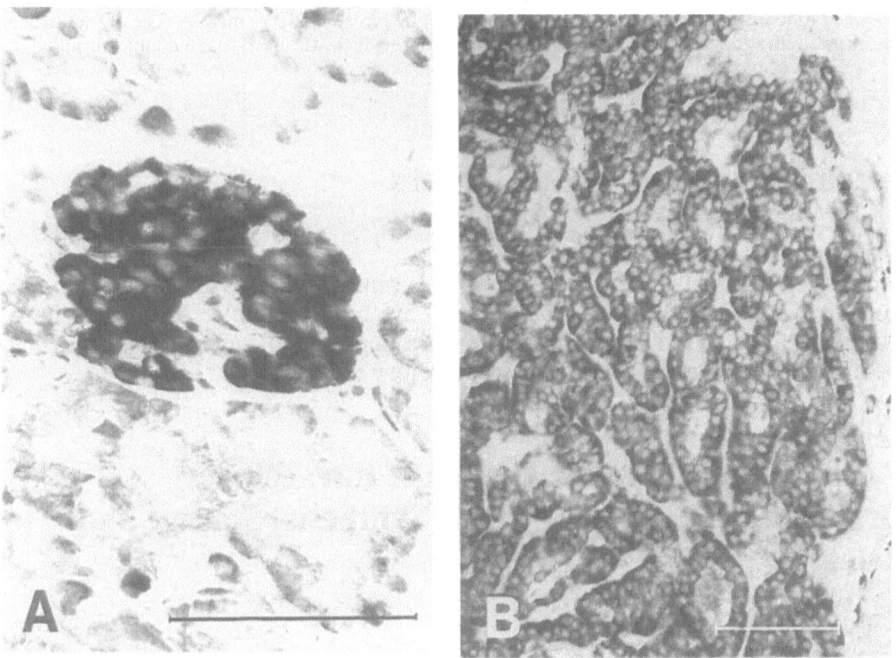

Fig. 1.8.a 7B2-immunoreactive islet in human pancreas. *p*-Benzoquinone vapour fixed, wax-embedded 5 μm section. Immunoperoxidase (PAP) technique, haematoxylin counterstain. Scale bar represents 100 μm. **b** 7B2-immunoreactive insulinoma in transgenic mouse pancreas. Bouin's solution fixed, wax-embedded 5 μm section. Immunoperoxidase (PAP) technique, haematoxylin counterstain. Scale bar represents 100 μm.

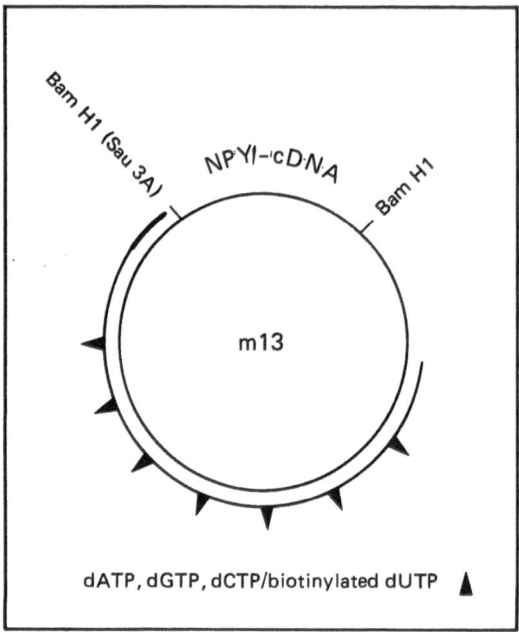

Fig. 1.9. Schematic representation of a single-stranded, biotinylated, complementary DNA (cDNA) probe which recognises part of the neuropeptide tyrosine (NPY) mRNA. The cDNA probe was inserted into the single-stranded vector plasmid M13 which was itself made double-stranded in the presence of biotinylated dUTP.

Specific Neuroendocrine Markers

Antibodies to regulatory peptides and amines (which can be used with conventionally fixed and embedded tissue) are fully available. Antibodies have also been raised to the various regions of pro-peptide molecules, thus increasing the chance of accurate localisation of secretory product.

Techniques for the Localisation of Intracellular Organelles Involved in Peptide Synthesis, Storage and Release

Visualisation of Messenger RNA Directing Peptide Synthesis

Advances in recombinant DNA technology have now made it possible to identify specific messenger RNA (mRNA) molecules by using cell-free translation systems. DNA probes, complementary to the specific mRNA molecules, can be constructed, and by the technique of in situ hybridisation histochemistry, mRNA can be-visualised (Coghlan et al. 1985). In combination with immunocytochemistry, this may give some information on intracellular messenger processing (for further details see Chapter 2).

The genomic DNA is transcribed into a nuclear heterogenous messenger RNA (hmRNA) which is then enzymically transcribed, clipped and reassembled into a cytoplasmic messenger product involved in directing peptide synthesis. Nascent secretory products are then assembled at the rough endoplasmic reticulum. This process occurs during or immediately after the initiation of biosynthesis.

Radiolabelled or biotinylated complementary DNA/RNA probes can now be constructed and may be used to visualise intracellular mRNA (see Fig. 1.9). We have carried out visualisation studies using a single-stranded DNA probe complementary to the RNA directing synthesis of the pro-neuropeptide tyrosine (NPY) system (Fig. 1.9) in phaeochromocytoma tissues (Varndell et al. 1984). Phaeochromocytomas are known to produce large concentrations of NPY (Adrian et al. 1983). A similar procedure has been used by us to detect mRNA directing somatostatin synthesis in cell lines known to produce large concentrations of somatostatin. The technique was used at both light and electron microscopical levels. In the latter application the classical avidin–biotin–peroxidase reaction product was detected at the rough endoplasmic reticulum. An oligonucleotide probe (30 mer) complementary to the mid-region of

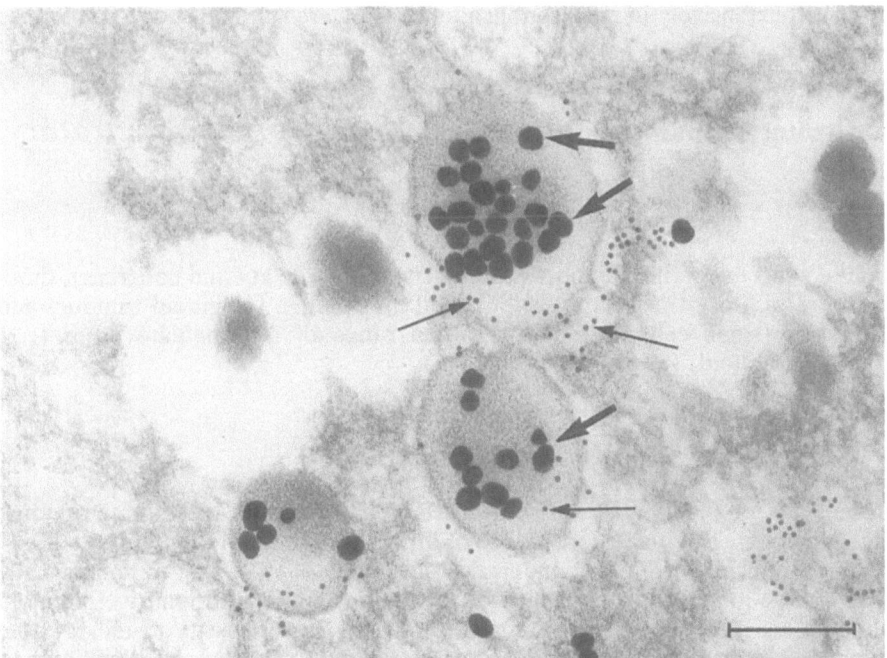

Fig. 1.10. Electron micrograph of glucagon (40 nm gold; *thick arrows*) and glicentin (10 nm gold; *thin arrows*) localised to different compartments within single pancreatic A cell secretory granules. Double immunogold staining procedure. Scale bar represents 250 nm.

mammalian bombesin mRNA was also used and labelled with ^{32}P by the T_4-polynucleotide kinase method. This probe was used on cultures of a small cell carcinoma of the lung.

Ultrastructural Features of Peptide Formation, Storage and Release

Electron immunocytochemistry using region-specific antibodies to active peptides and their precursor forms (Fig. 1.10) (Varndell and Polak 1985) has enabled the visualisation of stages in peptide formation, from early pro-peptide synthesis in the Golgi area to storage of the final product in mature secretory granules. Secretory phenomena have also been observed. This visualisation is improved when employed in combination with special ultrastructural procedures such as ultrathin frozen sections and low-temperature embedding media, measures designed to preserve the integrity of labile antigens.

Main Features of Peptide-producing Neuroendocrine Tumours

The main features of peptide-producing neuroendocrine tumours have been described extensively in many publications. They are summarised in Table 1.2.

Pathology of Neuroendocrine Tumours of the Respiratory Tract

Unlike neuroendocrine tumours of other sites (e.g. the gut and pancreas), those of the respiratory tract can be subdivided into benign (carcinoid tumour) and malignant (small cell carcinoma), with a range of intermediate types (e.g. atypical carcinoid) (Sheppard et al. 1985).

Carcinoid Tumours

About 12% of all carcinoids arise in the lung but less than 1% of lung tumours are carcinoids. The highest incidence of bronchial carcinoid occurs in the 31–40 years age group, with a preponderance in females (62%). The tumour usually arises in the main bronchi but may be located in the lung periphery. Carcinoid tumours are generally well demarcated and may either just protrude into the bronchial lumen or may be predominantly endobronchial in their growth pattern. Microscopically, carcinoids consist of small regular cells with vesicular nuclei and eosinophilic granular cytoplasm (Fig. 1.11). The cells are arranged in a mosaic, trabecular or alveolo-papillary pattern. Mitotic figures are usually

Table 1.2. Characteristics of neuroendocrine tumours

Site	Tumour nomenclature	Main peptide/ amine product(s)[a]	Approximate frequency[b]	Malignancy	Typical clinical features
Pancreas	Islet cell	Insulin	1:150000	10%	Hypoglycaemia
		Glucagon	1:10000000	60%	Skin rash, anaemia, diabetes
		Gastrin	1:450000	70%–90%	Zollinger-Ellison syndrome
		VIP	1:2000000	50%70%	Watery diarrhoea
		Somatostatin	<1:100000000	Not known	None
		PP	<1:100000000	One case[e]	None
Foregut	Carcinoid	5-hydroxytryptophan, histamine	0.2%–30%[d]	30%	Upper gastrointestinal bleeding
Midgut	Carcinoid	Serotonin, substance P	60%–90%[d]	40%–75%	Carcinoid syndrome
Hindgut	Carcinoid	Not known	0.5%[d]	8%–50%	None
Thyroid	Medullary carcinoma	Calcitonin, CGRP, katacalcin, somatostatin, ACTH, bombesin	1:250000	100%	Diarrhoea, carcinoid or Cushing's syndrome
Pituitary	Adenoma	ACTH, LH, FSH, TSH, GH	10%[e]	Rare	Endocrine syndrome
Adrenal	Phaeochromocytoma	Noradrenaline, adrenaline, NPY, met- and leu-enkephalin, galanin	0.5%†	6%–12%	Hypertension

[a] Per capita, unless stated.
[b] VIP, vasoactive intestinal polypeptide; PP, pancreatic polypeptide; CGRP, calcitonin gene-related peptide; ACTH, adrenocorticotrophic hormone; LH, luteinising hormone; FSH, follicle stimulating hormone; TSH, thyroid stimulating hormone; GH, growth hormone; NPY, neuropeptide Y.
[c] Only one case reported: Ljungberg et al. (1981).
[d] Percentage of gastrointestinal neoplasms.
[e] Percentage of intracranial neoplasms.
[f] Percentage of hypertensive patients.
Sources (for Approximate frequency and Malignancy): Klöppel and Heitz (1984), Wilander (1984), Schottenfeld and Gershman (1977), Doniach (1977), Ashley (1978).

infrequent or absent, but atypical variants characterised by cellular polymorphism, nuclear atypia and mitotic figures have been described. At the ultrastructural level the main feature associated with all carcinoids is the presence of large numbers of dense-cored neurosecretory granules in the cytoplasm of virtually all tumour cells (Fig. 1.11). The majority of carcinoids contain spherical neurosecretory granules (140–170 nm in diameter) similar to those found in endocrine cells of the normal adult respiratory epithelium. However, polymorphic and large spherical granules have also been described. Only one type of granule occurs in each cell, but tumours may be composed of one or more cell types. When the tumour cells line glands, they possess microcilia and the neurosecretory granules are frequently concentrated towards one pole of the cell. Bronchial carcinoids grow slowly and have a low malignancy potential. Atypical carcinoids have a worse prognosis.

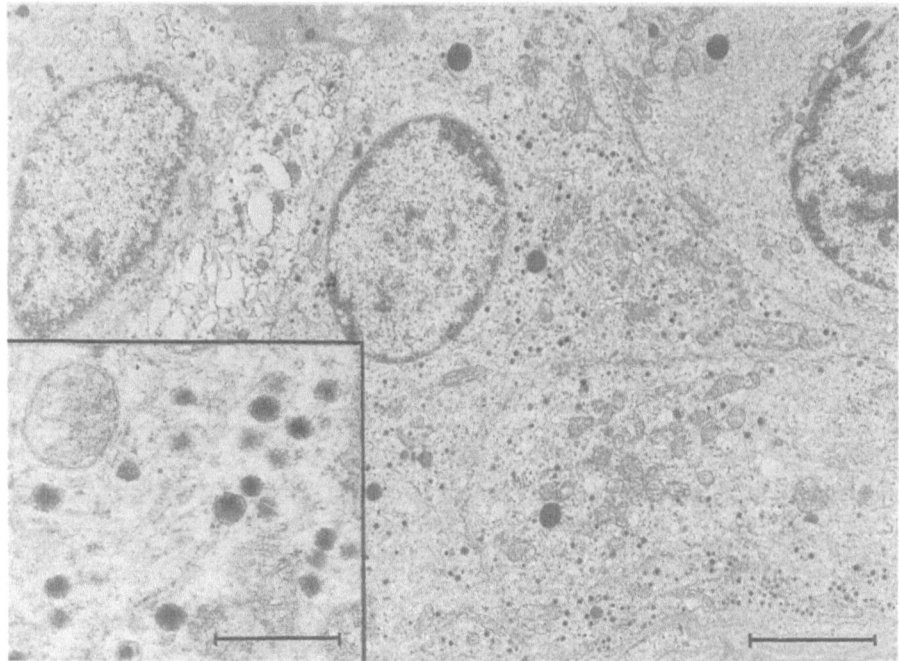

Fig. 1.11.   Electron micrograph of bronchial carcinoid, exhibiting cells with few, electron-dense, spherical granules (130–180 nm diameter). Glutaraldehyde/osmium fixation. Scale bars represent 2 μm and (insert) 750 nm.

Small Cell Carcinoma

Small cell carcinoma comprises about 20% of bronchial carcinomas. Many workers grouped them with other undifferentiated carcinomas until Azzopardi's classic paper (Azzopardi 1959) established them as a distinct entity. The revised WHO histological classification of lung tumours has divided them into two main types depending on cell size. The oat cell type (Fig. 1.12), consists of small oat-shaped cells with a finely granular chromatin pattern, an absence of nucleoli and a thin ring of cytoplasm. The intermediate cell type is composed of slightly larger cells with nuclei similar to the oat cell type but with more abundant cytoplasm. Secretory granules are not abundant and are scattered throughout the cytoplasm. In view of this the best general marker for the determination of neuroendocrine differentiation is the use of antibodies to NSE.

The cell of origin of neuroendocrine tumours of the lung has been suggested to be a mucosal endocrine cell from the lining epithelium of the respiratory tract, variously termed the Feyrter, Kultchizky or APUD cell. This cell occurs singly or in groups (neuroepithelial bodies of Lauweryns) (Lauweryns et al. 1972). Endocrine cells occur from the larynx down to the smallest bronchioli and alveoli and are principally found in the developing lung. The morphology of the electron-dense secretory granules permits subdivision into at least three separate cell types. Endocrine cells of the lung can be stained with antibodies to NSE (Wharton et al. 1981) and to PGP 9.5. In man, a subpopulation of these cells react to antibodies to mammalian bombesin (Wharton et al. 1978) (Fig. 1.13). Mammalian bombesin is a 27 amino acid peptide which shares C-terminus homology with amphibian bombesin and also with neuromedin C (see Fig. 1.14). The finding of a particularly large concentration of mammalian bombesin immunoreactivity in endocrine cells of the developing human lung (Wharton et al. 1978) led to the postulation of a growth-promoting role for this peptide. This was later supported by the finding of particularly low concentrations of bombesin immunoreactive material in hypoplastic lungs associated with the respiratory distress syndrome (Ghatei et al. 1983) (Fig. 1.15). The finding of a large concentration of immunoreactive bombesin in a rapidly growing small cell carcinoma of the lung further supported this contention (Moody et al. 1981, Sorenson et al. 1982). Evidence is now quite firm for mammalian bombesin playing a growth-promoting role (Cuttitta et al. 1985). This includes data from a number of experimental procedures on tumour cell lines, such as growth enhancement following the addition of bombesin to tumour cells in vitro (Rosengurt and Sinnett-Smith 1983), and growth suppression by the inclusion of specific monoclonal antibodies to bombesin (Fig. 1.16). Furthermore, receptors to bombesin on the surface of growing tumour cells have been demonstrated biochemically and by a novel visualisation procedure at the ultrastructural level (Lackie et al. 1985) (Figs. 1.17, 1.18). From these observations it has been postulated that the tumour cells produce bombesin which is released and which then stimulates its own specific receptors, thus inducing further cell growth (an autocrine effect).

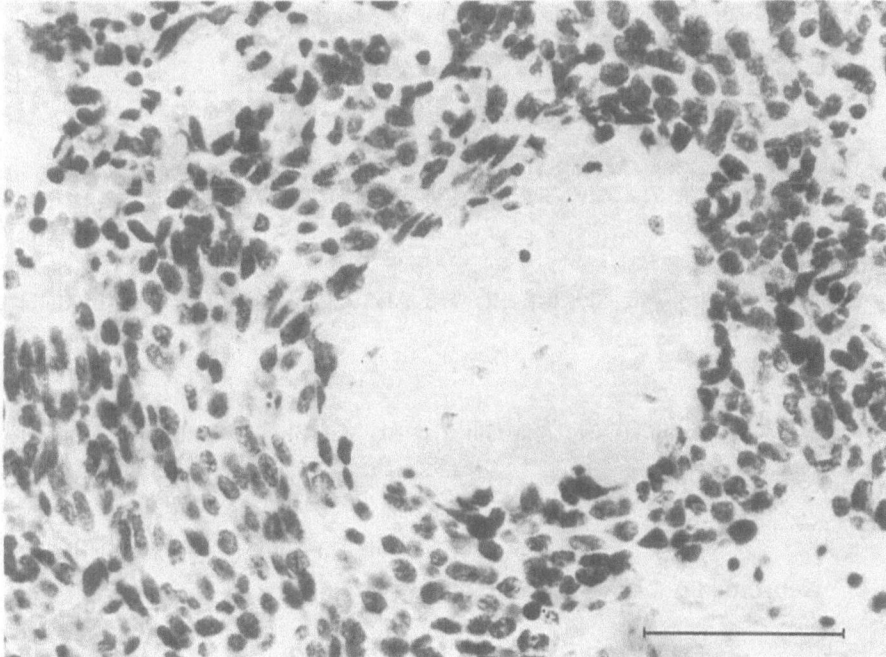

Fig. 1.12. Section of formalin fixed, wax-embedded lung tumour showing typical morphological features of oat cell carcinoma of lung. Haematoxylin and eosin stained. Scale bar represents 100 μm.

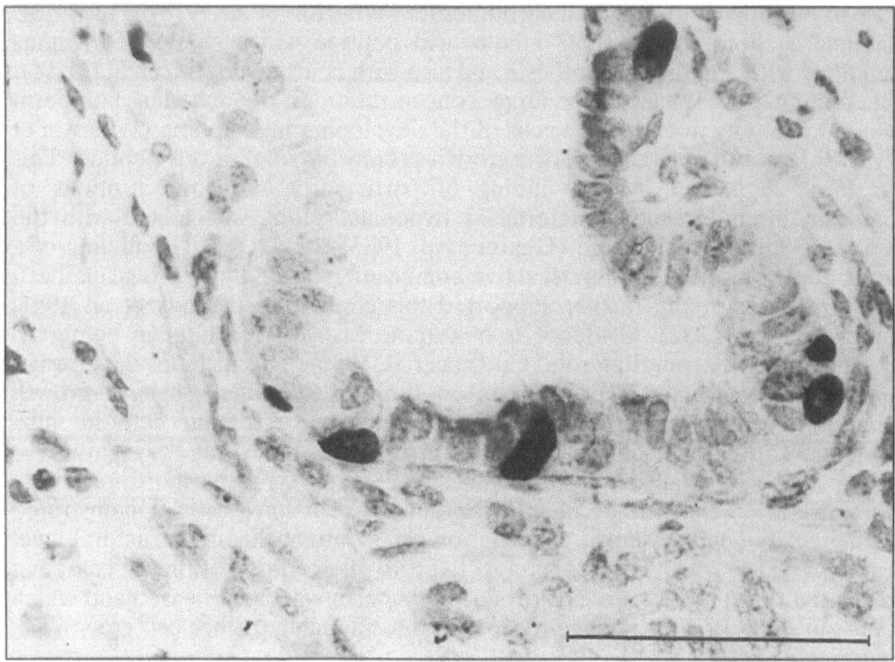

Fig. 1.13. Section (5 μm) of human foetal lung immunostained for bombesin by the peroxidase–antiperoxidase method, showing immunoreactive endocrine cells in the epithelium of a bronchiole. Benzoquinone fixed, wax-embedded tissue. Scale bar represents 100 μm.

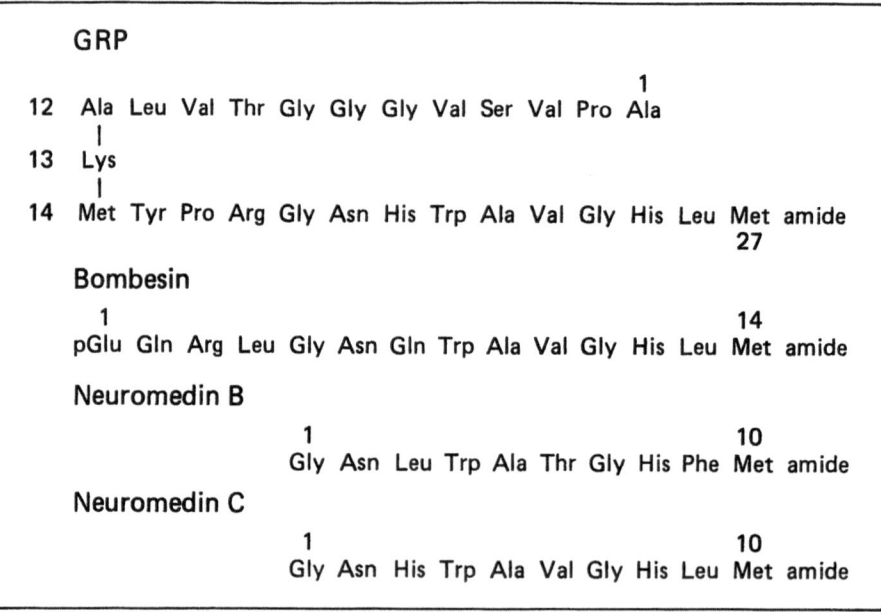

Fig. 1.14. Bombesin and related peptides.

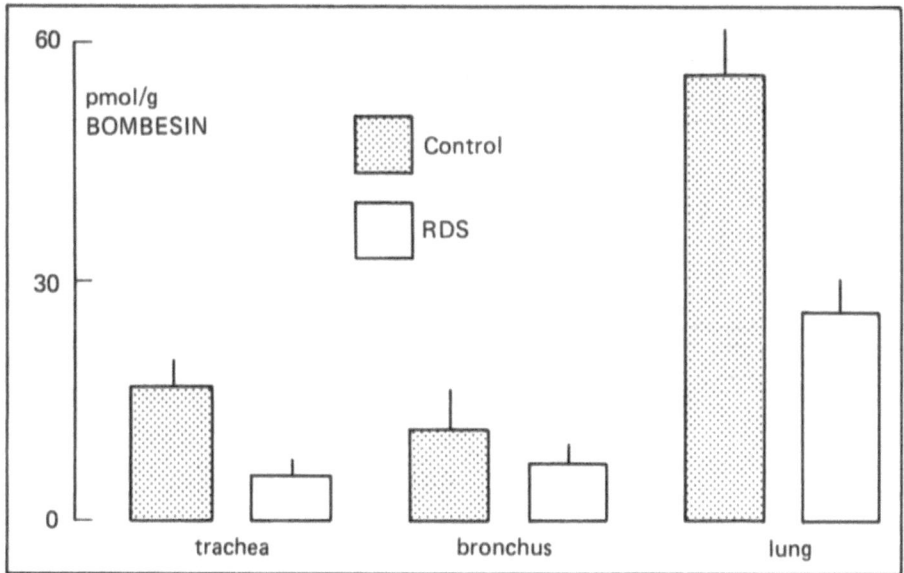

Fig. 1.15. Histogram showing decreased levels of bombesin in respiratory distress syndrome (RDS). Radioimmunoassay results from extracts of different regions of the respiratory tract. Error bar indicates the standard error of the mean. Data expressed in pmol/g of wet weight tissue.

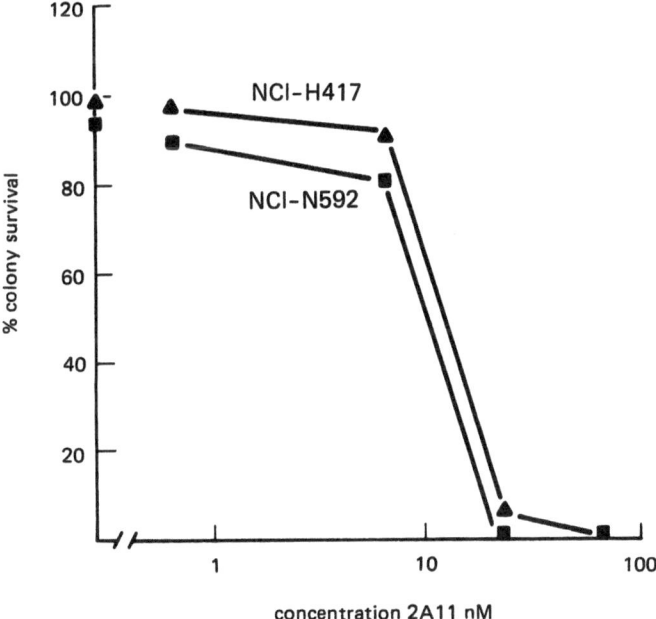

Fig. 1.16. Effect of specific monoclonal antibody to bombesin (2A11) on colony survival in vitro of cell lines from two small cell carcinomas of the lung. (Data from Cuttitta et al. 1985.)

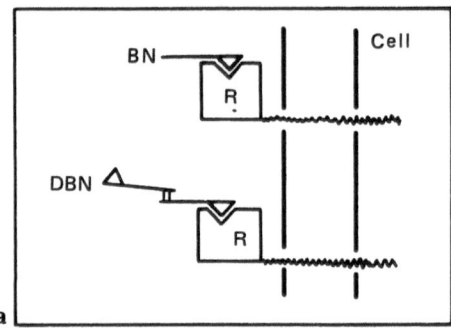

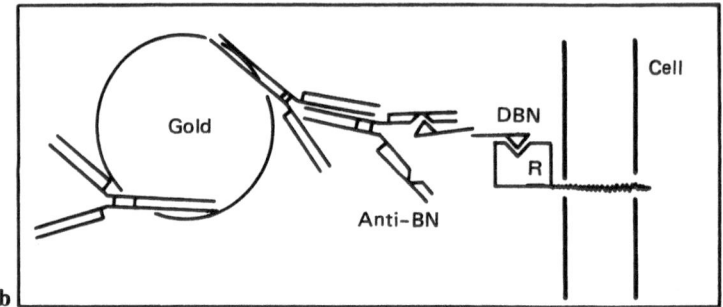

Fig. 1.17.a Diagrammatic representation of bombesin (BN) and a divalent bombesin ligand (DBN) binding to a cell surface receptor (R). **b** Diagrammatic representation of visualisation of divalent ligand using monoclonal antibody specific for bombesin (anti-BN) and a colloidal gold label.

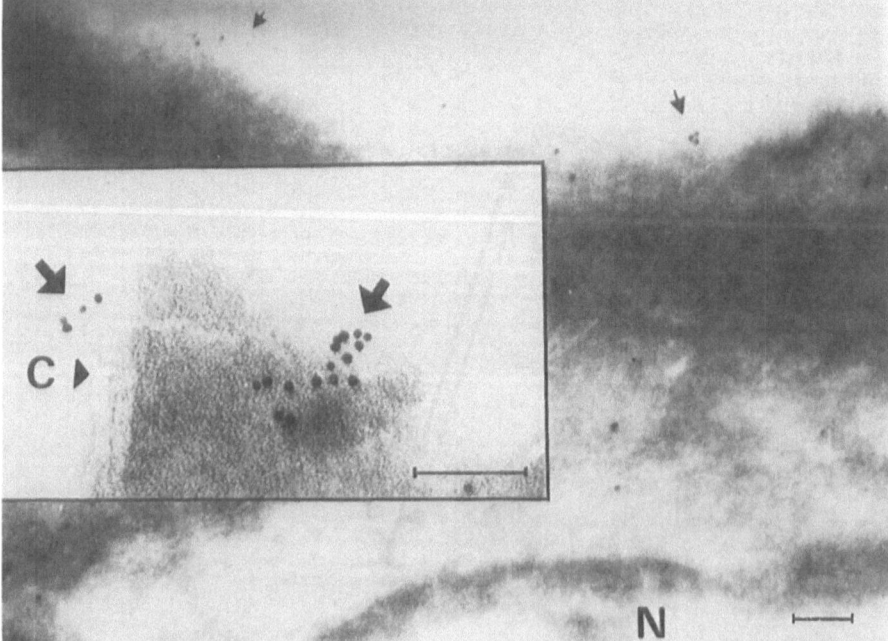

Fig. 1.18. Ultrathin frozen section of a small cell carcinoma of the lung with arrows showing binding of gold particles employed to localise bombesin receptors using dimeric bridge method. C, cell membrane; N, nucleus. Scale bar represents 100 nm.

Conclusion

Advances in morphological techniques have allowed the full recognition of neuroendocrine differentiation in tumours, even those whose clinical or biochemical features render them unremarkable or "silent". Furthermore novel technology permits a more complete understanding of tumour cell biology and its abnormal gene/peptide expression, as well as the distribution and number of growth receptors. A multidisciplinary collaborative approach to the study of tumour behaviour, its potential for treatment and for monitoring progress of the disease is now being adopted, and a future with better patient management is easy to predict.

This work was supported in part by the Cancer Research Campaign and the Council for Tobacco Research USA. Secretarial help of Miss Anita Williams is gratefully acknowledged.

References

Adrian TE, Allen JM, Terenghi G et al. (1983) Neuropeptide Y in phaeochromocytomas and ganglioneuroblastomas. Lancet II: 540–542

Ashley DJB (ed) (1978) Evan's histological appearances of tumours. Churchill Livingstone, Edinburgh

Azzopardi JG (1959) Oat cell carcinoma of the bronchus. J Pathol Bacteriol 78: 513–519

Ballesta J, Bloom SR, Polak JM (1985) Distribution and localisation of regulatory peptides. CRC Crit Rev Lab Sci 22: 185–217

Bishop AE, Carlei F, Lee C et al. (1985) Combined immunostaining of neurofilaments, neuron specific enolase, GFAP and S-100. Histochemistry 82: 93–97

Coghlan JP, Aldred P, Haralambidis J, Niall HD, Penschow JD, Tregear GW (1985) Hybridisation histochemistry. Anal Biochem 149: 1–28

Cuttitta F, Carney DN, Mulshine J et al. (1985) Bombesin-like peptides can function as autocrine growth factors in human small-cell lung cancer. Nature (Lond) 316: 823–826

Dahl D, Bignami A (1986) Intermediate filaments and differentiation in the central nervous system. In: Polak JM, Van Noorden S (eds) Immunocytochemistry: modern methods and applications, 2nd edn. Wright-PSG, Littleton, MA

Doniach I (1977) Histopathology of the anterior pituitary. Clin Endocrinol Metab 6: 21

Facer P, Bishop AE, Lloyd RV, Wilson BS, Hennessey RJ, Polak JM (1985) Chromogranin: a newly recognised marker for endocrine cells of the human gastrointestinal tract. Gastroenterology 89: 1366–1373

Facer P, Bishop AE, Ghatei MA, Bloom SR, Polak JM (1986) 7B2 in normal pancreas and pancreatic endocrine tumours. J Pathol 148: 91A

Ghatei MA, Sheppard MN, Henzen-Logman S, Blank MA, Polak JM, Bloom SR (1983) Bombesin and VIP in the developing lung: marked changes in acute respiratory distress syndrome. J Clin Endocrinol Metab 57: 1226–1232

Grimelius L, Wilander E (1985) Silver impregnation and other non-immunocytochemical staining methods. In: Polak JM, Bloom SR (eds) Endocrine tumours. Churchill Livingstone, Edinburgh, pp 95–115

Hacker GW, Polak JM, Springall DR et al. (1985) Antibodies to neurofilament protein and other proteins reveal the innervation of peripheral organs. Histochemistry 82: 581–593

Iguchi H, Chan JSD, Seidah NG, Chretien M (1984) Tissue distribution and molecular forms of a novel pituitary protein in the rat. Neuroendocrinology 39: 453–458

Klöppel G, Heitz PL (eds) (1984) Pancreatic pathology. Churchill Livingstone, Edinburgh

Lackie PM, Cuttitta F, Minna JD, Bloom SR, Polak JM (1985) Localisation of receptors using a dimeric ligand and electron immunocytochemistry. Histochemistry 83: 57–59

Lauweryns JM, Cokedaere M, Theunynck P (1972) Neuroepithelial bodies in the respiratory mucosa of various animals. A light optical, histochemical and ultrastructural investigation. Z Zellforsch 135: 569–592

Ljungberg O, Jarnerot G, Rolny P, Wickborn G (1981) Human pancreatic polypeptide (HPP) immunoreactivity in an infiltrating endocrine tumour of the papilla of Vater with unusual morphology. Virchows Arch A 392: 119–126

Moody TW, Pert CB, Gazdar AF, Carney DN, Minna JD (1981) High levels of intracellular bombesin characterise human small-cell lung carcinoma. Science 214: 1246–1248

Polak JM, Bloom SR (1985) (eds) Endocrine tumours. Churchill Livingstone, Edinburgh

Polak JM, Marangos PJ (1984) Neuron-specific enolase, a marker for neuroendocrine cells. In: Falkmer S, Hakanson R, Sundler F (eds) Evolution and tumour pathology of the neuroendocrine system. Elsevier, Amsterdam, pp 433–480

Polak JM, Van Noorden S (1983). In: Polak JM, Van Noorden S (eds) Immunocytochemistry, practical applications in pathology and biology. Wright-PSG, Littleton, MA

Rode J, Dhillon AP, Doran JF, Jackson P, Thompson RJ (1985) PGP 9.5: a new marker for human neuroendocrine tumours. Histopathology 9: 147–158

Rosengurt E, Sinnett-Smith J (1983) Bombesin stimulation of DNA synthesis and cell division in cultures of Swiss 3T3 cells. Proc Natl Acad Sci USA 80: 2936–2940

Schottenfeld D, Gershman ST (1977) Epidemiology of thyroid cancer: I. Clin Bull 7: 47–98

Sheppard MN, Corrin B, Bloom SR, Polak JM (1985) Lung endocrine tumours. In: Polak JM, Bloom SR (eds) Endocrine tumours. Churchill Livingstone, Edinburgh, pp 209–228

Sorenson GD, Bloom SR, Ghatei MA, Del Prete SA, Cate CC, Pettengill OS (1982) Bombesin production by human small cell carcinoma of the lung. Reg Pep 4: 59–66

Trojanowski JQ (1986) Neurofilaments and glial filaments in neuropathology. In: Van Noorden S, Polak JM (eds) Immunocytochemistry: modern methods and applications, 2nd edn. Wright-PSG, Littleton, MA, pp 413–424

Van Noorden S, Polak JM (1985) Immunocytochemistry of regulatory peptides. In: Bullock GR, Petrusz P (eds) Techniques in immunocytochemistry, vol 3. Academic Press, New York London, pp 116–154

Varndell IM, Polak JM (1985) Immunocytochemistry. In: Polak JM, Bloom SR (eds) Endocrine Tumours. Churchill Livingstone, Edinburgh, pp 1–20

Varndell IM, Polak JM, Sikri KL, Minth CD, Bloom SR, Dixon JE (1984) Visualisation of messenger RNA directing peptide synthesis by in situ hybridisation using a novel single-stranded cDNA probe: potential for the investigation of gene expression and endocrine cell activity. Histochemistry 81: 597–601

Varndell IM, Lloyd RV, Wilson BS, Polak JM (1985) Ultrastructural localisation of chromogranin: a potential marker for the electron microscopical recognition of endocrine cell secretory granules. Histochem J 17: 981–992

Wharton J, Polak JM, Bloom SR et al. (1978) Bombesin-like immunoreactivity in the lung. Nature (Lond) 273: 769–770

Wharton J, Polak JM, Cole GA, Marangos PJ, Pearse AGE (1981) Neuron-specific enolase as an immunocytochemical marker for the diffuse neuroendocrine system in human fetal lung. J Histochem Cytochem 29: 1359–1364

Wilander E (1984) Endocrine cells and hormones in gastrointestinal carcinoid tumours. Ups J Med Sci [Suppl] 39: 47–58

Wilson BS, Lloyd RV (1984) Detection of chromogranin in neuroendocrine cells with a monoclonal antibody. Am J Pathol 115: 458–468

2 New Molecular Techniques in Pathological Diagnosis: Visualisation of Genes and mRNA in Human Tissue

J. O'D. McGee, J. Burns and K. A. Fleming

Visualisation of Gene Products

In the past 50 years or so there has been great emphasis on the development of morphological techniques for the analysis of cell structure and function. The result has been that pathology has advanced considerably from a purely descriptive discipline into an era where statements can be made about the protein, enzyme, gene and messenger RNA (mRNA) complement of individual cells in intact tissue. The first major advance was the development of histochemical techniques for the identification of specific chemical residues and enzymatic activities in tissues. Electron microscopy then added further fine-structural detail to our knowledge of cell function. The single biggest technological advance which helped in the elucidation of the molecular nature of cell structure was, however, the introduction of immunohistochemistry in the 1940s (Coons et al. 1941).

It is worth recalling the various stages of development that immunohistochemistry has gone through, because similar stages of evolution are now evident in the development of techniques for the in situ analysis of the gene and transcript content of human cells. When Coons and others developed immuno-histochemistry they were limited to using polyclonal antibodies raised in rabbits (and other animals). These antibodies were, by today's standards, relatively crude since they were made against biological components which were chemically impure. The antisera, therefore, were usually absorbed with powdered extracts of tissues to absorb unwanted reactivities of the antisera, thus achieving better specificity. The sites at which antibodies bound to tissues were identified by immunofluorescent techniques after coupling the antibodies directly to fluorescent dyes. The coupling reaction, however, tended partially to destroy the reactivity of the specific antibody. This was circumvented by introducing an indirect immunohistochemical technique in which the antigen reacted with its primary (unlabelled) antibody and the site of the antigen–antibody reaction was identified by a fluorescent labelled second antibody directed against the immunoglobulins of the species in which the primary antibody was raised; the second antibody was made in large amounts and a little loss of reactivity on coupling to a fluorescent dye became less important. Since fluorescent antibodies required specialised microscopes for their visualisation and also because the fluorescence signal deteriorated on exposure to the light used for its visualisation, alternative ways of labelling antibodies were sought.

In the late 1960s the foundations were laid for the introduction of antibodies labelled with enzymes such as peroxidase and phosphatase (Nakane and Pierce 1966). Both of these enzymes are stable and simple histochemical techniques were available for their visual detection in tissues by conventional light microscopy. Enzyme-labelled antibody reaction products in general are stable and preparations can be stored for long periods under ambient laboratory conditions. Until the early 1970s most immunohistochemical studies were performed on freshly collected, rapidly frozen tissue, a restriction which limited their usefulness to specialised laboratories. The emphasis on fresh tissue was because it was thought that the universally used fixatives such as formaldehyde destroyed the antigenic structure of tissue proteins. It was then realised that fixation and processing to paraffin wax did not destroy the antigens, but rather that in the process of fixation they were masked by adjacent proteins which were cross-linked by formaldehyde to the antigen of interest. These "masked" antigens could be "unmasked" by treating the fixed tissue with proteolytic enzymes to remove occluding proteins; the antigen revealed by proteolysis could then be visualised by either fluorescence or enzyme immunohistochemistry (see Burns 1982 for a review). This development therefore opened up the possibility of using archival paraffin blocks in many investigations.

In spite of these advances, however, it was not always possible to produce polyclonal antibodies to all cellular components because of difficulties in isolating the component of interest. Even when proteins are purified to homogeneity as judged by gel electrophoresis (and other techniques) the final protein preparations may contain minor impurities which may be highly antigenic and thus produce a good antibody response. Great care, therefore, had to be taken in ensuring not only the purity of the starting material for antibody production but also the purity (and specificity) of the polyclonal antibody raised against the starting material. This drawback of immunohistochemistry was solved by the introduction of monoclonal antibody technology by Kohler and Milstein (1975). Monoclonal antibodies are made in bulk in vitro and react specifically with only one epitope of a cell component.

Since this discovery was made many monoclonal antibodies have been produced with the idea that they would serve as chemical reagents for identification of tissue components. This expectation has not been entirely fulfilled because monoclonal antibodies react with an epitope which may be the result of the chemical sequence and/or of the conformational domains of molecules. Because of this it has been found that some monoclonal antibodies react with cell structures other than the immunogenic material used in their production. For example, a monoclonal antibody against the cell surface antigen

Thy-1 reacts also with intermediate filaments (Dulbecco et al. 1981). This type of cross-reaction may signify functional or evolutionary relationships between proteins but may also reflect small areas of chemical conformational homology between proteins. Similar cross-reactivities with polyclonal antibodies may also be based on chemical homology; for example an antiserum against an *src* gene product (p60 src) reacts with a variety of cell structures which have small areas of amino acid sequence homology (four to six amino acids) with p60 src (Niggs et al. 1982). As will be shown below, the technology being developed for gene and mRNA identification is evolving along historically similar lines to immunohistochemical technology.

It is usual to equate antibody staining of a cell with the synthesis of the corresponding antigen by that cell. This interpretation, although sometimes correct, is not invariably so. Antibody staining of a cell simply indicates that it contains the epitope of interest. The epitope may have been synthesised by the cell but equally it may have been engulfed by the cell by phagocytosis or it may have been adsorbed by the cell from surrounding extracellular fluid. Several studies indicate that all three interpretations of antibody staining may be true depending on the cell or tissue investigated.

Visualisation of Genes and their Transcripts

With the advent of recombinant DNA technology it is now theoretically possible to identify and quantify unique DNA sequences (single copy genes) and their transcribed mRNAs. The mRNA, in conjunction with ribosomes and a series of other factors, forms the apparatus required for the synthesis of the product encoded by a gene.

Human genes, or bits of them, can be produced in bulk in vitro by inserting them into vectors such as plasmids which in turn are transfected into a bacterium such as *E. coli* (Glover 1985). The "infected" *E. coli* can then be grown in bulk and the plasmids, with their human gene insert proportionately amplified, purified by standard extraction and centrifugation procedures. The gene insert may have been derived directly from human DNA (i.e. a genomic probe) or indirectly by isolation of the mRNA of the gene which is copied (c) into DNA by reverse transcriptase (i.e. cDNA probe) before insertion into the vector. Naturally, if the whole human genome (or cDNA) is inserted into many plasmids those bacteria which contain the gene of interest are isolated by an appropriate screening procedure from single bacteria (clones). The cloned DNA combines (hybridises/anneals) with the native gene or the mRNA copy of the gene. For the detection of mRNA it is sometimes better to use an mRNA copy of the cloned gene. In the latter instance, the gene is cloned into a vector (e.g. pSP6) which in the presence of added reactants transcribes the inserted human DNA into mRNA. This will bind not only to native mRNA but also to DNA, since it is a ribonucleotide copy complementary to the former and one strand of the latter.

The principles of hybridising cloned DNA/mRNA to native nucleic acids, either in solution or bound to filters, are established (Hames and Higgins 1985).

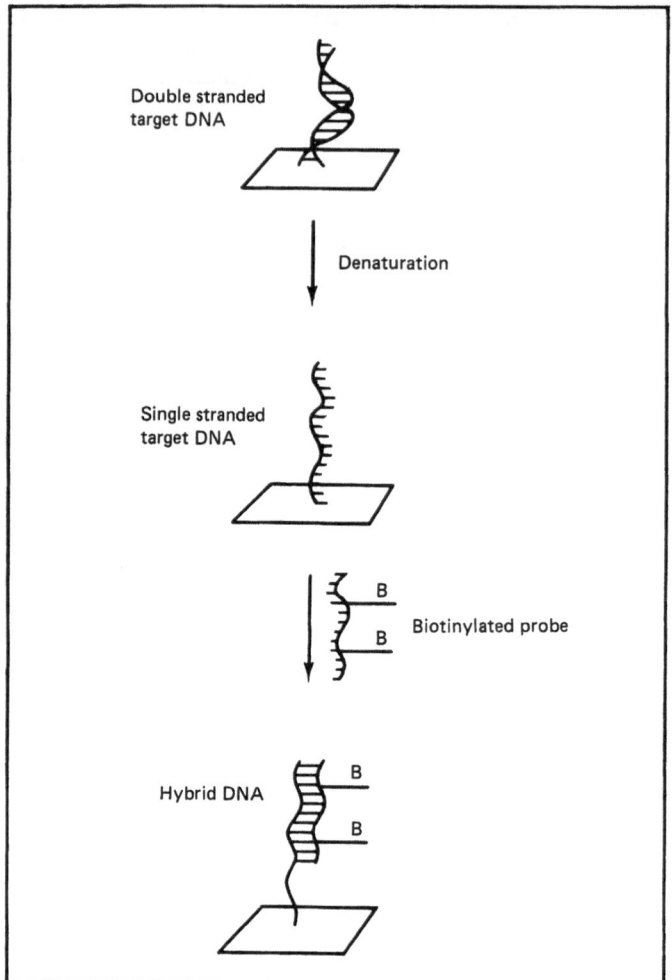

Fig. 2.1.   Schematic representation of in situ hybridisation protocol. B, biotin-dUTP.

The same principles, as far as is known, apply to hybridisation experiments on intact cells, although the conditions of the reaction usually are modified. These principles are outlined in Fig. 2.1. In essence, a gene within the nucleus is detected by first denaturing the DNA (because it is double stranded), and adding denatured labelled cloned gene the single strands of which combine with its complementary strands in the nucleus. When hybridisation of cloned DNA to intact cells (in situ hybridisation) was introduced the cloned DNA was labelled with ^{32}P because of the high proportion of phosphate residues in DNA. The intracellular site of the hybridisation event can be localised by autoradiography. Because of the short half-life and the high energy/long track length of ^{32}P, more recently ^{3}H has been used as a radioactive label. Tritium, having a shorter track length (approx. 1 μm) produces better resolution at the cellular level. However, even a track length of 1 μm is large in cellular terms for precise intracellular localisation when it is recalled that a lymphocyte has a diameter of approximately 8 μm. Additionally, the visualisation of tritium by autoradiography requires long exposure periods (days or months) to enable detection of unique DNA sequences or small amounts of intracellular mRNA.

To circumvent these disadvantages of radiolabelled probes (and also the hazards of radioactivity), considerable effort has been expended over the past 5 years to design ways of introducing non-radioactive labels (reporter molecules) into nucleic acids (Pereira 1986). The compound which has been most used for non-radioactive labelling of DNA is biotin, a naturally occurring vitamin. Biotin is incorporated into DNA probes very easily by nick translation, a reaction in which DNA is "nicked" with a DNAse and biotin-dUTP is incorporated (translated) into the nicks by DNA polymerase, restoring the DNA to nearly its original length. (dUTP is an analogue of thymidine, one of the constituent bases of DNA.) Biotin is a small molecule (molecular weight 365) and interferes little with the ability of a biotinylated DNA strand to combine with its complementary strand.

Biotinylated DNA probes hybridised in situ are detected by two systems (Fig. 2.2), viz. streptavidin/avidin or antiserum to biotin. Both avidins and antibody, conjugated directly or indirectly to peroxidase or alkaline phosphatase, can be

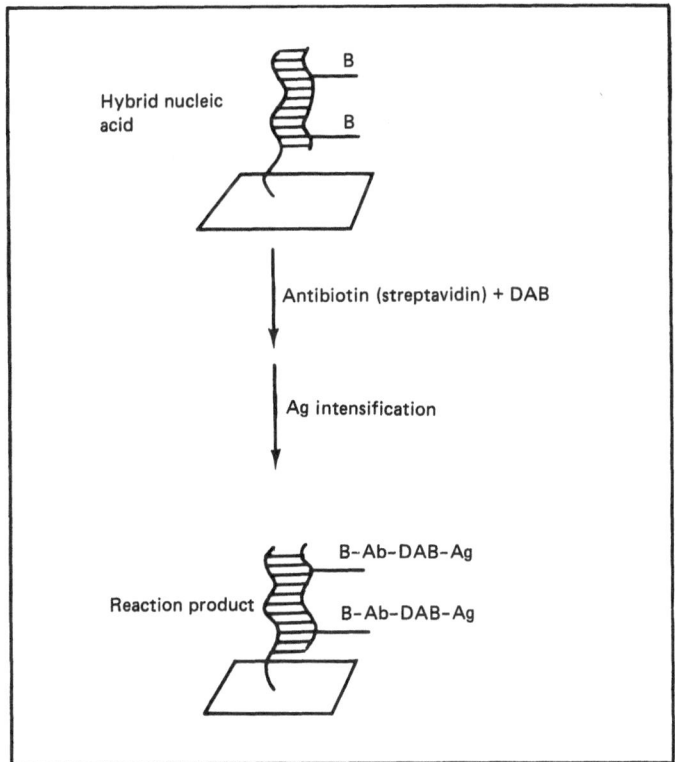

Fig. 2.2. Detection scheme for biotinylated DNA. Ab, antibody; DAB, diaminobenzidine; Ag, silver. (See Burns et al. 1985 for details.)

identified by the usual histochemical reactions which yield a coloured reaction product.

Applications of Hybridisation with Biotinylated Probes

Sex Determination

Using radioactive probes abundant DNA and mRNA species, and more recently unique DNA sequences, have been delineated in cells and chromosomes respectively. This approach to gene mRNA localisation will not be described further here; readers are referred to the review by Coghlan et al. (1985).

Of the various non-radioactive reporters available, biotin-labelled probes—which are easy to use—have been successfully used for visualising abundant DNA and mRNA species in *Drosophila*, and for abundant DNA copies such as cytomegalovirus and some repetitive human genes (Pereira 1986). Single copy genes have been identified on filter hybridisation with biotin-labelled probes (Leary et al. 1983; Chan et al. 1985). The overall defect with biotin-labelled probes, however, is that they have lacked the sensitivity of radiolabelled probes. This has been due to the inadequacy of the detection system for biotin, but this problem has now largely been overcome. Procedures have been developed which amplify the signal from biotinylated probes such that single copy genes can be visualised on human chromosomes and on filters (Chan et al. 1985; Burns et al. 1985). These techniques give results more rapidly than do radioactive probes and the resolution is much better.

The most sensitive method for visualising biotin-labelled probes hybridised in situ is based on various principles which have been established over the last 30 years (Burns et al. 1985, 1986a). In essence, the regular histochemical methods for biotin detection based on peroxidase histochemistry generate a brown reaction product of diaminobenzidine (DAB) polymer. This is sufficient to identify multiple copy genes. This approach will not visualise a highly repetitive single gene such as those found on the Y chromosome in male cells unless very large amounts of probe are used. However, DAB complexes bind heavy metals such as gold, which when converted into sulphide will reduce metallic silver in large quantities. Using these reactions the brown reaction product of DAB catalysed by peroxidase is converted to a black product by the superimposition of a silver precipitate at the same site, and the sensitivity of detection of biotin is raised many-fold. It is difficult to quantify the degree of amplification achieved in sections, but on filters about a 25-fold increase in sensitivity is achieved. In intact cells, however, it is likely that the amplification is much larger. Suffice it to say that this amplification procedure can visualise a single copy gene on a human chromosome.

This amplification technique was first used in a model system to distinguish between male and female cells (Burns et al. 1985). Cells of both sexes were hybridised with a biotinylated DNA probe which is relatively specific for the Y chromosome. Male cells are easily distinguished by the presence of a single black spot which is usually placed near the nuclear membrane (Fig. 2.3). Female cells

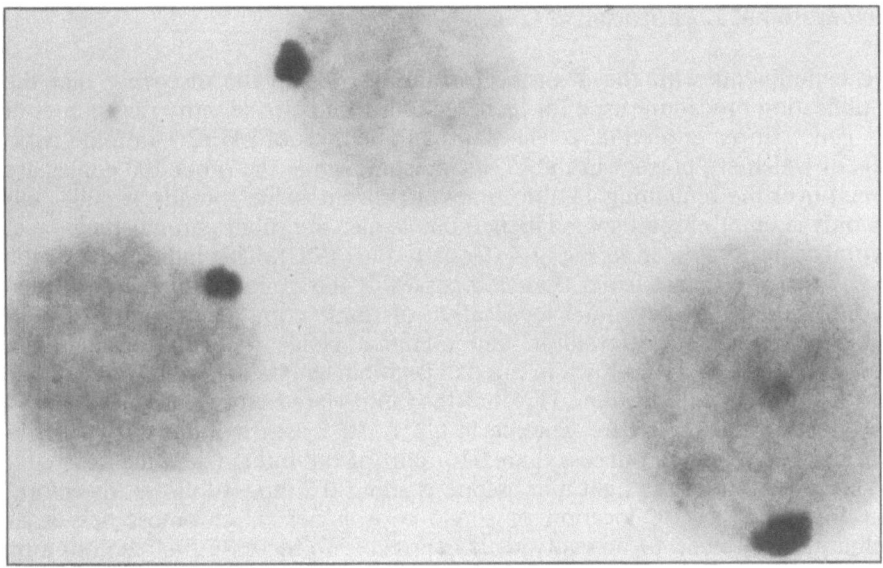

Fig. 2.3. Demonstration of the Y chromosome in male interphase nuclei by in situ hybridisation. The Y body is evident at the nuclear membrane as a black spot. The probe used was biotinylated pHY2.1, detected as described by Burns et al. (1986a).

lack this black Y body which is the equivalent in the interphase cell of the Y chromosome. This hybridisation procedure is the most accurate and rapid way of sexing cells in vitro. It has been applied to sexing unborn children by hybridising amniotic cells or chorionic villi with the Y-"specific" probe. This enables sex determination as early as 3–4 weeks after conception and may have applications in prenatal counselling of parents with a hereditary sex-linked disorder. With further refinement of the technology, no doubt, the same principles will be used for the identification of mutant single copy genes in specific hereditary disorders. In the latter, however, very small probes (about 20 bases long rather than 2100, as in the Y-specific probe) will be required; it is relatively easy to synthesise 20-base oligonucleotides. It is physically impossible for large probes (more than 100 bases) to distinguish a point mutation which is based on a single nucleotide difference from the normal gene.

The Y probe used in these experiments may also be able to discriminate at the 16-cell stage between male and female embryos fertilised in vitro. This observation is at the moment of only academic interest because the embryos used for sex determination are killed by the hybridisation procedure. It should be emphasised that these experiments were done on fertilised ova which by morphological criteria were destined to die in vitro and would not have survived in utero. In tumour pathology this probe is also being used for analysis of the sex of teratomas and other germ line tumours.

Chromosomal Localisation of Genes

The experiments with the Y probe fortuitously led to the discovery that the amplification procedure used for its detection would also identify rare copies of this gene (Burns et al. 1985). There are 2100 copies of pHY2.1 in male cells, 2000 of which are present in the Y chromosome while the other 100 copies are spread over the remaining 44 autosomes. In chromosome spreads of male cells not only is the Y chromosome labelled but so also are other chromosomes, e.g. chromosome 15 as seen in Fig. 2.4 (Cooke et al. 1982). This indicated that the procedures will detect fewer than 100 copies of this gene, and led to a formal investigation of chromosomal localisation of single copy genes such as the β-globin, α-globin, metallothionin and c-Ha-ras genes (Nicholls et al. 1986; McGee et al. 1986). As shown in Fig. 2.5 β-globin can be localised with relative ease to the tip of chromosome 11. Since the biotinylated probe used was only 4.4×10^3 bases and the entire genome is 6.3×10^9 bases it follows that in situ hybridisation can pick out less than $1/10^6$ part of the human genome.

The resolution of the light microscope is about 0.2 μm. It follows, therefore, that for more precise location of single copy genes or chromosomes other techniques will need to be evolved. It is possible to increase the resolution by scanning electron microscopy. To date, only multiple copy genes such as pHY2.1 have been visualised by this technique, but it should be possible to identify single copy genes using heavy metal probes of gold and silver and by visualising them by backscatter electrons (Ferguson et al. 1986).

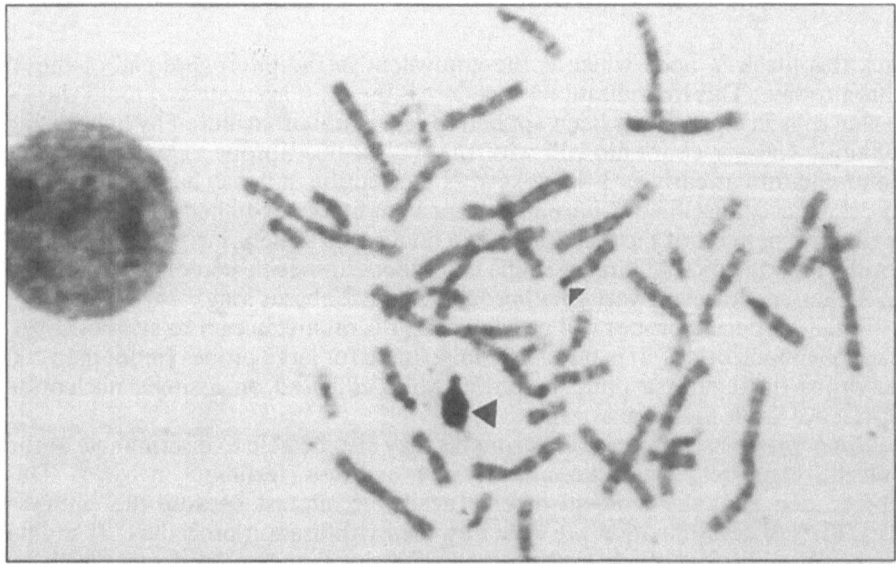

Fig. 2.4.   The Y chromosome in this chromosome spread is easily identified (*large arrowhead*) as are rarer copies of the pHY2.1 gene (*small arrowhead*). A Y body is also evident in the interphase lymphocyte. These chromosomes were banded after hybridisation with pHY2.1.

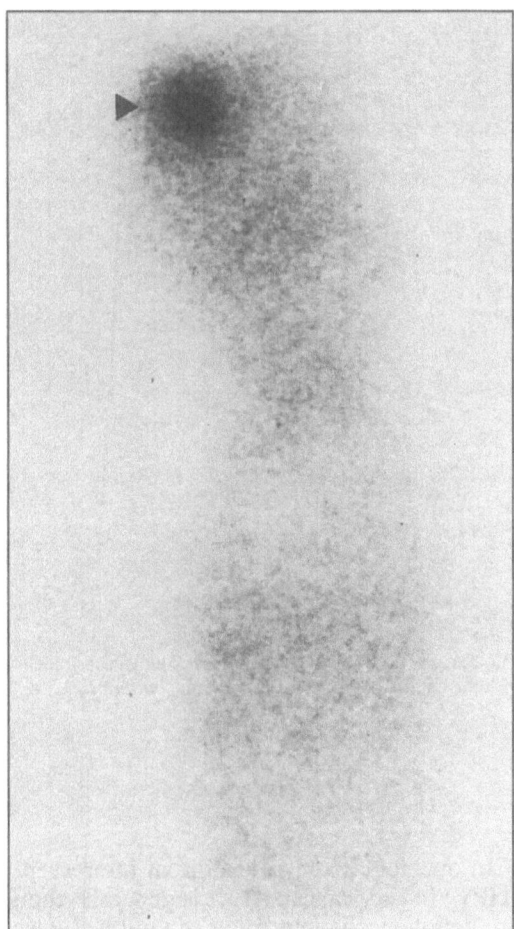

Fig. 2.5. The β-globin gene is present at the tip of chromosome 11 (*arrowhead*). The preparation was Giemsa banded after hybridisation with a biotinylated β-globin probe.

Gene Localisation in Paraffin Material

The evolution of in situ hybridisation techniques has, therefore, followed an analogous path to the development of immunohistochemistry, especially when it is noted that all of the studies referred to above have been done on fresh frozen, lightly fixed material. There is now great interest in identifying genes, particularly viral genes, in paraffin-embedded material. The techniques which have been developed for this purpose have used essentially the same principle which enables antibodies to gain access to paraffin-embedded tissue antigens, namely limited proteolysis. Cytomegalovirus, herpes (Burns et al. 1986b) and other viruses have been characterised by in situ hybridisation within intact cells in 8–24 hours (Pereira 1986). This is a considerable advance on routine virological culture methods which in most cases take weeks to complete. The technique will be of considerable importance in rapid viral diagnosis in patients who are immunocompromised.

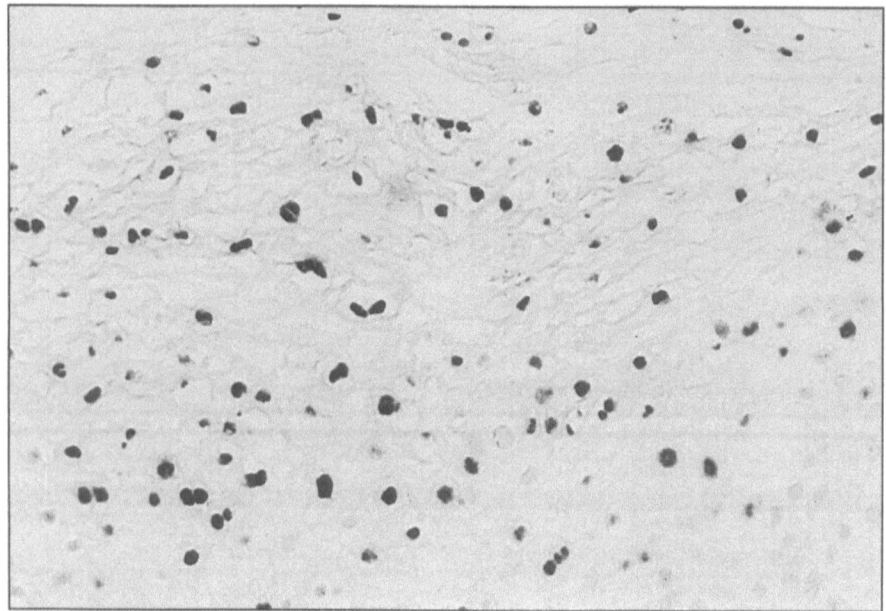

Fig. 2.6. HPV 11 in a cervical wart. The virus is black and the uninfected cells are evident because of light haematoxylin counterstaining (*bottom right*).

In oncology there is also great interest in the role of human papilloma virus (HPV) in cervical cancer. It is generally thought that only a few of these viruses are aetiologically important in viral neoplasia (Evered and Clark 1986). HPV 6 and 11 are found frequently in cervical/vulvar warts (Fig. 2.6), while HPV 16 and 18 are frequently associated with pre-invasive and invasive cervical cancer. These associations have been deduced mainly from isolation of HPV genomes from cervical cancers or cell lines derived therefrom. Now that archival paraffin blocks can be used for viral analysis by in situ hybridisation it may be possible to elucidate the question of the possible association between HPV, cervical preneoplasia and invasive cancer. Furthermore, if HPV 16 and 18 infections can be identified from cervical smears taken in the "well women" cervical screening programmes which operate in almost all developed countries, women carrying the virus could be selected and treated more rapidly, perhaps diminishing further the incidence of invasive cervical cancer.

Oncogene mRNA Expression in Human Tumours

The localisation of mRNA by in situ hybridisation with radiolabelled or biotinylated probes is more difficult than gene localisation. This is perhaps because mRNA has a very short half-life (usually minutes) so that much of it may be degraded in fresh tissue collected immediately after surgery. This cannot be the entire explanation since specific mRNAs can be demonstrated on filter hybridisations from the same tissues. Our view is that the present state of the art is such that the methods available are not good enough for general application to different organs. Some techniques obviously work well in sea urchin embryos but not in mouse or man. It should be noted that in situ hybridisation chemistry is much more complex than filter hybridisation. In the latter, nucleic acids are greatly purified from other cell components, whereas in intact cells nucleic acids (DNA and mRNA) are intimately admixed with numerous other cell proteins, lipids and carbohydrates which may interfere with the hybridising of probes with their complementary sequences.

Rous described a sarcoma of chickens caused by Rous sarcoma virus (RSV) in 1912, and a viral-induced rabbit papilloma was reported more than a decade later; viral-induced mouse tumours were then described. These observations were thought to have little relevance to the aetiology of malignancy in man until about the late 1960s or early 1970s. This was due to the fact that these tumours only occurred in inbred or rather specialised animal strains, but the discovery of viral-induced feline leukaemia in stray (outbred) cats indicated that viral tumours did occur sporadically in the wild. The *src* gene of RSV which induces sarcomas in chickens was then shown to have a homologue in normal DNA of uninfected chickens. These observations were primarily responsible for the growth in interest in cellular DNA homologues (c-oncs) of viral oncogenes (see Bishop 1985 for a review). More than 30 c-oncs have been described in the human genome. These human genes are not absolutely identical to the viral genes. Because of this, and because human cells contain these genes even in the absence of cancer, the concept has arisen that these c-oncs exist in a latent state as proto-oncogenes which need to be "activated" in some way before they can induce malignancy.

Most of these genes have been discovered in normal cells by transfecting NIH 3T3 cells (an established fibroblast line) with normal DNA. Some cells so infected transform mouse cells, and the human DNA isolated from them has been characterised and shown to share DNA homology with known oncogenic viruses. The puzzle has been to understand why these normal proto-oncogenes do not cause cancer in all cells. Essentially, it is now assumed that activation of these genes is necessary. Activation in this context implies that the genes are expressed in increased amounts (via mRNA) by a process of gene amplification or by translocation of the gene from its usual genomic environment to another chromosome where its expression is activated. The best-studied example of the latter is the translocation of the *c-myc* gene from chromosome 8 to chromosome 14 (or other chromosomes). It is assumed that the translocation of *c-myc* to the long arm of chromosome 14, where it is inserted nearby an immunoglobulin gene, is sufficient to induced increased expression of *c-myc*. An alternative way of c-onc activation is by point mutation within a c-onc. There are many examples of this in the *ras* gene family of cellular oncogenes.

It has been argued very cogently, however, that cellular oncogenes are neither sufficient nor necessary for the induction of neoplasia mainly because there is not complete homology between c-oncs and their viral counterparts; further, the viral genes act in a dominant fashion and induce neoplasia within weeks of infection (Cichutek and Duesberg 1986). The transfection assay used for c-onc definition is also not entirely satisfactory because NIH 3T3 cells are immortalised. However, it has now been demonstrated that the *c-Ha-ras* gene can immortalise primary (non-established) cell lines; in these cells, though, a second oncogene is necessary to establish complete transformation of the cells (Balmain et al. 1986). This hypothesis is the molecular equivalent of the initiation and promotion hypothesis of carcinogenesis put forward in the 1920s.

There have been very few studies on the isolation of c-onc mRNAs from primary human tumours as opposed to cell lines derived from them. All of the studies on actual tumours show that one (or more) c-onc is expressed in some human tumour biopsies, but so also are they expressed in the normal tissue from which they derive (Slamon et al. 1984). It should also be noted that several c-oncs are expressed in regenerating liver and that their expression is turned off before regeneration is complete, indicating that fleeting expression of these genes is not sufficient in vivo to induce neoplasia. The hypothesis that the c-oncs responsible for human neoplasia are mutated genes has been explored in human tumour biopsies with usually negative results, although mutant genes obviously occur in some cell lines derived from human tumours. Very recently it has been proposed that c-onc activation is not necessary for the induction of neoplasia but rather that these genes are expressed because of a hitherto unrecognised genetic aberration located close by the origin of the *c-Ha-ras* gene (Cichutek and Duesberg 1986).

The *ras* family of genes has been most extensively studied in human tumours. Activation of three members of this family—*c-Ha-ras* (bladder, breast, colon), *c-Ki-ras* (colon, lung, ovary) and *c-N-ras* (haemopoietic malignancy)—has been found in human tumours. Mutated versions of these genes probably occur in about 10%–15% of human tumours as measured by transfection assays. All of these genes encode proteins which may be cell-membrane-associated and have GTP binding and cleavage functions. They are assumed to participate in cell proliferation.

We have examined the expression of *c-Ha-ras* in hyperplastic, benign and malignant neoplasms of the human breast by in situ and filter hybridisations. This gene is expressed in malignant cells of human mammary cancers of the ductal, lobular and medullary types. Surprisingly, however, the gene is also expressed in fibroblasts and endothelial cells in the stroma of these tumours. The same gene is expressed in fibroadenoma and hyperplastic cystic disease in epithelial and stromal cells. We estimate that about 80% of the lesions of breast that we have examined express this gene. In situ hybridisation does not give quantitative information so it could be argued that there is more *c-Ha-ras* mRNA in malignant tumours than in benign lesions. Filter hybridisation experiments from three tumours and one fibroadenoma, however, demonstrated that there are about five to 17 copies of *c-Ha-ras* mRNA per cell in the cancers and about 17 copies per cell in the single fibroadenoma examined (McGee, unpublished).

In situ hybridisation using the probe employed in these experiments does not distinguish the mutant *c-Ha-ras* gene from its normal homologue. However, we have now examined three breast cancers and two benign lesions by restriction enzyme and Southern blot analysis and the *c-Ha-ras* gene is not mutated in any of these lesions at either codon 12 or 61 (McGee, unpublished).

It is apparent from these results, therefore, that *c-Ha-ras* expression is not an exclusive property of malignant cells, as the gene is expressed in benign and malignant lesions and also in the benign stromal cells of cancers. It is therefore not an absolute or a necessary correlate of malignancy. It would also seem unlikely that mutation of this gene is a common occurrence in human mammary cancer. The functional significance of the expression of this gene is not clear from these or other studies. Recently it has also been shown by a monoclonal antibody to the ras p21 protein that this protein is also found in the same mammary cells and lesions detailed above (Ghosh et al. 1986). It is clear, therefore, that further work is necessary to examine other putative oncogenes in breast cancer.

Conclusions

In summary, in situ and filter hybridisation give qualitatively different information from studies using monoclonal and polyclonal antibodies. The types of data generated by each technique are probably complementary. Some applications of in situ hybridisation technology have been referred to, and it is self-evident that the procedure will be used increasingly in the future in combined pathological and clinical studies.

The original work reported in this chapter is supported by the Cancer Research Campaign, UK.

References

Balmain A, Quintanilla M, Brown K, Ramsden M (1986) An approach to the molecular mechanisms of cancer induction. J Pathol 149: 3–8
Bishop JM (1985) Viral oncogenes. Cell 42: 23–38
Burns J (1982) The unlabelled antibody peroxidase–antiperoxidase method (PAP). In Bullock GR, Petrusz P (eds) Techniques in immunocytochemistry, vol 1. Academic Press, London, pp 91–105
Burns J, Chan VTW, Jonasson JA, Fleming KA, Taylor S, McGee JO'D (1985) Sensitive system for visualising biotinylated DNA probes hybridised in situ: rapid sex determination of intact cells. J Clin Pathol 38: 1085–1092
Burns J, Chan VTW, Jonasson JA, Fleming KA, Taylor S, McGee J'O'D (1986a) Sensitive system for visualising biotinylated DNA probes hybridised in situ. J Clin Pathol 39: 230–231
Burns J, Redfern D, Esiri M, McGee JO'D (1986b) Human and viral gene detection in routine paraffin embedded tissue by in situ hybridisation with biotinylated probes. J Clin Pathol 39: 1066–1073
Chan VTW, Fleming KA, McGee JO'D (1985) Detection of subpicogram quantities of specific DNA sequences on blot hybridisation with biotinylated probes. Nucleic Acids Res 13: 8083–8091
Cichutek K, Duesberg PH (1986) Harvey ras genes transform without mutant codons, apparently activated by truncation of a 5' exon (exon-1). Proc Natl Acad Sci USA 83: 2340–2344
Coghlan JP et al. (1985) Review. Hybridisation histochemistry. Anal Biochem 149: 1–28
Cooke HJ, Schmidtke J, Gosden JR (1982) Characterisation of a human Y chromosome repeated sequence and related sequences in higher primates. Chromosoma 87: 491–502
Coons AH, Creech HJ, Jones RN (1941) Immunological properties of an antibody containing a fluorescent group. Proc Soc Exp Biol Med 47: 200–202
Dulbecco R, Unger M, Bologna M, Battifora H, Syka P, Okada S (1981) Cross reactivity between Thy-1 and a component of intermediate filaments demonstrated using a monoclonal antibody. Nature (Lond) 292: 772–774
Evered D, Clark S (eds) (1986) Papilloma viruses. Ciba Foundation Symposium 120. Wiley, New York

Ferguson DJP, Harrison D, Burns J, Jonasson J, McGee JO'D (1986) Chromosomal localisation of genes by scanning electron microscopy using in situ hybridisation with biotinylated probes: Y chromosome repetitive sequences. Histochem J 18: 266–270

Ghosh AK, Moore M, Harris M (1986) Immunohistochemical detection of ras oncogene p21 product in benign and malignant mammary tissue in man. J Clin Pathol 39: 428–434

Glover DM (1985) DNA cloning, vols 1 and 2. IRL Press, Oxford

Hames BD, Higgins SJ (1985) Nucleic acid hybridisation. IRL Press, Oxford

Kohler G, Milstein C (1975) Continuous cultures of fused cells secreting antibody of predefined specificity. Nature (Lond) 256: 495–497

Leary JJ, Brigati DJ, Ward DC (1983) Rapid and sensitive colonimetric method for visualising biotin-labelled probes hybridised to DNA or RNA immobilised in nitrocellulose bioblots. Proc Natl Acad Sci USA 80: 4045–4049

McGee JO'D, Burns J, Jonasson J, Chan VTW, Dickson M (1986) Chromosomal assignment of unique sequences by in situ hybridisation using biotinylated probes β-globin, α-globin and metallthiomine. (Submitted)

Nakane PK, Pierce GB (1966) Enzyme labelled antibodies: preparation and application for the localisation of antigens. J Histochem Cytochem 14: 929–931

Nicholls RD, Jonasson JA, McGee JO'D, Patel S, Ionasescu VV, Weatherall DJ, Higgs DR (1986) High resolution gene mapping of the human α-globin locus. J Med Genet (in press)

Niggs EA, Watler E, Singer SJ (1982) On the nature of cross reactions observed with antibodies directed to defined epitopes. Proc Natl Acad Sci USA 99: 5939–5943

Pereira HG (1986) Non-radioactive nucleic acid probes for the diagnosis of virus infections. BioEssays 4: 110–113

Slamon DJ, DeKernion JB, Verma IM, Cline MJ (1984) Expression of cellular oncogenes in human malignancies. Science 224: 256–262

3 Statistical Methods of Evaluating and Comparing Imaging Techniques

Laurence S. Freedman

Introduction

Over the past 20 years several new methods of generating images of internal organs and the anatomy of the body have been developed and used to enhance the accuracy of diagnosis and treatment. These include ultrasonic scanning, radioisotope scanning, computerised X-ray tomography (CT) and magnetic resonance imaging (MRI). The new techniques have made a considerable impact on radiological practice in hospital departments, not least on the investigational process for patients suspected or known to have malignant disease.

As a consequence of the increased range of imaging techniques now available, there has developed a need to evaluate and compare their usefulness. Over the past 10 years formal studies of the application of imaging technology have been conducted and many reports have appeared in the literature. These studies cover a range of clinical situations. Likewise, the methodologies employed for evaluating and comparing the techniques in question have differed widely.

While not attempting an exhaustive review of the clinical studies which have been reported, this paper aims to examine the statistical designs and analyses which have been used. First a brief review of the different types of study is given. Examples of each type are then chosen to illustrate statistical issues related to their design and analysis. In the final sections it is argued that a form of classification for these different types of study might be helpful in clarifying relationships between them and bringing a perspective to the field. A classification based upon a limited analogy with clinical trials is suggested.

Study Designs Employed to Evaluate Imaging Techniques

Table 3.1 lists five broad descriptions of designs of studies that have been conducted to evaluate or compare imaging techniques.

Table 3.1. Types of study design for evaluating imaging techniques

1.	Pilot
2.	Diagnostic accuracy
3.	Clinical value
4.	Randomised comparisons
5.	Before-and-after

1. Pilot studies are concerned with the feasibility of a new technique and address questions such as the acceptability of the method to patients and hospital staff, the quality of the images and the training required to achieve adequate levels of interpretation of the images. These studies may include some case studies to illustrate the potential use of the new technique but do not comprise any formal evaluation. Necessary as they are, their statistical content is negligible and they will not be dealt with here in more detail. A good example is to be found in the early papers on MRI (Hawkes et al. 1980).

2. Studies to evaluate the diagnostic accuracy of a technique are the most common form of assessment. Patients are assessed by the imaging technique under study and the radiologist's diagnosis is compared with a final or "gold-standard" diagnosis. The same design may be used to evaluate the accuracy of an imaging technique for clinical staging of disease.

3. Some studies aim to evaluate the contribution of an imaging technique to the clinical management of the patient. We will refer to these as "clinical value" studies. A typical experiment consists of the clinician making two assessments of a case, one before and one after receiving the radiologist's report. The impact of the technique on both the diagnostic and therapeutic process may be studied in this way. A particularly interesting application has been the study of the impact of CT on radiotherapy.

4. Randomised comparisons have only rarely been conducted to evaluate imaging techniques. Typically, the patient is allocated one of two imaging techniques or policies by randomisation and is then followed to assess the subsequent diagnosis, treatment and outcome. The two groups of patients are then compared with respect to these measures.

5. Before-and-after studies may be conducted when an imaging policy is replaced by a new one in a particular hospital. The typical study is a comparison of diagnostic practice before and after the introduction of a major new technology such as CT scanning.

The following four sections examine more closely each of these types of design, excluding pilot studies. Since studies of diagnostic accuracy are the most commonly performed, these will be treated in the most detail.

Studies of Diagnostic Accuracy

A typical example of this type of study is reported by Foster et al. (1984), in which ultrasound scanning, CT and an oral pancreatic function test were compared prospectively for the diagnosis of 107 patients with suspected pancreatic disease. Various aspects of study design and analysis will be considered in the context of their report.

Final Diagnosis

As mentioned in paragraph 2 above, diagnostic accuracy is measured in relation to a final "gold standard" diagnosis. The rules for establishing the final diagnosis are most important. Foster and colleagues report: "The final diagnosis was made *independently* of the three tests under evaluation, on the basis of radiology, operative and histological findings and follow-up" (this author's italics). Foster et al. express an essential principle here: that the final diagnosis must be established independently from the imaging technique under evaluation. The reason is quite obvious. Allowing the technique to contribute to the final "gold standard" diagnosis is no different from allowing a candidate to mark some of his own examination papers. It is surprising at first sight how often this simple principle is forgotten. However, in studies carried out retrospectively (e.g. Sostre et al. 1978) it is difficult if not impossible to meet the independence principle. In prospective studies, many reports do not say explicitly whether the final diagnosis was independent of the imaging technique. Even in the paper by Foster and coworkers, immediately following the sentence quoted above we read: "In addition, endoscopic retrograde cholangiopancreatography and a Lundh test were performed when not contra-indicated or rendered superfluous by the results of *other investigations*" (this author's italics). The reader is left to wonder whether these "other investigations" included the test results, and to speculate on the effect of allowing the tests partially to determine what other investigations are required to establish the final diagnosis.

In summary, the independence principle strictly requires that the results of the imaging techniques are not given to the clinician in charge before diagnosis has been established, so that they do not influence the diagnostic process.

In many clinical situations a definite final diagnosis may be difficult to obtain. Sharp et al. (1985) cite suspended liver metastases as an example. For imaging studies it is important to avoid reliance on another imaging technique, since this itself may not be completely reliable. The ideal, particularly in oncology, is to use autopsy or histological evidence. Otherwise, two strategies have been used in the face of this difficulty. The less radical solution (Reid et al. 1983) is to grade the reliability of the final diagnosis by introducing a diagnostic rating. Such a rating on a nine-point scale is shown in Table 3.2. A simple way of using the scale is to exclude from analysis all patients with a particularly doubtful rating; e.g. excluding patients rated between 2 and 5 on the scale would be equivalent to demanding biopsy, laparotomy or post-mortem proof. More sophisticated uses of the ratings are possible but have not been developed.

Table 3.2. Rating of final diagnosis of liver disease (adapted from Reid et al. 1983)

Rating	Results from biopsy, laparatomy or post-mortem	Other evidence
0	Negative	Negative
1	Negative	Positive or conflicting
2	None available/equivocal	Negative
3	None available/equivocal	Conflicting but probably negative
4	None available/equivocal	Conflicting
5	None available/equivocal	Conflicting but probably positive
6	None available/equivocal	Positive
7	Positive	Negative or conflicting
8	Positive	Positive

The other strategy for meeting difficulties with the final diagnosis has been to dispense altogether with an "objective" measure of diagnostic accuracy and to use another measure in its place. For example Hauser and Gottschalk (1978) compared a tomographic camera with a gamma camera technique by eliciting the preferences of nuclear medicine physicians for one or another set of images in a series of patients. The results from these studies, although of some use, do not allow strong conclusions about the accuracy of the techniques and the design is limited to a comparison of techniques.

Selection of Patients

How should one select the patients to be entered into a study of diagnostic accuracy? Foster and coworkers included in their study "all patients who were referred for investigation of suspected pancreatic disease" except those with a history of exocrine pancreatic disease or those who were jaundiced. These investigators consciously chose to select their patients on clinical grounds only, even though they knew that this would yield relatively small numbers of patients who were finally found to have pancreatic disease. In fact, out of 107 patients in the study, only 17 (16%) had a final diagnosis of chronic pancreatitis (11 patients) or pancreatic neoplasm (6 patients). There were 15 other patients with pancreatograms showing minimal changes (10) or an unfused ventral pancreas (5). Naturally these small numbers reduce the precision with which diagnostic accuracy may be measured. However, the authors claim that "other investigators have assessed the tests in populations comprising 25–50% of patients with disease" which "necessarily implies an element of selection . . . and artificially enhances sensitivity and specificity" (two measures of diagnostic accuracy to be defined later in this section).

Ranshoff and Feinstein (1978) emphasise a similar point when they discuss the spectrum of patients to be entered into these types of study. They point out that within the "diseased" groups of patients (e.g. colonic cancer) the accuracy of the test may vary with the pathological type of disease and clinical stage. Similarly within the comparative "non-diseased" group (that is, the group without the disease in question) the accuracy of the test may differ according to the patient's condition; in particular the test may be more likely to yield false positives for patients with conditions similar to the disease (e.g. colitis or carcinoma of the breast).

The important principle which underlies these comments is that, ideally, the imaging technique should be tested in patients who are representative of the target population, that is, the patients for whom the technique is intended in the future. Failing this, an effort should be made to include a wide enough spectrum of patients to cover the composition of the target population. Even though the study group may not contain the various subgroups of the population in the same proportion, it is possible to make corrections once the distribution of subgroups in the target population is ascertained.

Performance of the Imaging Technique

Foster et al. (1984) report that "all the investigations were performed as part of the hospital's routine diagnostic service". The authors note in their discussion that the lower estimates of diagnostic accuracy resulting from their study, in comparison with seven other reports, might have been partly due to differences in operator skill. Sharp et al. (1985) remark that results obtained by a highly skilled operator in a research environment are likely to overestimate the diagnostic accuracy of a new technique. The critical test for the technique will be in routine hospital service and the study should therefore evaluate it in such an environment.

It is usual in these studies for the radiologist (or nuclear medicine physician) to make the diagnosis based on the technique and essential that this is not reported to the clinician until after the final diagnosis (see section on final diagnosis above). While this requirement is necessary for the proper evaluation of diagnostic accuracy, it is at the expense of the introduction of an artificiality into the study, namely that the technique is performed but not used in the clinical management of the patient. The above comments do not imply, however, that the radiologist should have any other evidence, such as medical history, withheld from him before his diagnosis is made. A good rule here is to give the information in accordance with normal clinical practice.

Comparative Studies

Although a study of diagnostic accuracy is both feasible and informative when applied to a single imaging technique, studies comparing two or more techniques will generally yield more useful information. The study of Foster et al. (1984) is an example of a comparative study. Although this is not stated explicitly, it can be assumed that they intended to give each patient all three diagnostic tests. They report that only 97 out of 107 patients were examined by ultrasound, 86 by CT and 99 by the oral pancreatic function test. The practical difficulties of organising three separate diagnostic tests for a large number of patients can be appreciated.

Assessing each patient with all the imaging techniques under study is, therefore, one option which may have associated practical disadvantages. If this option is used, in what order should the techniques be performed? In an ideal study where all organisational difficulties were overcome and all patients received all the techniques under study, with a negligible time interval between the performance of the techniques, the order would not matter. However, in reality, it might be safer to randomise the order for two reasons. First, to try to avoid more drop-outs occurring from one particular technique because it was always placed last in the order. Second, to reduce the risk of systematic time trends in the case of rapidly developing disease. It is probable, however, that if there is difficulty in performing all the techniques there will be even more difficulty in complying with the order of tests determined by randomisation!

If diagnostic tests have been missed in a considerable proportion of cases, the investigators should consider the possible effect on the results. The report by Foster and coworkers indicates that 20% of the patients had no CT but does not mention why this occurred or whether it could have biased the final results in any way.

Just as the results of the imaging technique should not be allowed to influence the final diagnosis, so one technique under study should not be allowed to influence the performance of a competing technique. Thus Abrams et al. (1982), in a comparison of CT and ultrasound, were wrong to permit that "in some patients who had CT first, with definitely negative or positive results, ultrasound was omitted".

An alternative design which avoids the organisational complexity of arranging two or more imaging investigations for each patient, is to allocate to each patient just one of the techniques using a randomisation method (Reid et al. 1983). However, the investigator pays for this organisationally simpler option by the need to include substantially more patients to achieve the same accuracy of comparison (Hanley and McNeil 1983).

Measures of Diagnostic Accuracy: Sensitivity, Specificity and Predictive Value

The most commonly used measures of diagnostic accuracy are sensitivity and specificity. Take the simplest case where the result of an imaging technique is reported as either negative or positive for a particular disease and the final diagnosis is that the patient is either diseased or disease-free (that is, has or does not have the disease under study). Sensitivity is then defined as the proportion of diseased patients who are reported positive; specificity is the proportion of disease-free patients who are reported negative.

Table 3.3 presents data taken from a study by Brion et al. (1985) who reported on the ability of CT to detect metastatic involvement of the mediastinal lymph nodes in patients with carcinoma of the lung. From these data the sensitivity of CT is calculated as 48/54 (89%) and its specificity as 46/99 (46%). It can be seen that, in this study, there were a large number of false positives (i.e. positive results in disease-free patients) leading to low specificity. This finding suggests that the authors' criterion for evidence of metastatic involvement (a node diameter greater than 5 mm) may have been too liberal.

Sensitivity and specificity have the statistical property that their values are independent of the prevalence of the disease, that is how commonly patients present with that disease. This property has peculiar advantages and disadvantages. The principal advantage is that the results of studies carried out in patient populations with different prevalences of the disease under study can, theoretically, be compared using sensitivity and specificity. This perceived

Table 3.3. Evaluation of mediastinal lymph node involvement by CT against final staging (at surgery) (data from Brion et al. 1985)

Final staging	CT evaluation		Total no. of patients
	No involvement	Involvement	
No involvement	46	53	99
Involvement	6	48	54
Total no. of patients	52	101	153

Sensitivity = 48/54 = 89%
Specificity = 46/99 = 46%
Positive predictive value = 48/101 = 47%
Negative predictive value = 46/52 = 88%
Prevalence = 54/153 = 35%

advantage has recently been weakened by the realisation that differences in the spectrum of patients in a study can indeed affect the estimates of sensitivity and specificity (see the section on selection of patients above). The principal disadvantage in the use of sensitivity and specificity is that they cannot by themselves tell the investigator how useful the imaging technique will be in practice. Two measures of accuracy which do provide this information are the positive and negative predictive values. The positive predictive value is defined as the proportion of patients reported positive who are diseased. The negative predictive value is the proportion of patients reported negative who are not diseased. If we return to the data in Table 3.3 we see that the positive predictive value is 48/101 (47%) while the negative predictive value is 46/52 (88%). These values give us direct information about how much reliance can be placed on the imaging result. If there is a positive result there is roughly a 1 in 2 chance (47%) that the patient has involvement of the mediastinal lymph nodes. This is strong enough to make the clinician suspicious but not enough to make him certain. With a negative result there is a 7 in 8 chance (88%) of there being no mediastinal lymph nodal involvement, which is strong but not conclusive evidence.

The positive and negative predictive values depend upon sensitivity and specificity and also upon the prevalence of the disease. Thus the predictive values calculated from any study will only apply in an environment with the same prevalence. Table 3.4 gives the formulae which are needed to calculate the positive and negative predictive values in an environment with a different prevalence. For example, in the report by Brion et al. (1985) about one-third (35%) of the patients had mediastinal lymph node involvement. How would the same test apply to a hospital department to which two-thirds (67%) of the patients presented with involved nodes? In this case the positive predictive value would increase from 47% to 77% and the negative predictive value would decrease from 81% to 67% (see Table 3.4). A positive result is now more strongly predictive than a negative result.

More dramatic changes in predictive value occur when transferring a test from teaching hospital to district hospital and thence to a screening centre. Phillips et al. (1983) demonstrate that the positive predictive value of hip arthrography for femoral compartment loosening can reduce from 97% as a diagnostic test in a teaching hospital population to 3% as a screening test for the general

Table 3.4. Formulae linking sensitivity, specificity, prevalence and predictive value

$$\text{Positive predictive value} = \frac{\text{Sensitivity}}{\text{Sensitivity} + [(1 - \text{Specificity}) \times (1 - \text{Prevalence}) \div \text{Prevalence})]}$$

$$\text{Negative predictive value} = \frac{\text{Specificity}}{\text{Specificity} + [(1 - \text{Sensitivity}) \times \text{Prevalence} \div (1 - \text{Prevalence})]}$$

If, for example, we apply the Sensitivity and Specificity of Table 3.3 to a Prevalence of 2/3 (0.67) we obtain:

$$\text{Positive predictive value} = \frac{0.89}{0.89 + [(1 - 0.45) \times (1 - 0.67) \div 0.67]} = 77\%$$

$$\text{Negative predictive value} = \frac{0.45}{0.45 + [(1 - 0.89) \times 0.67 \div (1 - 0.67)]} = 67\%$$

population, simply as a result of the difference in prevalence of the disease in the two populations.

Measures of Diagnostic Accuracy: ROC (Receiver Operating Characteristic) Curves

In the preceding section it was assumed that the result of the imaging technique must be negative or positive. However, for most techniques levels of positivity can be distinguished. To define sensitivity or specificity an arbitrary level of positivity must be chosen. All images falling on one side of the chosen level are then designated negative and all others positive. A good example is in the paper by Brion et al. (1985), mentioned earlier, in which mediastinal nodes less than 5 mm in diameter were called negative and those greater than 5 mm, positive. Naturally investigators must define their criteria for positivity carefully to enable proper comparison of results.

Table 3.5. Comparison of CT and mediastinoscopy in evaluation of mediastinal lymph node involvement (adapted from Brion et al. 1985)

Final staging at surgery	CT evaluation		Mediastinoscopy evaluation	
	No involvement	Involvement	No involvement	Involvement
No involvement	46	53	99	0
Involvement	6	48	18	36
Sensitivity = 48/54 = 89% Specificity = 46/99 = 46%			Sensitivity = 36/54 = 67% Specificity = 99/99 = 100%	

A typical problem of interpretation caused by the arbitrary choice of a cut-off point is shown in Table 3.5 (Brion et al. 1985). The data indicate that CT has greater sensitivity than mediastinoscopy to mediastinal lymph node involvement, but less specificity. Which is the better test?

This problem may be avoided by defining a scale of positivity and reporting the distribution of scores on this scale for diseased and disease-free subjects. In the detection of mediastinal node involvement a natural scale of positivity would be the maximum diameter of lymph nodes seen on the scan. This would give rise to a continuous scale. More commonly the scale is chosen to be discrete with five

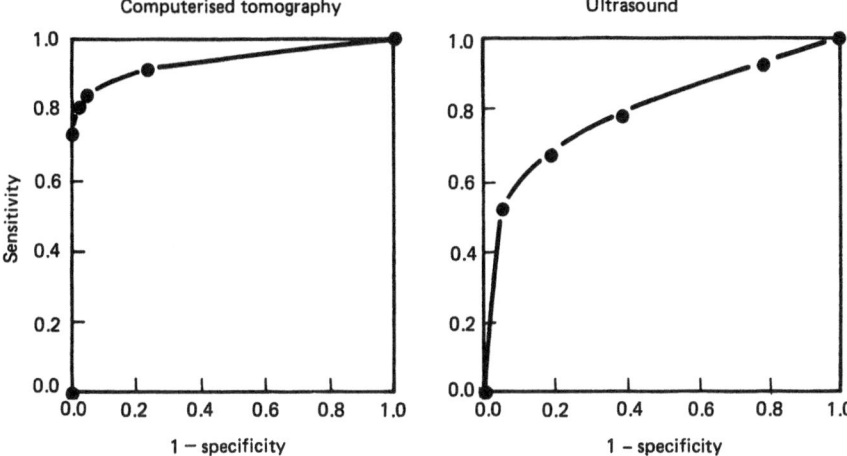

Fig. 3.1. ROC curves comparing CT with ultrasound. Note the degree to which the CT curve moves to the upper left-hand corner of the graph, indicating greater diagnostic accuracy. (Adapted from Abrams et al. 1982.)

or six points, based on a subjective judgement of the confidence of the radiologist in the diagnosis (e.g. 1 = definitely negative, 2 = probably negative, 3 = possibly positive, 4 = probably positive, 5 = definitely positive: cf. Abrams et al. 1982).

The ROC curve is constructed by considering, in turn, each point on the scale as the cut-off point for the definition of positivity and plotting the sensitivity against (1 − specificity) for each point. Some results for CT and ultrasound for patients with suspected adrenal disease (Abrams et al. 1982) are shown in Fig. 3.1. A smooth curve has been drawn through the points on the basis of some statistical assumptions. When there is no predictive worth in the imaging technique the curve will tend to a straight line joining the origin with the top right-hand corner of the graph. A perfect technique will be represented by a vertical line from the origin to the top left-hand corner and a horizontal line from left to right at the top of the graph. The most commonly used summary of the ROC curve is the area under the curve, which will tend towards 0.5 for a useless technique and 1.0 for a perfect technique. The larger the area the more accurate is the technique and different techniques may be compared by means of the areas under their ROC curves.

However, this methodology has not yet gained wide acceptance. The meaning of the ROC curve is not easy to master, and assigning a diagnostic image to one of the points of the scale is difficult and may vary considerably from one occasion to the next, even for the same radiologist. Furthermore, the area under the curve does not have the direct interpretation that is enjoyed by sensitivity or predictive value.

Numbers of Patients

Studies of diagnostic accuracy conventionally include somewhere between 30 and 500 patients with a median figure of about 100. On the other hand there is almost never any mention in reports of the reasons for choosing the particular size of sample adopted. The reason is probably that standard sample size methodology cannot be applied to these studies without the investigators specifying values for quantities of which they are largely uncertain.

The simplest way of determining sample size would be to ask how precise an estimate of the sensitivity and specificity of the technique is needed. It would be reasonable to give an answer to this question by specifying the magnitudes of the standard errors. However, in most situations little more than an educated guess at the appropriate standard errors is possible.

Nevertheless, some guidance can be given on the matter of sample size. An investigator will often be able to dismiss a range of standard errors as too large and another range as unnecessarily small. Thus a standard error of 10% will lead to 95% confidence intervals of width approximately 40%, which will usually be too wide for useful interpretation. A standard error of 1%, on the other hand, giving a confidence width of 4%, will sometimes provide more precision than is required for decision making.

Table 3.6 shows the standard error of sensitivity (specificity) achieved by a given number of diseased (normal) patients. The standard error is affected by the level of sensitivity (specificity) as well as the sample size and the table includes sensitivities ranging from 50% to 99%. An investigator may use this table in the following way. First he should specify a few sample sizes that are within the bounds of practicality. Secondly he should ascertain the likely prevalence of the disease in his study population and so calculate for each sample size the numbers of diseased and normal patients available for study. Thirdly he should make realistic guesses at the levels of sensitivity and specificity of the technique under evaluation. Finally, for each sample size he should read off from the table the standard errors of sensitivity (using the number of diseased patients) and specificity (using the number of normals), using interpolation where necessary. He may then consider whether the samples are inadequately small or unnecessarily large for the study. Investigators should demand smaller standard errors for sensitivities or specificities near the extremes of 0 and 100%; as a rule of thumb standard errors should be less than half the difference between the expected sensitivity and the scale extremity (e.g. for a sensitivity of 95% the standard error should be less than 2.5% ((100%−95%)/2).

Hanley and McNeil (1982, 1983) give formulae and tables for sample sizes of studies using ROC curve analysis.

Table 3.6. Standard error (%) of the estimate of sensitivity (or specificity)

No. of diseased (normal) patients	Expected sensitivity (specificity) (%)						
	50	70	80	90	95	98	99
25	10.0	9.2	8.0	6.0	4.4	2.8	2.0
50	7.1	6.5	5.7	4.2	3.1	2.0	1.4
75	5.8	5.3	4.6	3.5	2.5	1.6	1.1
100	5.0	4.6	4.0	3.0	2.2	1.4	1.0
150	4.1	3.7	3.3	2.4	1.8	1.1	0.8
200	3.5	3.2	2.8	2.1	1.5	1.0	0.7
300	2.9	2.6	2.3	1.7	1.3	0.8	0.6
500	2.2	2.0	1.8	1.3	1.0	0.6	0.4
1000	1.6	1.4	1.3	0.9	0.7	0.4	0.3

Excluding 'Uninterpretable' Test Results

Foster et al. (1984) report that "Ninety-seven patients were examined by ultrasound and the pancreas visualised in 83 (86%)". The measures of diagnostic accuracy described above do not take into account the proportion of "uninterpretable" test results. Harris (1981) notes that authors may exclude results that are "inconclusive", do not have observer agreement or are associated with "technical" failure. He warns that this is a potential source of bias and that if results are to be excluded the criteria for exclusion should be specific and widely accepted. He suggests that "authors . . . should begin to consider whether any failures, other than those owing to equipment malfunction, can be excluded from data analysis". One way of including "uninterpretable" results in the analysis would be to introduce an extra category between the normal and diseased categories and conduct an ROC curve analysis. The most important point, however, is to report clearly the definition and the number of uninterpretable results for the imaging technique.

Summary of Statistical Points in the Design of Diagnostic Accuracy Studies

1. The imaging technique under evaluation should not influence the final diagnosis, either directly or indirectly.
2. The final diagnosis should, ideally, be based on autopsy or histological evidence, particularly in oncology.
3. Patients selected for study should be as nearly representative of the target population as possible.
4. The imaging technique should be performed and reported in a routine hospital service environment.
5. To assist his diagnosis, the radiologist should be presented with clinical information in accordance with normal clinical practice.
6. When comparing two or more techniques it is most economic (in terms of patient numbers) to assess each patient with each of the techniques in turn.
7. The order of the techniques should, ideally, be randomised, although this may be impractical.
8. If techniques are sometimes missed the investigators should consider the possible effect on their results.
9. No imaging technique should be allowed to influence the performance of a competing technique.
10. Predictive value is of more direct relevance to the performance of a test than sensitivity or specificity.
11. Predictive value can change dramatically with an alteration in the prevalence of the disease.
12. If there is a problem of interpretation which is partly or wholly caused by an arbitrary choice of cut-off point to separate negative from positive results, ROC curve analysis offers a possible solution.
13. Numbers of patients should be chosen in relation to the standard errors required for estimating sensitivity or specificity.

14. Uninterpretable test results should be reported and could be included formally in the analysis using an ROC curve approach.

Clinical Value Studies

As mentioned above, diagnostic studies require that the investigator deliberately takes the imaging technique out of clinical context so as to evaluate it. The result of the technique is, ideally, not allowed to influence the management of the patient in any way, at least until the final diagnosis has been established. A different sort of study is to enquire how an imaging technique contributes to the diagnostic and therapeutic process in real-life conditions, particularly when the result of the technique is reported directly to the clinician in charge. This question may be split into three components: How does the technique affect (i) diagnosis, (ii) treatment and (iii) patient outcome? Clinical value studies may be designed to answer questions (i) or (ii) or both. Only randomised comparisons can provide a direct answer to question (iii). In this section we describe the

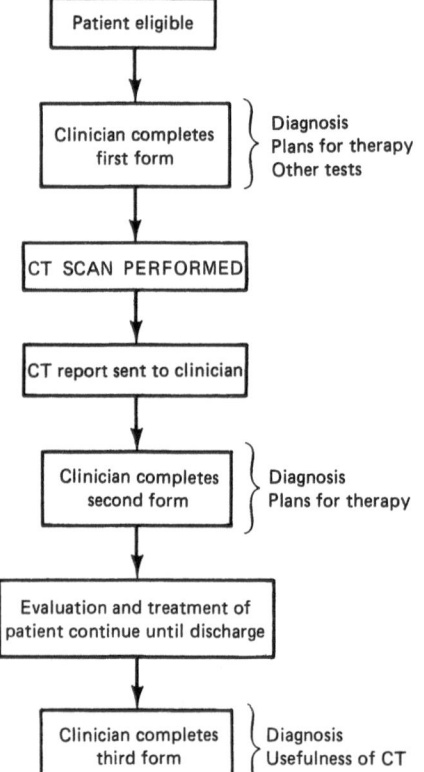

Fig. 3.2. Flow diagram of the design of a clinical value study. (Adapted from Wittenberg et al. 1980.)

design of a clinical value study, drawing heavily on the report of Wittenberg et al. (1980).

The essential feature in the design of clinical value studies is that assessments are made firstly without the information contributed by the imaging technique and then again with that information. Fig. 3.2, adapted from Wittenberg et al., shows the design of their study to evaluate the efficacy of body CT. If a patient was deemed eligible, the clinician was first asked to complete a form giving differential diagnostic probabilities together with a provisional treatment plan as well as any contemplated additional diagnostic tests. CT was then performed and the result reported to the clinician, at which point he completed the form for a second time. At the time of the patient's discharge from hospital (or for outpatients, several weeks later) the clinician completed the form for a third time. In addition he gave a grading to the overall usefulness of CT in diagnostic understanding and choice of therapy. The scales for usefulness of CT are shown in Table 3.7. Using this study design, for a total of 623 patients in ten sub-protocols, the investigators were able to report a perceived improvement in diagnostic understanding in 52% of patients, and beneficial change of therapy in 14%.

Table 3.7. Scale for usefulness of CT (adapted from Wittenberg et al. 1980)

Diagnostic understanding

1.	CT *confused* my understanding of this patient's disease and *led* to investigations I would not otherwise have done
2.	CT *confused* my understanding of this patient's disease but *did not* lead to any additional investigations
3.	CT had *little or no effect* on my understanding of this patient's disease
4.	CT provided information which *substantially* improved my understanding of this patient's disease
5.	My understanding of this patient's disease depended upon diagnostic information provided *only* by CT (unavailable from any other non-surgical procedure)

Choice of therapy

1.	CT led me to choose therapy which in retrospect was *not* in the best interests of the patient
2.	CT was of *no influence* in my choice of therapy
3.	CT did not alter my choice of therapy but did *increase my confidence* in the choice
4.	CT contributed to a *change* in my chosen therapy but other factors (underline which: other imaging tests, other diagnostic tests, changes in patient status) were *equally* or *more* important
5.	CT was very important compared to other factors in leading to a beneficial change in therapy

The investigators of this carefully designed study recognise in their report that the results are based on the subjective impressions of the participating clinicians. However, by recording opinions at three points during patient management they were able to check retrospectively on the consistency of the clinical course and the final assessment. They note that they are unable using this design to evaluate the ordering of CT among a battery of diagnostic tests. They also note that the scale for choice of therapy may be insensitive to improvements in therapy such as CT-guided percutaneous biopsies.

In oncology there has been particular interest in the effect of CT on precision rather than choice of treatment, with particular reference to CT-assisted radiotherapy planning. Several studies of this particular aspect of CT have been conducted and the design used by Prasad et al. (1981) is typical. First routine diagnostic information was used to select a treatment plan with no CT result available. Then the treatment was replanned with the CT information. The plans were compared and it was decided whether the CT resulted in a modification of treatment. This design is another example of a simulated study, but where the limited objective of the study allows a more specific and objective measure of CT effect to be used. This strengthens confidence in the results.

Some of the statistical problems mentioned in connection with diagnostic studies apply equally to clinical value studies. First, the patients should be selected to represent the population for whom the technique is intended in the future. Secondly the performance and interpretation of the imaging technique should be done in the usual clinical setting and not in a specially funded research environment. A special problem arises from the reaction of the clinician to information from a new imaging technique. Wittenberg et al. (1980) show that as their study progressed the clinicians found CT more useful. The learning curve needs to be considered when designing and analysing studies of this kind. However, this problem should not exist for radiotherapy planning studies.

With regard to sample size, the same considerations as with diagnostic studies apply. Mostly we are interested in estimating proportions. That is, the proportions of patients for whom CT improved diagnostic understanding, or led to beneficial change of therapy, or led to more precise radiotherapy. If the investigator has a feel for the appropriate standard error of such a proportion, then Table 3.6 may be used. To employ Table 3.6 a guess at the true proportion (in terms of a percentage) will have to be made, although in the range 20%–80% the standard errors are rather insensitive to the variation in this figure. For percentages (P) below 50% the column corresponding most closely to $(100-P)\%$ should be used.

Assessment of Patient Outcome and Randomised Studies

The benefits of a new imaging technique are excessively difficult to measure. Wittenberg's study and general experience suggest that CT is able to improve diagnostic understanding in many conditions; can avoid the performance of more invasive diagnostic tests; and can give the clinician confidence in a treatment plan or suggest a change to a more beneficial treatment. These benefits may in themselves justify the expense of purchasing and running the new equipment, but in the presence of doubt about the relative costs and benefits some information on the effect of a new technique on patient outcome would be welcome. However, reliable information about even the crudest measure of outcome, survival time, is nearly always absent from the cost/benefit equation. Two approaches to measuring the effect of a diagnostic technique on patient outcome have been described.

First, Goitein (1979) has taken data from simulated studies of the effect of CT on radiotherapy planning and has fed these into a model to predict the clinical results of the increased precision of radiotherapy. This model is based upon an average dose–response relationship for the tumour and involves estimating the change in the probability of tumour control when part of the tumour is underdosed. Bearing in mind all the reservations that one must have over these extrapolations, Goitein estimates that CT improves the probability of local tumour control by an average of 6%, and 5-year survival by 3.5%.

Goitein's approach represents an attempt to measure the effect of imaging on patient outcome in an indirect way, using the results of clinical value studies which by their nature cannot provide a direct answer. The only type of study which can provide a direct answer is the randomised trial. The design requires that a patient is allocated to one of two alternative investigational policies. One policy will include the use of the new imaging technique, the other will not. By comparing the progress of the two groups of patients, the effects of the new technique on diagnosis, treatment, quality of life, response to treatment and length of survival may all be evaluated. Unfortunately ethical and logistic problems abound and these trials have only rarely been attempted. Reid et al. (1983) conducted a randomised trial of scintigraphy with and without tomography for 245 patients, but restricted the analysis to effect on diagnosis. Dronfield et al. (1977) compared endoscopy with radiology for 318 patients with acute upper gastrointestinal tract bleeding. Dixon et al. (1981) compared CT with conventional imaging for 53 patients with an abdominal mass. While Dronfield detected no difference in management or survival, Dixon found that CT reduced the period of in-patient observation.

The ethical difficulties of randomised trials of imaging techniques appear to be greater than for trials of therapy. In most trials of therapy a new treatment is usually associated not only with potential benefit, but may also have potential toxicity. Doubts over the toxicity allow the firm possibility that the current standard may be better than the new treatment and make the study ethically justifiable. Thus, disagreements over the reality of the hazard from multivitamins taken during pregnancy have led to arguments over the ethics of a Medical Research Council trial (*Lancet* editorial 1982).

In imaging studies the element of risk is usually considered to be minimal, otherwise the technique would not have reached the clinic. Thus once a technique has shown promise in a diagnostic study it is difficult to deny its potential benefits to a patient. In a local study it was recently proposed to compare CT and ultrasound for the diagnosis of suspected abdominal abscess, using a randomised design. However, the proposal foundered over the problem of having to deny CT to those whose ultrasound result was "suggestive" or "equivocal", and equally to deny ultrasound to those with an equivocal CT result.

A randomised trial is ethically sound if the new treatment is in short supply and available only to a limited number of patients, as in the pioneering Medical Research Council trial of streptomycin for pulmonary tuberculosis (Medical Research Council 1948). There may also be occasions when an imaging technique is available to only limited numbers of patients. Could one then justify a randomised study by claiming that even outside the study many patients would not be able to benefit from the technique? From a practical point of view this argument would not usually hold, since once the technique is available in a hospital it would naturally be available for all patients in that hospital. One would therefore have to randomise hospitals rather than patients—a grand design, but one which may prove both unpopular and unworkable!

A major practical problem for a randomised study is highlighted by Goitein's estimate of a 3.5% increase in 5-year survival following the use of CT in radiotherapy, for to detect an increase of this order reliably would require tens of thousands of patients. Russell and Williams (1983) have extensively reviewed the problems awaiting the investigator who embarks on a randomised trial of imaging techniques.

In conclusion, the occasions when a randomised study is a feasible method of evaluating imaging techniques will be fairly rare. However, since it is theoretically the best method, its feasibility should always be considered at the design stage.

Before-and-After Studies

The introduction of a new imaging technique into routine clinical use in a hospital affords an opportunity to study subsequent changes in diagnostic practice and results. While such studies are useful for monitoring changes in the use of diagnostic facilities, they are uncontrolled and as such are unreliable for drawing conclusions about the direct impact of a new technique. An example of the use of this type of study for monitoring is the report by Dixon (1985), who investigated the practice of lymphography before, during and after the introduction of CT. He found a reduction in the number of lymphograms performed and considered the factors which may have been responsible, including the introduction of CT. Appropriately the Discussion section in his paper accounted for half the length of the article! Ambrose et al. (1976) are less circumspect about the conclusions of their before-and-after study of the impact of brain CT on the management of head injuries. Russell and Williams (1983) criticise this study because, although reductions in the number of technetium scans, arteriograms and exploratory operations were observed, no information was given on the trends which would have been expected in the absence of CT. In addition the introduction of CT itself may have caused a change in the pattern of referral.

The Clinical Trial's Classification

Participants and organisers of research in therapeutic intervention have, over the years, developed a nomenclature for the various stages of investigation which may be required to introduce a new treatment (particularly a drug) into clinical practice. Table 3.8 shows the four phases in chronological order with brief definitions of each. Phase I trials are concerned with establishing a safe dose of the drug and the range and frequency of side-effects which are to be expected with that dose. Phase II trials aim to determine the efficacy of the drug in a quick and preliminary manner. In oncology this is done by selecting patients with measurable tumours and observing the change in size of tumour after treatment with the drug. Phase III trials are concerned with evaluating the use of

Table 3.8. Clinical trials' classification

Phase I	Toxicity, feasibility
Phase II	Screening for activity against disease
Phase III	Randomised controlled comparison in a clinical setting
Phase IV	Monitoring routine use and outcome

the drug, possibly in combination with other therapies, in a clinical setting, and including a comparative group of patients chosen by randomisation to receive the standard therapy. Phase IV studies are concerned with monitoring the long-term effects of a therapy which has been newly adopted as routine treatment.

The above classification has been useful in sorting out the different possible investigations available and relating the appropriateness of a particular type of study to the aims of the research worker. The classification implies an order in which the questions relating to the drug should be tackled, and a strategy, partly based on common sense, for providing answers to the questions. Thus, for example, phase II trials involving 15–50 patients, which are relatively quick to perform, are a preliminary screening measure for the identification of the more promising therapies. For such therapies one may sensibly proceed to spend considerable resources in mounting a more complex phase III study to try to establish the place of the therapy in routine practice. The existence of the classification therefore provides suitable advice to the investigator not to undertake a difficult and expensive study without first obtaining good objective evidence of the worth of the treatment. At the same time it also provides a rein on the imagination of the enthusiastic investigator who would like to recommend his new treatment for routine use following a promising preliminary study. Thus, classifications are not simply convenient categorisations, but can influence the broad strategy of research.

Classification of Imaging Studies

Table 3.9 shows a suggested classification of imaging studies which is somewhat analogous to the clinical trials classification.

Table 3.9. Classification for imaging studies

Phase I	Feasibility, promise
Phase II	Diagnostic accuracy studies
Phase III	Clinical value studies (*or* randomised comparisons where feasible)
	Endpoints: diagnosis, treatment, patient outcome
Phase IV	Before-and-after studies for monitoring routine use

Phase I incorporates pilot studies which assess the feasibility of a technique or make a very preliminary assessment of its promise.

Phase II corresponds to diagnostic accuracy studies. These are placed early in the classification because, as explained, they assess the use of the imaging technique out of clinical context. While one would hope the results of diagnostic studies would transfer to clinical practice this cannot be guaranteed. The discovery by Wittenberg et al. (1980) of a clinician's learning curve in the use of CT shows that transferral into clinical practice is not a simple matter. The experience with studies of carcinoembryonic antigen (CEA), which showed great promise in initial diagnostic accuracy studies but turned out to be of very limited value in the clinic, underlines the general problem. Nevertheless, nearly all investigators currently stop their research at this level.

Phase III comprises studies of the contribution of the technique to clinical management. Occasionally a randomised comparison will be possible, but usually the more feasible clinical value studies should be the design of choice. Where the imaging technique affects treatment an attempt should be made to assess indirectly the consequent change in patient outcome, as has been done for CT. In this author's opinion the major new effort in the evaluation of imaging techniques should be at the phase III level, particularly in view of the increasing interest in expensive techniques such as MRI.

Phase IV corresponds exactly to the monitoring of routine use of a newly introduced technique.

Finally, acknowledging on the one hand the difficulty and cost of running good diagnostic studies with large numbers of patients, and on the other hand the increasing expense of diagnostic equipment and the consequent need for careful evaluation, it is worth considering a remark of McNeil et al. (1981) in relation to one of their diagnostic studies. They stated "We spent 17 months collecting data from two major teaching institutions. Full time research assistants at each institution tried to obtain all cases in random order. Yet even this concerted effort produced only 156 cases and then only 50% of them included objective proof of disease. Now is the time to think about the administration, organization and financing of such studies."

I would like to thank Drs D. Spiegelhalter, I. Sutherland and A. Dixon for stimulating discussions and advice, and Professor N. M. Bleehen for encouraging my interest in this topic.

References

Abrams HL, Siegelman SS, Adams DF, et al. (1982) Computed tomography versus ultrasound of the adrenal gland: a prospective study. Radiology 143: 121–128

Ambrose J, Gooding MR, Uttley D (1976) EMI scan in the management of head injuries. Lancet I: 847–848

Brion JP, Depauw L, Kuhn G, et al. (1985) Role of computed tomography and mediastinoscopy in preoperative staging of lung carcinoma. J Comput Assist Tomogr 9: 480–484

Dixon AK (1985) The current practice of lymphography: a survey in the age of computed tomography. Clin Radiol 36: 287–290

Dixon AK, Fry IK, Kingham JGC, McLean AM, White FE (1981) Computed tomography in patients with an abdominal mass: effective and efficient? Lancet I: 1199–1201

Dronfield MW, McIlmurray MB, Ferguson R, Atkinson M, Langman MJS (1977) A prospective, randomised study of endoscopy and radiology in acute upper-gastrointestinal-tract bleeding. Lancet I: 1167–1169

Foster PN, Mitchell CJ, Robertson DRC, et al. (1984) Prospective comparison of three non-invasive tests for pancreatic disease. Br Med J 289: 13–16

Goitein M (1979) The utility of computed tomography in radiation therapy: an estimate of outcome. Int J Radiat Oncol Biol Phys 5: 1799–1807

Hanley JA, McNeil BJ (1982) The meaning and use of the area under a receiver operating characteristic (ROC) curve. Radiology 143: 29–36

Hanley JA, McNeil BJ (1983) A method of comparing the areas under ROC curves derived from the same cases. Radiology 148: 839–843

Harris JM (1981) The hazards of bedside Bayes. J Am Med Assoc 246: 2602–2605

Hauser MF, Gottschalk A (1978) A comparison of the Anger tomographic scanner and the 15 inch scintillation camera for gallium imaging. J Nucl Med 19: 1074–1077

Hawkes RC, Holland RN, Moore WS, Worthington BS (1980) NMR tomography of the brain: a preliminary clinical assessment with demonstration of pathology. J Comput Assist Tomogr 4: 577–586

Lancet Editorial (1982) Vitamins to prevent neural tube defects. Lancet II: 1255–1256

McNeil BJ, Sanders R, Alderson PO et al. (1981) A prospective study of computed tomography, ultrasound and gallium imaging in patients with fever. Radiology 139: 647–653

Medical Research Council (1948) Streptomycin treatment of pulmonary tuberculosis. Br Med J ii: 769–782

Phillips WC, Scott JA, Blasczcynski G (1983) How sensitive is 'sensitivity'; how specific is 'specificity'? AJR 140: 1265–1270

Prasad SC, Pilepich MV, Perez CA (1981) Contribution of CT to quantitative radiation therapy planning. AJR 136: 123–128

Ranshoff DF, Feinstein AR (1978) Problems of spectrum and bias in evaluating the efficacy of diagnostic tests. N Engl J Med 299: 926–930

Reid A, Dendy PP, Gemmell HG, Smith FW (1983) Value of tomographic section views in identifying liver abnormalities by scintigraphy. Acta Radiol [Diagn] (Stockh) 24: 107–111

Russell I, Williams A (1983) Evaluation of computerized tomography: a review of research methods. In: Culyer AJ, Horisberger B (eds) Economic and medical evaluation of health care technologies. Springer-Verlag, Berlin Heidelberg New York, pp 298–379

Sharp PF, Dendy PP, Keys WI (1985) Radionuclide imaging techniques. Academic Press, New York London, chapt 9

Sostre S, Ashare AB, Quinones JD, Schieve JB, Zimmerman JM (1978) Thyroid scintigraphy: pinhole images versus rectilinear scans. Radiology 129: 759–762

Wittenberg J, Fineberg HV, Ferrucci JT, et al. (1980) Clinical efficacy of computed body tomography: II. AJR 134: 1111–1120

4 Digital Subtraction Angiography

Duncan Irving

Introduction

Photographic subtraction has been used in angiography for many years. The technique depends on the effect that if a positive photographic image containing certain information is superimposed on a negative image containing the same information, the result will be a blank film. If further information is added to the second image, the image common to both will disappear, and leave only a picture of the additional image in the second film. Thus in an area where arteries are superimposed on bone, and additional information is gained by arterial injection, the bone will be subtracted resulting in much clearer definition of the arteries.

In digital subtraction angiography (DSA) the same result is achieved by computer-assisted electronic subtraction. With the addition of computer assistance to the process, however, the image is capable not only of subtraction but also of electronic enhancement. This enables a diagnostic image to be obtained at a much lower concentration of contrast medium, allowing for the use of smaller amounts of contrast medium than in conventional arteriography. This reduces the risk; and cost, of contrast medium in selective techniques. It also allows many procedures involving a flush intravenous injection of contrast medium resulting in total opacification of arteries to be performed on an outpatient basis. A drawback of DSA is that the image is taken from an image intensifier through a television chain, and the quality of the final image is limited by the comparatively poor spatial resolution of these systems as compared with that of film. However, in most clinical situations the enhanced subtracted image

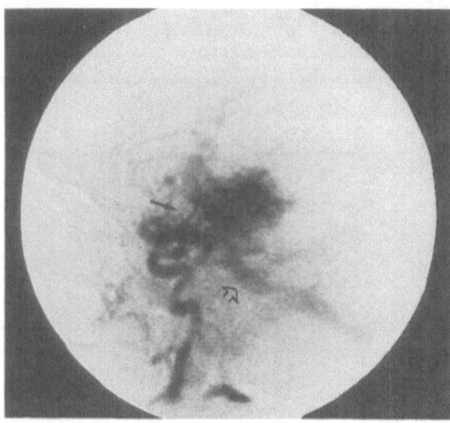

Fig. 4.1. Intracranial angioma shown by intravenous DSA. Note arterial supply (*arrow*) and early venous drainage (*open arrow*).

with increased contrast resolution compensates for this, and the clear demonstration of arteries 1 mm or less in diameter is not critical to diagnosis.

A further drawback of intravenous DSA is that all arteries are opacified and the resultant overlap can make diagnosis difficult if not impossible. Whereas an intravenous injection is adequate in the demonstration of the carotid and vertebral arteries in the neck, it is of limited value in intracranial vasculature distal to the circle of Willis, unless there is a highly vascular tumour such as an angioma (Fig. 4.1). However, these drawbacks can largely be overcome with selective arterial injection in which only the arteries of the area of interest are opacified. Even with the use of much smaller quantities of dilute contrast medium than in conventional radiography, the increased contrast resolution results in very comparable diagnostic images (Brant-Zawadzki et al. 1983, Weinstein et al. 1983, Stadnik et al. 1985).

Principles of Digital Subtraction Angiography

The patient is positioned so that the area under examination is projected on to an image intensifier. Depending on the amount of anatomical information desirable an appropriate intensifier field size is chosen; this varies in modern X-ray sets from a 5 inch to a 14 inch field. Obviously the smaller the field size the greater the magnification, and the more clearly the small arteries are seen. If too large a field size is selected, the diameter of the small arteries can approximate to the pixel size of the computer system, resulting in less sharpness of the image. Therefore, for examination of a limited area, the smaller the field the better.

The image is then conveyed through a television chain to the computer. Here the information is converted to digital form. The initial image taken before arrival of contrast medium is stored in a memory, and is then subtracted from subsequent images, so that all remaining images are viewed in a subtracted form. The images obtained are recorded on either a magnetic disc or magnetic tape where they are available for subsequent viewing or reprocessing. They are also simultaneously displayed on a television monitor.

If there is patient movement during acquisition of the image, imperfect subtraction may result in non-diagnostic images. These can be improved by reprocessing techniques. If an image containing contrast is rematched in the computer against subtracted images without contrast, great diagnostic improvement is possible (Fig. 4.2). Further improvement can sometimes be obtained by electronic shifting of the image to produce better matching. A permanent record of diagnostic images is made on film using a multiformat camera.

DSA using an intravenous injection of contrast medium is usually performed as an outpatient procedure. The contrast may be injected into a peripheral vein, but better results are achieved if the injection is given through a fine catheter (5 FG) introduced from the arm into the low superior vena cava or right atrium. If no arm vein can be found, the catheter can be introduced into the femoral vein at the groin. Between 25 and 40 ml of contrast medium containing 350 mg/ml iodine are injected at 15–25 ml/s. Although perfectly adequate results can be obtained with ionic contrast media, the lesser degree of discomfort following the injection of non-ionic contrast medium makes patient movement less likely. There is also the slightly lesser risk of allergic reaction favouring the latter. Just before the arrival of the contrast medium in the field of interest, the initial exposure (the mask) is made, together with, preferably, one or two subtracted images without prior arterial filling which can subsequently be used for reprocessing. When the medium is seen to have left the arteries under examination the X-ray exposures are terminated.

Intra-arterial DSA involves the use of selective arterial catheters. A flush aortic injection is rarely used since the aorta and the origins of its main branches can usually be shown adequately with an intravenous injection. However, when more distal arteries need to be demonstrated, the non-opacification of other vessels obscuring the field necessitates selective injection of the artery under examination. DSA does have certain advantages over conventional arteriography. Since low-density contrast only is needed, the concentration and total dose

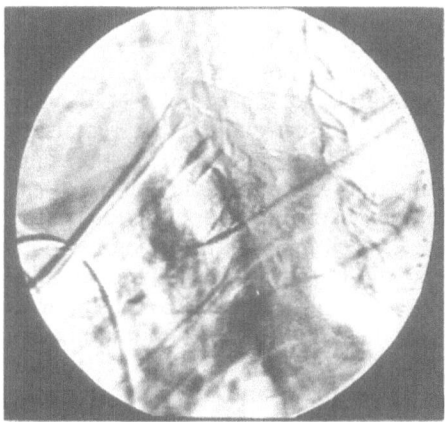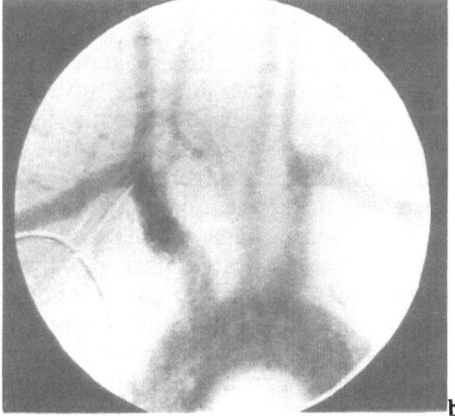

a b

Fig. 4.2. This demonstrates the effect of reprocessing. All the information in **b** is present in **a** and obtained by rematching with a subtracted image without contrast.

of contrast medium is significantly reduced, and adequate images can be achieved with 80–100 mg/ml of iodine, as opposed to 300–350 mg/ml with conventional arteriography. Furthermore, since much lower flow rates (usually 5 ml/s will suffice, finer catheters can be used with less risk of recoil. Immediate production of the image on the television screen, rather than having to wait while a series of films is developed, significantly reduces the time taken to complete an examination, and allows a much shorter procedure for the patient. In addition, the immediate viewing of the image during the procedure enables the operator to terminate the exposures as soon as the relevant information has been stored. This reduces the radiation dose to the patient. Also since the injection is given directly into the artery, not only can a higher degree of contrast resolution be achieved but also the time taken for the contrast medium to reach the field of examination is shortened, reducing the likelihood of movement artefact. A drawback is that the television field is usually smaller than that used in conventional arteriography, but two DSA examinations are both quicker to perform than one conventional examination and use less contrast medium than a single arteriographic series. DSA may be difficult or impossible in the uncooperative patient, but reprocessing of stored images will sometimes allow for adequate diagnosis even without patient cooperation (Fig. 4.2).

As the function of DSA is to demonstrate blood vessels its place in oncology is really the same as that of arteriography. The only differences are in the reduction of the amount of contrast medium used; the lessened radiation hazard to the patient; and in the saving of time and expense. Obviously if all procedures could be performed by intravenous injection the saving could be even greater since they could be done on an outpatient basis. The use of intravenous DSA is limited, however, to highly vascular tumours and to tumours involving major vessels not obscured by other vessels, both of which conditions limit the usefulness of the intravenous approach.

Tumours of the Head and Neck

Arteriography for the diagnosis of intracranial tumours has fallen into comparative disuse since the advent of computerised tomography (CT). The only intracranial space-occupying lesion in which intravenous DSA remains a valuable diagnostic technique is the large aneurysm or angioma. At the same time, the use of intravenous DSA in conjunction with ultrasonic angiology has increased the application of angiography in demonstrating arterial disease in the investigation of transient ischaemic attacks. Occasionally in this type of patient extracranial and large intracranial vessels are normal, but a hypervascular intracranial tumour may be demonstrated (Fig. 4.3). For this reason it is important that the intracranial circulation be included in the examination.

Chemodectoma is a vascular tumour of the head and neck in the investigation of which DSA or arteriography continues to be important. In the case of the carotid body tumour, intravenous DSA is adequate to either demonstrate or exclude its presence. Also, in view of the fact that these tumours are known sometimes to be multiple, it is important to cover all possible sites in the

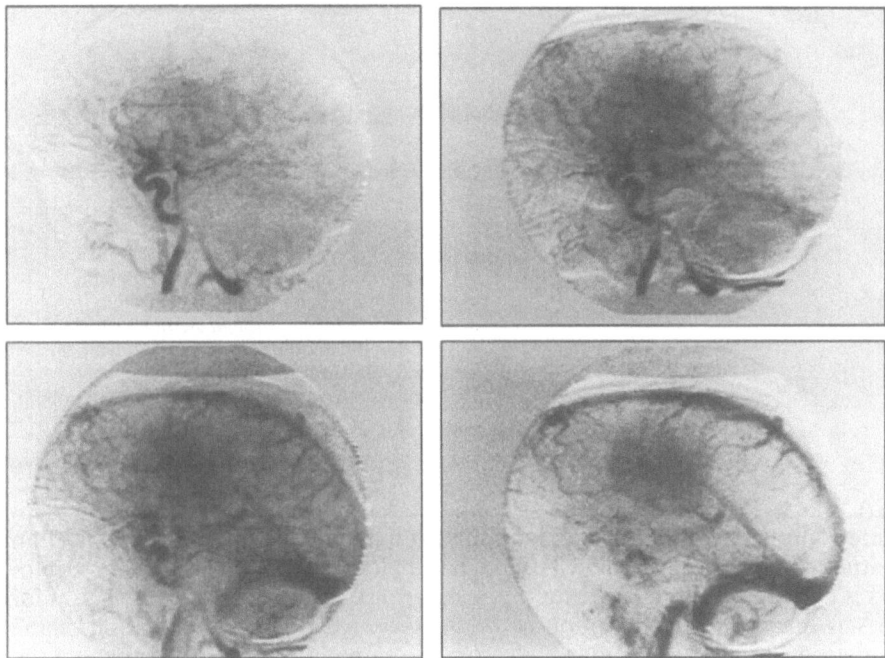

Fig. 4.3. Meningioma shown by intravenous DSA during examination for transient ischaemic attacks.

investigation (Fig. 4.4). For this purpose intravenous DSA constitutes the best screening examination. However, in patients with pulsatile tinnitus and suspected chemodectomas of the jugular or tympanic body, slightly imperfect subtraction can result in the intravenous examination providing a false negative result. In these patients, therefore, the ear should be examined by intra-arterial

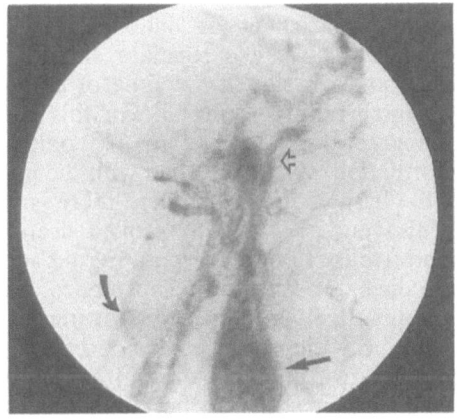

Fig. 4.4. Intravenous DSA showing tumours of the left carotid body (*straight arrow*) and left jugular body (*open arrow*). There is also a small right vagal body chemodectoma (*curved arrow*) clearly shown subsequently with intra-arterial DSA. A right carotid body tumour had been removed 10 years earlier. A sister of the patient also had a carotid body tumour.

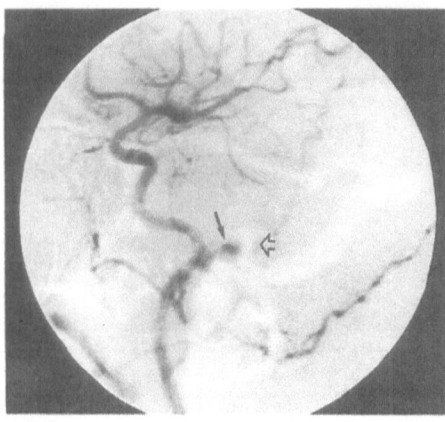

Fig. 4.5. Intra-arterial DSA, common carotid injection. A high jugular bulb (negative image, *straight arrow*) is shown within the middle ear, and a small tympanic body chemodectoma anteriorly (positive image, *open arrow*) indenting the jugular bulb.

DSA. The common carotid artery is catheterised with a 5 FG catheter, 6–8 ml of dilute contrast medium injected, and the ear examined in an oblique projection (Ratnesar and Irving 1979/80). Although the blood supply of aural chemodectomas is derived from the branches of the external carotid artery, the injection for DSA is made into the common carotid artery. This allows delineation of the cranial sinuses and the jugular bulb from the same injection, and as part of the same series of films. The tumour and its blood supply can be identified in the arterial phase, but as tumours may arise either from the tympanic or jugular body, the exact relation of the tumour to the jugular bulb can be shown. Whether or not the jugular bulb is actually invaded can also be demonstrated (Fig. 4.5). An anatomical variant important in the differential diagnosis and which produces similar symptoms to those of chemodectoma, is elevation of the jugular bulb into the middle ear due to dehiscence of the floor of the hypotympanum—a variant found in 6% of 257 dissections performed by Overton and Ritter (1973). Demonstration of this variant, which has been seen in conjunction with a tympanic body chemodectoma (Fig. 4.5), avoids the danger of biopsy, and diminishes the risk of surgery.

Arterial DSA is of considerable value in carotid embolisation techniques (Moret 1984). The anatomical display on the television monitor facilitates the accurate placement of balloons for balloon embolotherapy. Angiographic embolisation using particulate emboli requires many angiographic studies to assess at each step the degree of embolisation achieved and to help prevent unwanted reflux of emboli. For this purpose DSA is superior to conventional angiography and fluoroscopy. Not only is it considerably quicker, but also more information is obtained than with the unsubtracted film, especially in the region of the base of the skull where there is a considerable thickness of bone.

Intravenous DSA has proved useful in studies of the neck for the pre-operative localisation of parathyroid adenomas. Although a negative examination does not exclude their presence, a positive examination is of considerable pre-operative assistance. Following exploration of the neck with negative results, ectopic mediastinal parathyroid adenomas have been demonstrated by non-selective injection of contrast medium into the aortic arch (Krudy et al. 1984). Again it should be emphasised that in the localisation of parathyroid adenomas their presence cannot be excluded by arteriographic techniques; other techniques such as CT or venous sampling may prove most effective. However, if arteriography is used, the image enhancement inherent in DSA makes it a better technique than conventional arteriography.

Intrathoracic DSA

Intrathoracic DSA is useful in the investigation of the thoracic aorta and its main branches; in selected cases it is also of considerable value in excluding the possibility of pulmonary embolus. It has little part to play, though, in the diagnosis of intrathoracic neoplasia. More useful information on pulmonary tumours, with the exception of arteriovenous malformations, can always be obtained by CT or even plain radiography. As a rapid and simple screening technique in the investigation of paramediastinal masses, and for the differentiation between tumours and vascular structures, intravenous DSA is, however, very helpful (Fig. 4.6).

It is possible that in the future dual energy subtraction or selective enhancement of sections of an electronic image of the chest may add to the range of chest radiography. At present, however, contrast digital chest radiography is at a very early stage of development.

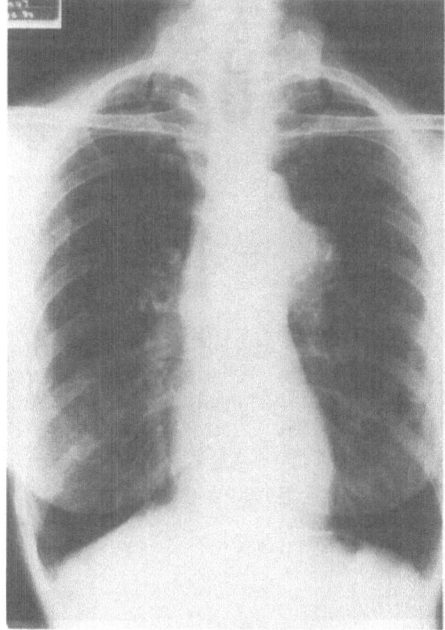
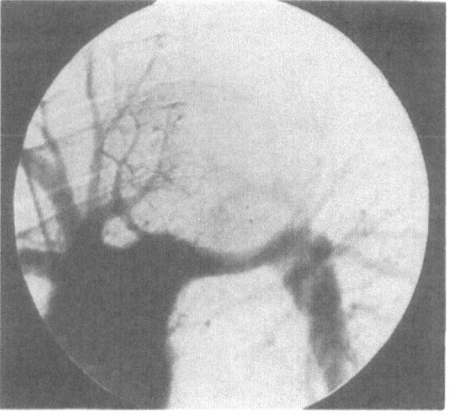

Fig. 4.6.a Chest X-ray showing left paramediastinal mass. **b** Intravenous DSA showing encasement of left pulmonary artery by bronchial carcinoma. (The descending aorta was normal.)

Urinary Tract

The principal use of DSA in the urinary tract is in the diagnosis of renovascular hypertension by intravenous injection, since the renal arteries can be demonstrated and stenosis diagnosed. This has proved a much more accurate method than intravenous urography (Hillman et al. 1982, Gomes et al. 1983).

In renal tumours, although intravenous DSA may demonstrate a large hypervascular neoplasm, the presence of subtraction artefacts may make an injection examination unreliable. Aortic or selective intra-arterial injection, however, has the same accuracy as conventional arteriography with the additional advantage of a saving in the time taken and the contrast material used. The anatomy of the blood supply is clearly seen, and a search for an arterial supply other than the renal artery can be rapidly and simply performed (Fig. 4.7). Occasionally in the less vascular tumours, the facility for subtraction and contrast enhancement can give information which would be less clearly defined by standard arteriography. This may then provide information not easily supplied by other methods and suggestive of a diagnosis (Fig. 4.8).

Selective DSA also contributes significantly to the saving of time in renal embolisation, since the artery which has been catheterised can immediately be visualised on the television monitor. If embolic materials such as alcohol or small particles are used this should diminish the risk of distal embolisation of a lumbar

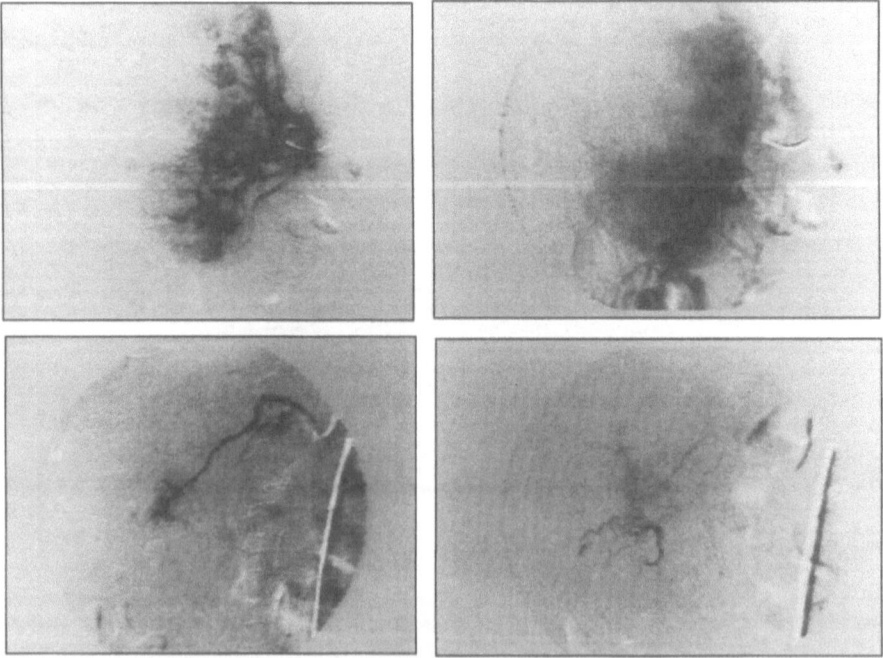

Fig. 4.7. Carcinoma of the right kidney showing tumour supplied by the right renal artery (upper images) and right first lumbar artery (lower images).

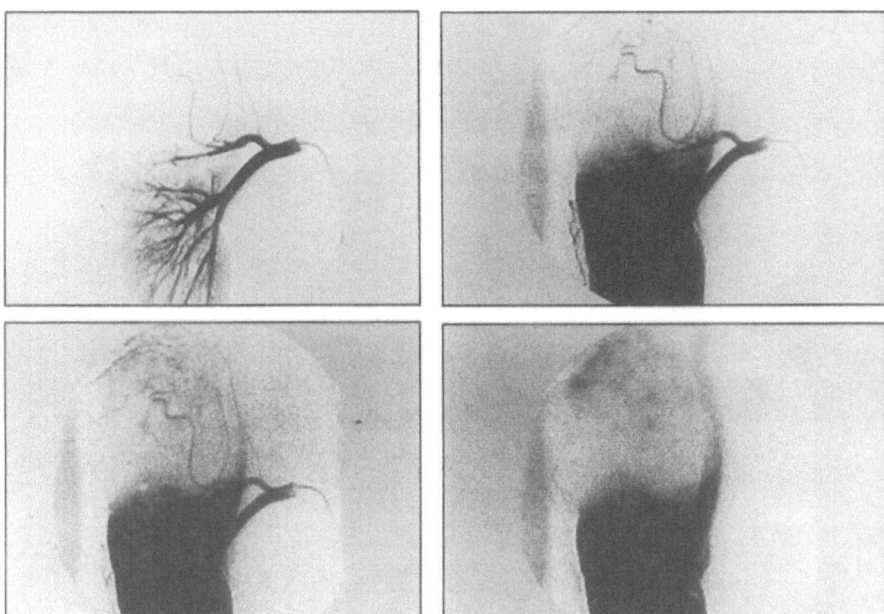

Fig. 4.8. Female of 21 years suspected of a right renal abscess. Attempted percutaneous drainage was unsuccessful, but aspiration biopsy suggested a simple tumour. Intra-arterial DSA showed sparse pathological circulation and tumour blush. At operation an apparent abscess was found but histologically this was a clear cell carcinoma.

or mesenteric artery (Cox et al. 1982). The risk of reflux from partially embolised arteries may also be diminished, since the flow pattern can be visualised clearly with slow injection of opacified emboli in dilute contrast medium.

Although suprarenal tumours are now best shown by CT, arteriography and therefore DSA can be extremely useful in delineating the blood supply and vascularity. The examination should include selective catheterisation of the renal and inferior phrenic arteries. In the presence of a large vascular adrenal carcinoma, lumbar arteries, as well as the splenic artery on the left or the hepatic artery on the right, should be visualised to define the full extent of the tumour.

Since the advent of ultrasound and CT arteriography has no place in the staging of bladder tumours. However, in the presence of intractable or severe bleeding from a bladder tumour or following radiotherapy, selective catheterisation of the anterior division of the internal iliac artery and its embolisation can be of considerable use in controlling blood loss, at least in the short term. Again accurate catheterisation and embolisation is facilitated by the use of selective intra-arterial DSA.

Retroperitoneal tumours are easily visualised and delineated by ultrasound or CT. However, in vascular tumours, selective arteriography using DSA provides a safe and rapid method of delineating the blood supply prior to surgery or embolisation. The technique was used in a 24-year-old West Indian with a large left retroperitoneal tumour, thought at CT to be a large angioma supplied by a

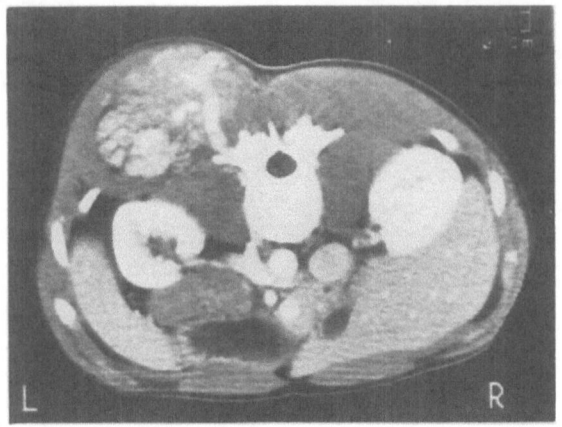

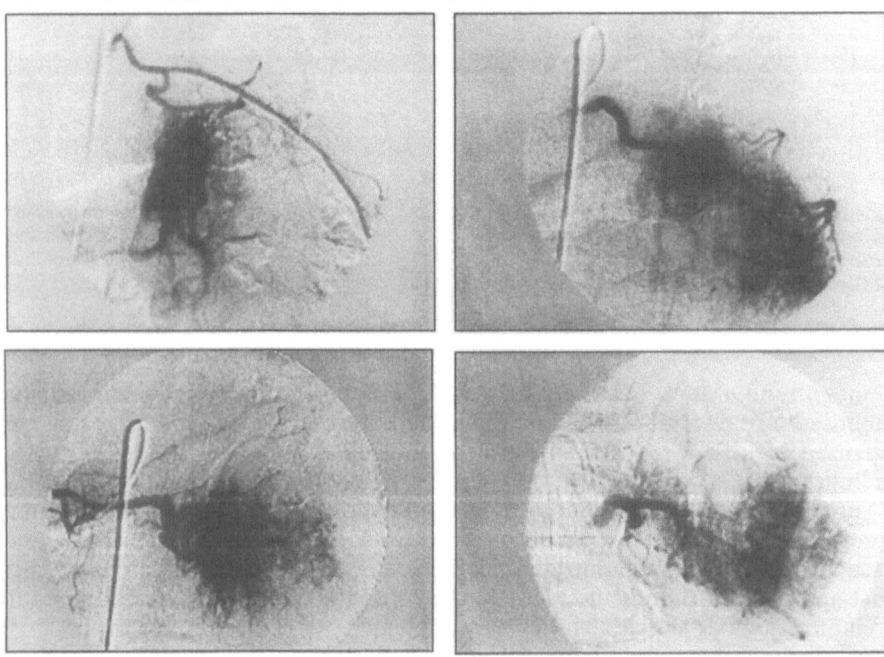

Fig. 4.9. Patient presenting with a large vascular tumour of the posterior abdominal wall. **a** CT shows hypervascularity and apparently large supplying vessel. **b** Selective intra-arterial DSA shows tumour to be supplied by multiple intercostal and lumbar arteries, with no single large feeding artery.

single large artery (Fig. 4.9a). This was not found on arteriography, and selective DSA examination of the ninth intercostal to the fourth lumbar artery showed a large vascular tumour supplied by the eleventh and twelfth intercostal and the first, second and third lumbar arteries. Large draining veins were demonstrated (Fig 4.9b). Embolisation was therefore not practicable. Fine needle biopsy showed a connective tissue tumour, with no evidence of malignancy.

Liver

It is in the management of tumours of the liver by interventional radiological techniques that intra-arterial DSA has proved to be of most value. A complete examination including hepatic arteriography and arterial portography by conventional angiography can necessitate the use of large amounts of contrast medium. Clear definition of the portal circulation may need 60–70 ml of contrast medium, possibly assisted by the use of vasodilators in order to increase the flow rate through the superior mesenteric arterial bed. With DSA a comparable result can be obtained using only 10–15 ml of contrast medium.

Although highly vascular tumours such as carcinoid metastases are clearly shown by conventional angiography and DSA, the facility for contrast enhancement inherent in the latter provides a much denser opacification (Fig. 4.10). For this reason these tumours are more clearly visible with considerably less contrast medium: 5 ml containing 300 mg/ml of iodine diluted to 10 ml will usually suffice, and very small deposits may be seen more easily. Furthermore DSA is considerably better than standard arteriography in the demonstration of "avascular" metastases. The hepatogram phase of a normal liver is homogeneous, and large metastases on conventional arteriography show as avascular filling defects. With the contrast enhancement of DSA, filling defects are seen to consist of a central avascular area surrounded by a hypervascular halo within the rather less vascular normal liver (Fig. 4.11). Ultrasound, CT or isotope techniques usually demonstrate at least the larger metastases, but deposits have been shown by DSA that were not visualised by other techniques. However, arteriographic techniques are now less frequently used in the diagnosis of liver tumours. Nevertheless in the presence of many hypervascular

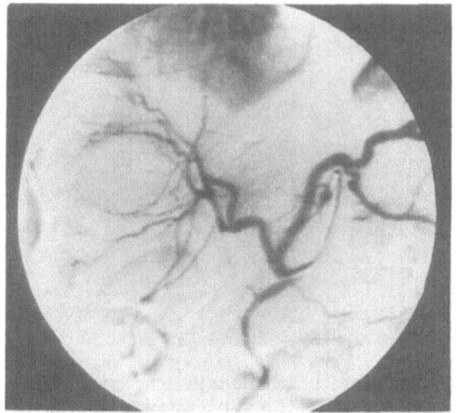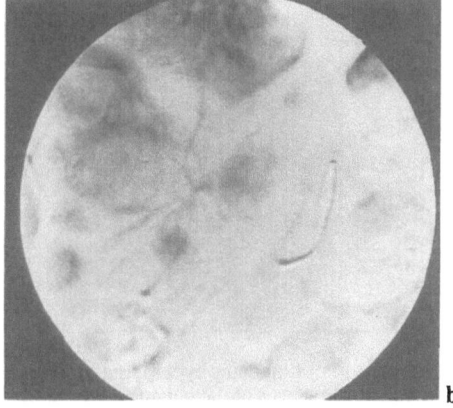

a   b

Fig. 4.10. Multiple carcinoid metastases in right lobe of liver: **a** arterial, **b** hepatogram phase.

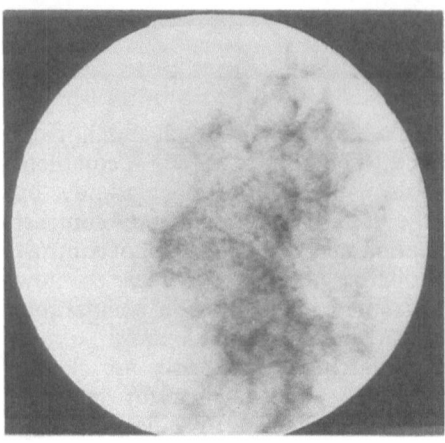

Fig. 4.11. Multiple adenocarcinoma "avascular" metastases in the right lobe of the liver. Note the hypervascular ring and clear avascular centre.

tumours such as carcinoid metastases, contraceptive pill adenoma or symptomatic focal nodular hyperplasia (Fig. 4.12) the treatment of choice will be by embolisation, and arteriography is therefore necessitated.

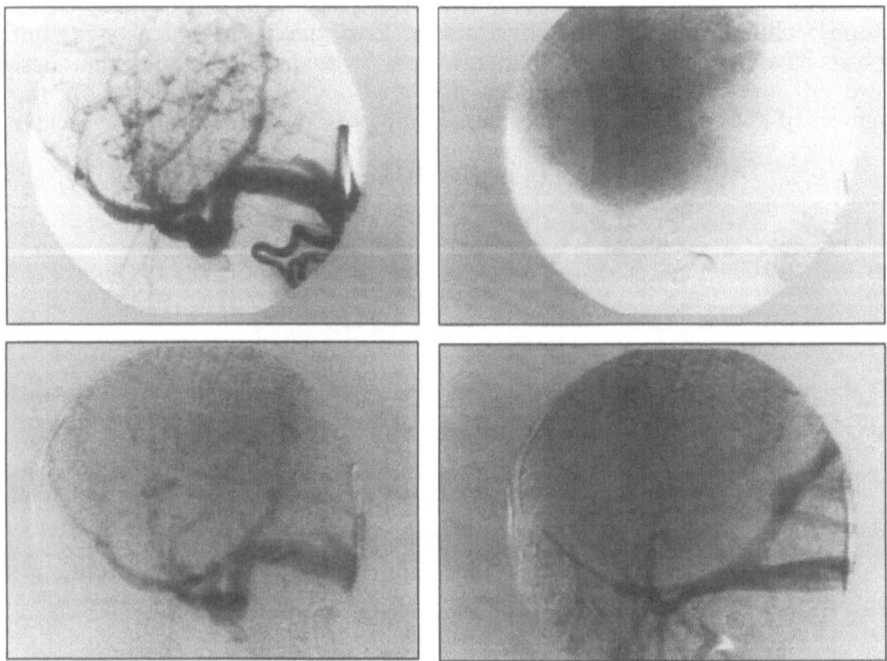

Fig. 4.12. Focal nodular hyperplasia of liver. Single highly vascular tumour in right lobe of liver, supplied by branches of the hepatic artery displaced over its surface. It is also displacing branches of the portal vein. Film obtained with hand injection into the coeliac axis of 10 ml of contrast medium containing 300 mg/ml of iodine.

The pre-embolic diagnostic arteriogram involves not only full delineation and diagnosis, but also an adequate demonstration of the portal circulation by portal venography. This is essential since normal liver tissue receives the greater part of its blood supply from the portal circulation whereas intrahepatic neoplasms are supplied largely by the hepatic artery. It was thought that neoplasms were virtually entirely vascularised from the hepatic artery (Breedis and Young 1984), and even though more recent work suggests that the portal vein plays a greater part in vascularisation than originally believed (Lin et al. 1984), nevertheless symptomatic relief can be obtained by arterial embolisation. However, since avoidance of the risk of necrosis of liver tissue depends on a good portal supply, it is necessary to show portal circulation by arterial portography prior to embolisation. The amount of contrast medium used in film angiography may make embolisation on a subsequent occasion advisable, whereas with DSA all necessary information can usually be achieved with not more than 100 ml of contrast medium. This makes it reasonable to proceed immediately to embolisation, thus subjecting the patient to a single procedure only.

Pancreas

Localisation of islet cell tumours of the pancreas can be extremely difficult. The larger tumours may be shown by CT or occasionally by ultrasound. However, it will often be impossible to demonstrate smaller tumours. Many of them are vascular and can be shown by superselective arteriography. Since a dense tumour blush is rare, however, DSA is probably more accurate for localisation, although superselective arteriography is still advisable (Fig. 4.13) since the very small tumour can be completely obscured by extrapancreatic arteries if these have been filled. As already stated, liver metastases from these tumours, when malignant, are all hypervascular and therefore hepatic arteriography should always be done as part of the DSA examination. However even with the contrast enhancement of DSA not all primary tumours will be visible, and a negative

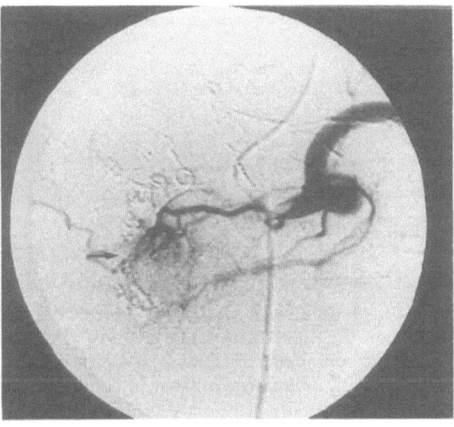

Fig. 4.13. Insulinoma in the head of the pancreas shown by dorsal pancreatic injection.

examination does not exclude their presence. In the functioning tumour perhaps the most accurate method of localisation is by transhepatic portal vein catheterisation and selective catheterisation of the pancreatic veins for venous sampling and hormone assay (Reichardt and Ingmansson 1980). However, even with a map of veins provided by DSA, this is liable to be an extremely protracted procedure. Arteriography with DSA should therefore be done first, in the hope not only of demonstrating a tumour but also of providing a map of the intrahepatic portal vein prior to transhepatic sampling.

Islet cell tumours can grow to a considerable size and may need transarterial intrahepatic procedures. This was seen in a female patient aged 53 who had been explored for a large unresectable non-secreting tumour in the head of the pancreas. Three and a half years later she was re-admitted with severe gastrointestinal bleeding which was seen endoscopically to originate from

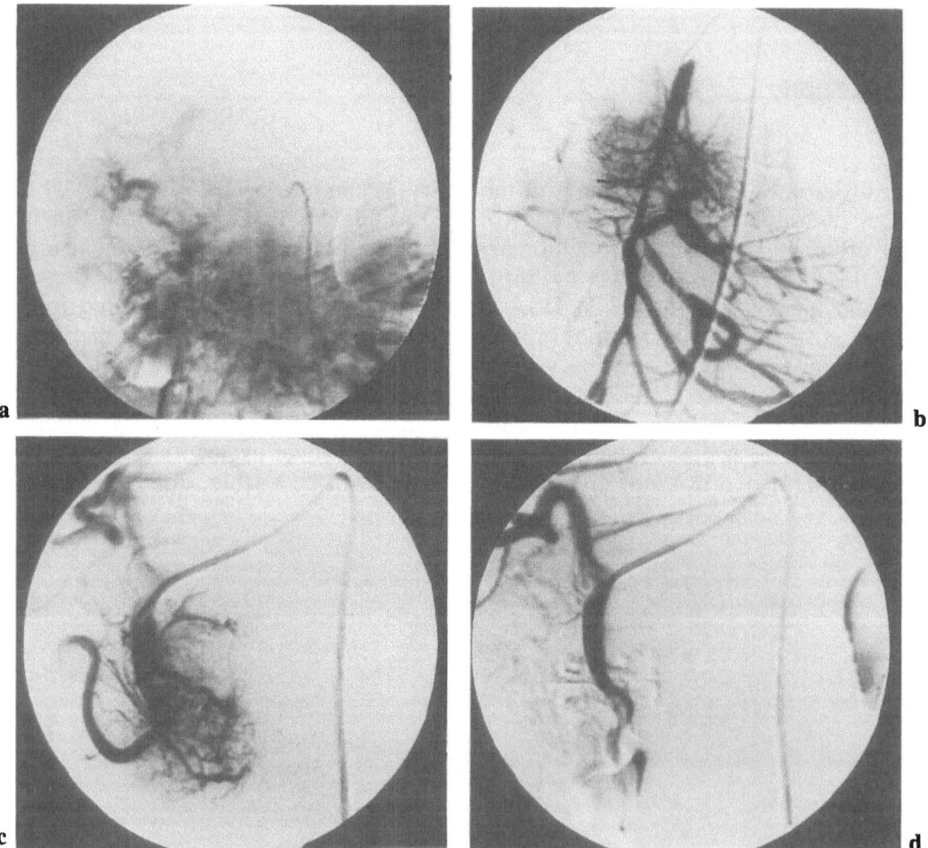

Fig. 4.14. Patient with islet cell tumour of the pancreas. **a** Large vascular tumour blush seen after injection of the superior mesenteric artery. There are multiple draining collateral veins, the superior mesenteric vein being occluded. **b** Main trunk of the superior mesenteric artery encased by hypervascular tumour (*arrow*). **c** Injection of the gastroduodenal artery showing hypervascular tumour filling. **d** After embolisation with microspheres, no tumour filling can be seen.

ulceration of the tumour into the duodenum. Using DSA, multiple hypervascular metastases were demonstrated in the liver, chiefly in the right lobe. DSA examination of the superior mesenteric artery showed occlusion of the superior mesenteric vein, and encasement of the upper part of the superior mesenteric artery (Fig. 4.14a,b). Selective catheterisation of the gastroduodenal artery provided a map showing clear tumour filling from the superior pancreatic duodenal arteries (Fig. 4.14c). These were catheterised selectively and embolised with microspheres (Fig. 4.14d). The bleeding was controlled but recurred after some weeks. Tumour was again seen to fill from the gastroduodenal artery which was completely embolised with wire coils, with further control of bleeding. At the same time the liver metastases were embolised with microspheres and a coil. When bleeding recurred some months later, considerable tumour opacification was seen from the superior mesenteric artery, but unfortunately it was impossible to catheterise the inferior pancreaticoduodenal arteries selectively and no further embolisation was possible. As these procedures involved multiple superselective catheterisations the saving in both time and contrast medium using DSA was considerable.

DSA in the Management of Pancreatic Carcinoma and Obstructive Jaundice

Malignant obstructive jaundice is not uncommon and in many cases the results of surgery are poor. A survey of survival statistics (Gudjonsson et al. 1978) found an operative mortality of 22% in patients with malignant jaundice (including that from palliative and exploratory surgery). Out of a total of approximately 15 000 patients, the 5-year survival was only 0.4%. It is the author's practice in these cases not only to provide percutaneous palliation of the jaundice by endoprosthesis, but also, using intra-arterial DSA, to attempt to select those patients with unresectable tumours.

Obviously in patients in whom curative surgery is precluded, because of old age or medical unfitness for major surgery, the bile ducts are drained by percutaneous biliary endoprosthesis and nothing further is done. However, there is a significant number of younger persons who are otherwise fit for resection of the tumour. In these patients insertion of a biliary endoprosthesis is followed by fine needle aspiration biopsy. It is of course not possible to prove resectability by radiological methods, since tumours are often considerably more extensive than radiology suggests. Inoperability may have been proved by ultrasound or CT, as for example by the demonstration of hepatic metastases. However if these modalities do not demonstrate an inoperable tumour, arteriography using DSA provides a quick, simple and safe screening technique. A tumour which extends to involve a major extrapancreatic vascular structure is not going to be resectable, and DSA examination is performed to show the hepatic, splenic and superior mesenteric arteries and the splenic, superior mesenteric and portal veins. Encasement (Fig. 4.15) or occlusion (Fig. 4.16), especially of the superior mesenteric or portal vein, will indicate complete irresectability, and enable the patient with a limited life expectancy to avoid

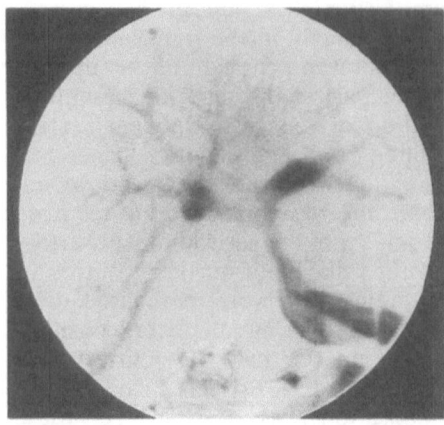

Fig. 4.15. Encasement of the extrahepatic portal vein by cholangiocarcinoma indicating inoperability. Ten millilitres of contrast medium were injected by hand into the splenic artery.

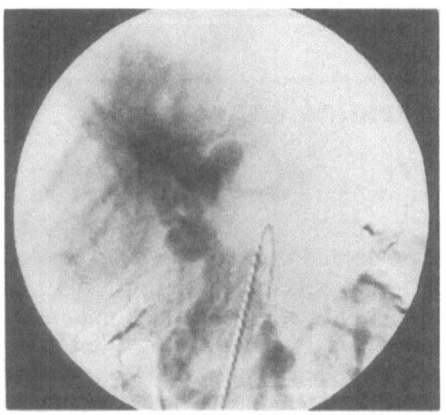

Fig. 4.16. Occlusion of the upper part of the superior mesenteric vein and extrahepatic portal vein by pancreatic carcinoma. Note the multiple collateral veins in the porta hepatis. Twelve millilitres of contrast medium were injected by hand into the superior mesenteric artery.

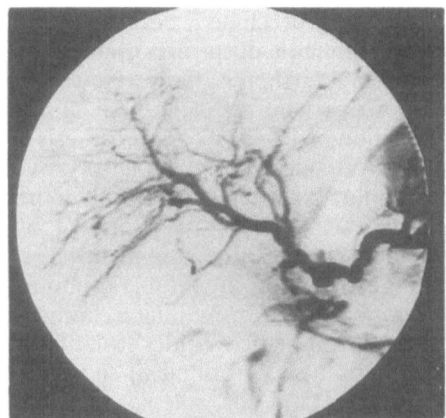
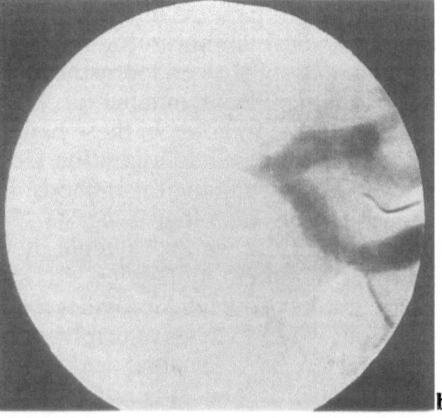

a   b

Fig. 4.17. Patient with carcinoma of the pancreas. **a** Extensive encasement of splenic, gastroduodenal and common hepatic arteries by carcinoma of pancreas. Five millilitres of contrast medium were injected by hand into the coeliac axis. **b** Total occlusion of the splenic vein.

laparotomy. Palliation without surgical exploration often allows the patient to leave hospital within a week or so.

In carcinoma of the body or tail of the pancreas the DSA examination concentrates initially on the splenic artery and vein. However, the hepatic artery and portal vein should always be included in the examination since pancreatic carcinoma can be much more extensive than expected (Fig. 4.17).

Gastrointestinal Tract

Arteriography in diseases of the gastrointestinal tract is used in the diagnosis, and sometimes the treatment, of gastrointestinal bleeding. As the commonest causes of bleeding are ulceration, angiodysplasia and diverticular disease they are not included in the scope of this paper. However some tumours such as leiomyoma or leiomyosarcoma (Kande et al. 1972) are highly vascular, and may be diagnosed by arteriography if beyond the reach of the endoscope.

Occasionally information may be obtained by DSA which radically changes the management of gastrointestinal tumours. A patient aged 58 had had a laparotomy as an emergency. A large apparently unresectable pancreatic mass was found and biopsied. The results of histology were inconclusive but suggested a renal neoplasm. The results of selective renal DSA were normal. Selective superior mesenteric DSA showed displacement of the superior mesenteric branches only. An injection into the coeliac axis gave no definite information. However when the gastroduodenal artery was catheterised a selective injection did not show a pancreatic tumour; a faint tumour blush was seen though, arising from the right gastro-epiploic artery (Fig. 4.18). On the strength of this the abdomen was re-explored and gastrectomy resulted in the complete removal of a leiomyoblastoma of the greater curve of the stomach. Although conventional arteriography was not done it was arguable whether the diagnosis would have been made without DSA, since even with contrast enhancement the tumour blush was not striking.

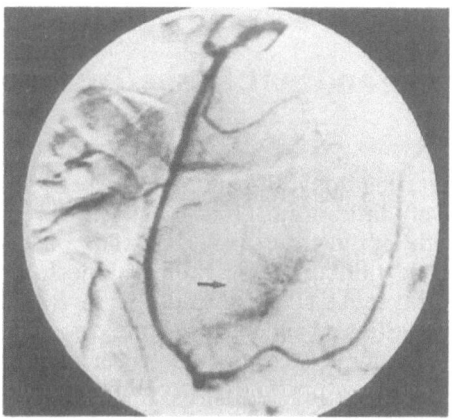

Fig. 4.18. Tumour blush seen after selective injection of 3 ml of contrast medium into the right gastro-epiploic artery (*arrow*) showing a tumour of the greater curve of the stomach. A leiomyoblastoma was removed.

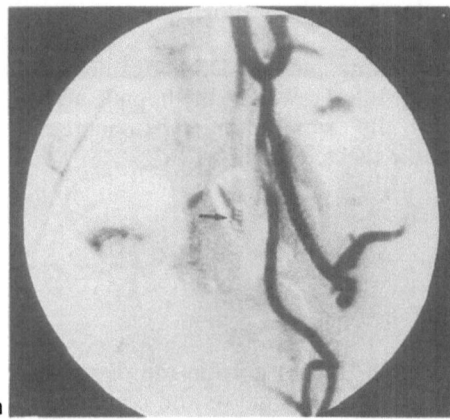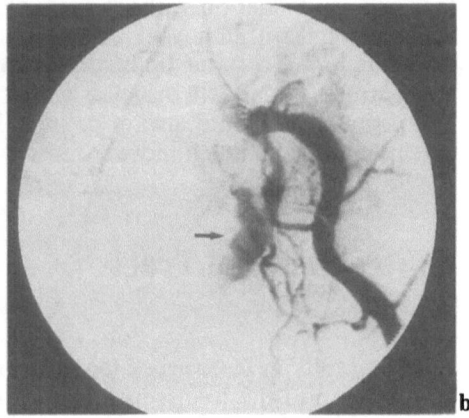

a   b

Fig. 4.19. A patient with an extensive adenocarcinoma in the pelvis presented with severe bleeding. The bleeding stopped after embolisation of the superior haemorrhoidal artery with a single Gianturco coil, then recurred. **a** Selective inferior mesenteric arteriogram shows superior haemorrhoidal occlusion. Note the image of the incompletely subtracted coil (*arrow*), and patent left colic artery. **b** Internal iliac arteriogram shows further bleeding from anterior division (*arrow*), which was then embolised.

DSA is of more limited use in the investigation of gastrointestinal bleeding, since catastrophic bleeding can easily be seen during normal fluoroscopy, and especially in small or large intestine subtraction artefacts can mask minor haemorrhages. However in certain instances where selective catheterisation is used, time can be saved by using DSA. A patient with a large sigmoid carcinoma presented with catastrophic rectal haemorrhage. An inferior mesenteric arteriogram showed bleeding of such severity that no films were needed. The superior haemorrhoidal artery was embolised with a coil and the bleeding stopped. Less severe haemorrhage recurred about an hour later and DSA examination showed complete occlusion of the superior haemorrhoidal artery, but active bleeding from the internal iliac artery (Fig. 4.19). This in turn was embolised with complete control of the haemorrhage.

Bone and Soft Tissue Tumours

Arteriography, though potentially useful in vascular bone tumours, is comparatively little used. Occasionally intravenous DSA may give useful information without the necessity for arterial puncture. For example a 2-year-old boy with a cystic tumour in the humeral neck was biopsied and only blood obtained. Intravenous DSA showed a highly vascular tumour with rapid venous drainage suggestive of aneurysmal bone cyst. This diagnosis was subsequently confirmed surgically. Osteosarcoma has a high vascularity and both the extent of the tumour within and beyond bone, and its blood supply, can be shown by intravenous DSA.

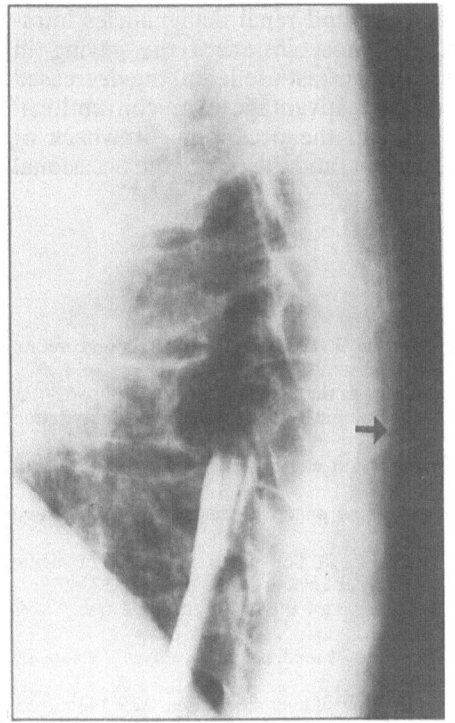
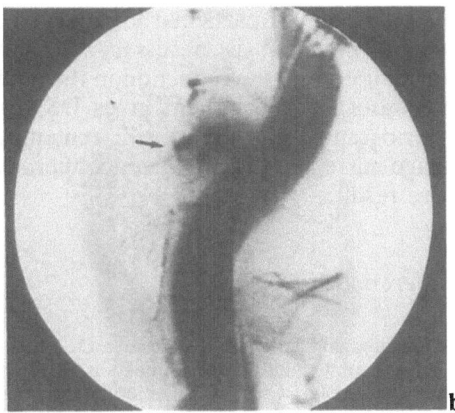

Fig. 4.20. Patient with renal carcinoma and paraplegia. **a** Myelogram showing complete spinal block and erosion of the posterior margin of the body of the tenth dorsal vertebra. **b** Injection into the thoracic aorta shows a highly vascular deposit (*arrow*). A second injection into the abdominal aorta demonstrated a renal carcinoma.

Occasionally arterial and selective injection is better, as is shown by the case of a patient who developed paraplegia due to a spinal block at the level of the tenth dorsal vertebra. CT suggested high vascularity, and a selective DSA examination showed a vascular deposit supplied by the ninth and tenth intercostal arteries (Fig. 4.20). The possibility of a metastasis was considered, and despite lack of preparation an injection into the abdominal aorta using DSA demonstrated the presence of a renal carcinoma. This was removed and the spinal metastasis treated with radiotherapy.

Conclusion

In summary, it must be said that for the most part DSA has little to offer in oncology that is not provided by conventional arteriography. But as has been shown, most vascular tumours, particularly those in head and neck and in bone, can be demonstrated by intravenous injection followed by DSA. Since this offers a simple and rapid outpatient procedure, distinct advantages can be seen.

In abdominal, particularly hepatic, pancreatic and renal malignancies intra-arterial injection is necessary. However in most instances the saving in procedure time, the reduction in the amount of contrast used, and the decreased discomfort to the patient gives DSA a distinct advantage over conventional arteriography. One must still remember though the occasional drawback of image misregistration in the uncooperative patient, and the risk of the occasional false result.

References

Brant-Zawadzki M, Gould R, Norman D, Newton TH, Lam B (1983) Digital subtraction cerebral angiography by intra-arterial injection. AJR 140: 347–353

Breedis C, Young G (1984) The blood supply of neoplasms in the liver. Am J Pathol 30: 969–985

Cox GC, Lee KR, Price HC, Gunter K, Noble MJ (1982) Colonic infarction following embolisation of renal cell carcinoma. Radiology 145: 343–345

Gomes AS, Pais SO, Barbarie ZL (1983) Digital subtraction angiography in the evaluation of hypertension. AJR 140: 779–783

Gudjonsson B, Livston EM, Spiro HM (1978) Cancer of the pancreas: diagnostic accuracy and survival statistics. Cancer 42: 2494–2506

Hillman BJ, Ovitt TW, Theron WO, Capp MP et al. (1982) The potential impact of digital subtraction angiography on screening for renovascular hypertension. Radiology 142: 577–579

Kande J, Selseth C, Tyler U (1972) Angiography in myomas of the gastrointestinal tract. Acta Radiol [Diagn] (Stockh) 12: 691–704

Krudy AG, Doppman JL, Miller DL et al. (1984) Detection of mediastinal parathyroid glands by non-selective digital arteriography. AJR 142: 693–695

Lin G, Hagerstrand I, Lunderquist A (1984) Portal blood supply of liver metastases. AJR 143: 53–55

Moret J (1984) Digital subtraction angiography regarding interventional radiology. Paper presented at the Symposium on Digital Subtraction Angiography, Westminster Hospital, 25 February 1984

Overton SB, Ritter FN (1973) A high placed jugular bulb in the middle ear: a clinical and temporal bone study. Laryngoscope 83: 1986–1991

Ratnesar P, Irving JD (1979/80) Arteriography in the diagnosis and management of chemodecto-mas, and extracranial meningiomas of the head and neck. J Oto-Laryngol Soc Aust 4: 335–338

Reichardt W, Ingmansson S (1980) Selective vein catheterisation for hormone assay in endocrine tumours of the pancreas. Acta Radiol [Diagn] (Stockh) 21: 177–187

Stadnik TW, Kersschot EAJ, de Schepper Amap (1985) Intracranial tumours examined by intraarterial DSA: comparative angiographic study. Radiology 154: 671–675

Weinstein MA, Pavlicrek WA, Modie MT, Duchesneau PM (1983) Intra-arterial digital subtraction angiography of the head and neck. Radiology 147: 717–724

5 Interventional Radiology in Oncology

James McIvor

Introduction

Interventional radiology has a useful role in the management of patients with malignant disease. Many of the currently used techniques have been developed or substantially improved during the last decade, and improvements continue. The procedures are both diagnostic and therapeutic. The main diagnostic procedure is guided aspiration or biopsy and the main therapeutic procedures are arterial embolisation and the relief of obstruction. Although time-consuming and often technically difficult, such techniques have the advantage of a low morbidity when compared with open surgery.

Fluoroscopically Guided Aspiration and Biopsy

Fluoroscopy may be used to direct a needle into a lesion in the chest or skeleton, and is particularly useful in obtaining samples from small lesions. Ultrasound and computerised X-ray tomographic scanning (CT) are more effective in soft tissue organs such as the liver and pancreas and are outside the scope of this paper.

Thin needles (20G–22G) are commonly used in the chest, as cutting and biopsy needles carry an increased risk of pneumothorax and intrapulmonary haemorrhage. Specimens obtained with thin needles are smeared on slides and examined cytologically, whereas specimens obtained with cutting needles are fixed, sectioned and examined by conventional histological techniques. Although modern cytological techniques can detect primary and secondary malignancies, particularly carcinoma, with a high degree of accuracy, the technique is less accurate than histology. In the skeleton cutting or biopsy needles are preferred, as complications are extremely rare and biopsy specimens provide more diagnostic information than tissue smears obtained by aspiration.

Lung

Guided lung aspiration and biopsy under local anaesthesia can obtain material from intrapulmonary lesions for cytological, histological and microbiological examination. The technique is often an alternative to thoracotomy and has a very low morbidity, particularly if a thin 20G or 22G needle is used.

The diagnosis of malignancy by aspiration or biopsy allows the patient to be managed without thoracotomy. This is of considerable value in patients considered to be poor surgical risks; in patients with extensive unresectable disease in the chest; and in those with evidence of widespread disease but no tissue diagnosis. A positive result should be reliable and justify treatment with chemotherapy or radiotherapy. The value of detecting localised malignancy in a patient fit for thoracotomy is much more doubtful, unless the lesion is an anaplastic small cell carcinoma for which chemotherapy is the treatment of choice.

Technique and Complications

The lesion must be accurately localised before aspiration. Large lesions are usually adequately shown on posteroanterior and lateral films; small lesions and those situated close to the hilum or chest wall may require tomography or even CT scanning for precise localisation.

If the distance from the skin surface to the lesion is accurately known then single-plane fluoroscopy is satisfactory. The patient is placed prone or supine on the screening table to allow aspiration by the shortest route, the skin and subcutaneous tissues are infiltrated with local anaesthesia and the skin is punctured with a scalpel directly over the lesion. The aspiration needle is then passed vertically through the skin for a measured distance.

The earlier aspirations were carried out with 16G or 18G needles (Dick et al. 1974; Sinner 1976; Sinner and Zajicek 1976; Berquist et al. 1980), but more recently thin-walled 20G or 22G Chiba needles have been used (Chin and Yee 1978; Westcott 1981; Frable 1982) as they seem to incur a lower morbidity. It is sometimes difficult to pass a flexible needle into a deep-seated lesion, as the needle tip is carried sideways by the bevel, but the flexibility means that parallax can be used to check the position of the needle tip in relation to the lesion. If the needle is correctly placed the tip will move with the lesion during respiratory movement (Fig. 5.1), but if the needle is short of the lesion, or has been passed through it, the tip will move away from the lesion during inspiration and expiration.

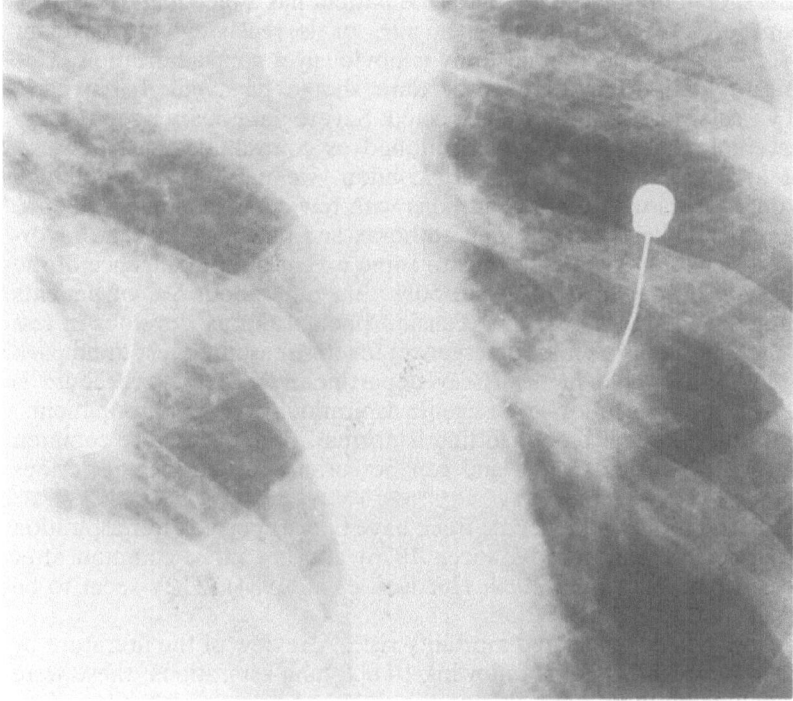

Fig. 5.1. Diagnostic aspiration of an intrapulmonary mass in a 64-year-old male unfit for thoracotomy due to respiratory failure. A posterior approach was used as the mass was situated posteriorly. The needle tip moved with the lesion indicating that it was correctly placed. The aspirate contained undifferentiated malignant cells.

When the needle tip has been correctly placed, the stillette is removed, a 20 ml syringe connected to the hub, and suction applied by withdrawing the piston to the 10 ml mark. A specially designed pistol grip is available for single-handed aspiration. The needle is oscillated up and down five to ten times, the pressure is gently released and the needle withdrawn. The contents of the needle are smeared onto a series of slides which are dried and immediately fixed. It is usual to repeat the aspiration two or three times to obtain samples from different parts of the lesion.

An ingenious screw device has been described which obtains material by drawing tissue into the needle. This can usually be relied upon to obtain good specimens (Allison and Hemingway 1981).

Biplane screening is helpful if the needle has to be passed obliquely and is of some help in entering small lesions, as the needle can be visualised in two planes. However, most small opacities (less than 2 cm in diameter) cannot be seen on lateral screening, so the technique is often unhelpful when it is most needed. It can be difficult to visualise a very small lesion on anteroposterior screening, but it is often possible to sample it by careful localisation of the lesion in relation to the bones of the thoracic cage and by guiding the needle into the lesion using the bony landmarks.

Aspirations should not be carried out if the patient has a bleeding disorder, a platelet count of less than 100 000 per ml^3, or is receiving anticoagulant treatment. Contralateral pneumonectomy is obviously a contraindication, as is severe respiratory failure, and the procedure should be avoided if hydatid disease or a vascular malformation is suspected. Severe pulmonary hypertension and bullous emphysema have been mentioned as contraindications in some papers, but at Charing Cross Hospital, London, we have carried out lung aspirations on patients with these conditions with few complications.

The common complications are pneumothorax and haemoptysis. The reported incidence of pneumothorax depends to some extent on the diligence of the search. It has varied between 10% and 50%, but only about 5% of patients require treatment with a chest drain. Tension pneumothorax develops in less than 1% of patients and is a major emergency; for this reason a chest drain pack should be readily available in the X-ray department when the procedure is carried out. Haemoptysis follows thin needle aspiration in 5%–10% of patients, but should not be serious if blood clotting is normal. It is much more common after biopsy with a cutting needle and can be serious in deep-seated lesions (Harrison et al. 1984).

Metastatic deposits along the needle track have been reported after aspiration with an 18G needle (Sinner and Zajicek 1976) and are more common after biopsy (Wolinsky and Lischner 1969; Harrison et al. 1984). They seem to be unknown after thin needle aspiration.

The procedure has an associated mortality risk. A review of the literature by Sinner in 1976 reported 9 deaths following 10 000 lung aspirations; these were due to tension pneumothorax (3), air embolism (3) and pulmonary haemorrhage (2). In 1 case no cause of death was found at autopsy. Berquist et al. (1980) reported 2 further deaths from severe haemorrhage into the bronchial tree following 430 aspirations, and it may be significant that an 18G needle was used in these cases.

Results

The accuracy of needle aspiration in detecting malignant disease depends as much on the quality of the cytological examination as on the quality of the specimen. The reported sensitivity in primary bronchial carcinoma has varied between 80% and 95% and seems to be highest with squamous cell carcinoma (Payne et al. 1979). At Charing Cross Hospital the sensitivity is 86%. The specificity is often 100%, indicating few false positive results. The sensitivity for metastatic disease and malignant lymphoma is much lower, usually 40%–50%. The accuracy of cutting and drill biopsy is higher but carries an increased risk of tension pneumothorax and serious haemorrhage (Harrison et al. 1984).

Results of cell typing following thin needle aspiration compared with histological examination have varied widely. Flower and Verney (1979) found 57% agreement in 77 lesions. Thornbury et al. (1981) reported 86% agreement for squamous cell carcinoma, adenocarcinoma and small cell anaplastic carcinoma, but Payne et al. (1979) found only 50% agreement for adenocarcinoma and oat cell carcinoma. Tru-cut biopsy will determine cell type with a much higher degree of accuracy and Harrison et al. (1984) reported complete agreement between biopsy and subsequent histology in 18 consecutive cases.

Thin needle aspiration has been used to diagnose infections in patients with malignant disease with a success rate of 42% (5/12) (Zavala and Schoell 1981). The procedure is often contraindicated in immunosuppressed patients owing to the low platelet count and the risk of haemorrhage, but Greenman et al. (1975), using an 18G needle, reported 35% treatable infections in 78 immunocompromised patients, with one death due to haemothorax.

In conclusion, thin needle aspiration of the lung will detect primary malignant tumours with a sensitivity in excess of 80%, secondary tumours with a sensitivity of 40%–50% and infections with a similar sensitivity. The accuracy of percutaneous biopsy is higher but so is the morbidity.

Bone

Fluoroscopically guided needle biopsy is an alternative to open bone biopsy. The technique can diagnose malignant bone tumours with an accuracy approaching 90%, and benign tumours and infections with a slightly lower accuracy. The morbidity and mortality are extremely low and the procedure can often be carried out under local anaesthesia.

Technique and Complications

The lesion should be accurately localised with plain films, and tomography is necessary. There is general agreement that the best results are obtained with cutting or trephine needles. The second-generation Jamshidi needle (Jamshidi and Swaim 1971) is widely used; it was preferred by Shaltot et al. (1982) and Stoker and Kissin (1985) for all lesions, and by Ayala and Zornosa (1983) for most lesions. The advantages are twofold: first, the absence of teeth on the cutting edge means that the core is not fragmented; and second, the core is removed by ejecting it backwards through the hub of the needle which causes less fragmentation than ejection through the slightly narrowed cutting end. The Ackerman and Craig needles have serrated cutting edges and are easier to use where access is difficult, but the core is more likely to fragment. The former provides a core measuring 1.5 mm in diameter and the latter a core 3.5 mm in diameter. A special trephine biopsy needle for use in the spine was described by Maclarnon (1982). Tru-cut biopsy needles have been used for lytic lesions by de Santos et al. (1979) and Ayala and Zornosa (1983) and thin 20G aspiration needles have been used with some success for detecting carcinoma cells in lytic lesions.

In the USA local anaesthesia combined with sedation is most frequently used, but in the UK general anaesthesia is often used, particularly for children and those unable to keep still during the procedure. Single-plane fluoroscopy is usually adequate, although Shaltot et al. (1982) used biplane fluoroscopy in most cases.

The most important contraindication to bone biopsy or aspiration is a bleeding defect, particularly a low platelet count (less than 100 000 per ml^3). Lesions suspected of being vascular malformations should not be biopsied owing to the risk of haemorrhage, but aneurysmal bone cysts can safely be biopsied.

The procedure is commonly used to provide a tissue diagnosis, but it has also been used to assess the response of malignant bone tumours to chemotherapy and radiotherapy (Ayala and Zornosa 1983). Needle biopsy has been used in the spine, pelvis, scapula, ribs and long bones.

Stoker and Kissin (1985) have described the technique of spinal biopsy with a Jamshidi needle in some detail. The patient is placed in a lateral decubitus position and the skin is infiltrated with local anaesthesia 6–8 cm from the midline. A 19G–20G spinal needle is advanced at an angle of 30°–45° to the sagittal plane, anterior to the transverse process of the selected vertebra, and local anaesthetic is infiltrated into the soft tissues and periosteum. The Jamshidi needle is passed through the skin and advanced in a similar direction until the tip is in contact with the posterolateral surface of the vertebral body. The trocar is used to penetrate the cortex and is then removed before the main part of the needle is advanced into the vertebra with a gentle to and fro rotating movement. At least two cores are taken from the vertebral body through the same cortical defect before the needle is withdrawn. Shaltot et al. (1982) recommend firm suction with a syringe, while rocking the needle (Fig. 5.2).

In most cases the core of tissue is fixed, decalcified and sectioned before being histologically examined, and this takes a few days. Cytological examination is sometimes helpful, particularly in metastatic carcinoma, and it is worth making a few slides of any liquid aspirate if this diagnosis is suspected.

Complications are rare. In a review of 9500 bone biopsies Murphy et al. (1981) found 2 deaths (0.02%) and 1 case of permanent paraplegia (0.01%), giving a serious morbidity of 0.03%. Four cases of spinal cord injury with complete recovery and 3 cases of temporary foot drop were also reported. The other complications included pneumothorax (7), pneumonia (1), tuberculous sinus tract (2) and paravertebral haematoma (1), giving a total morbidity of 0.2%. Spread of malignancy through the needle tract has not been reported.

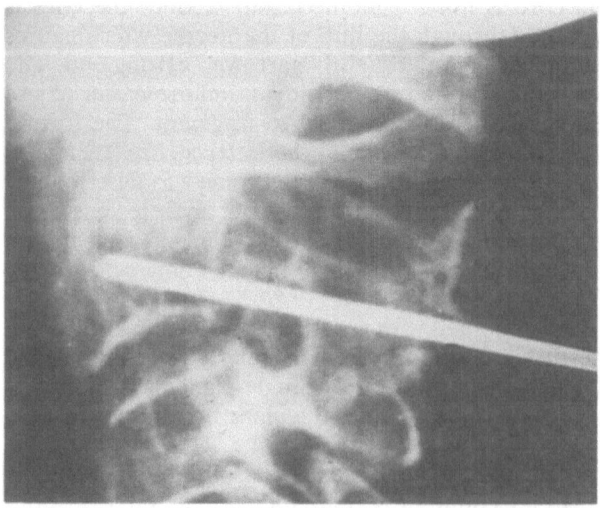

Fig. 5.2. Diagnostic biopsy of a solitary plasmacytoma in the body of the second cervical vertebra, using a Jamshidi needle. (Courtesy of Dr. D.J. Stoker, The Institute of Orthopaedics, London.)

Results

Ayala and Zornosa (1983) reported 83% sensitivity of the technique for 136 primary bone tumours and 64% sensitivity for 42 benign bone tumours. Stoker and Kissin (1985) achieved an overall accuracy of 89% in 135 mixed spinal lesions. In both these series the Jamshidi needle was used in the majority of cases. Most of the failures were due to undetected infection. Murphy et al. (1981) reported an overall diagnostic accuracy of 94% in 169 needle biopsies carried out on a series of malignant tumours, benign tumours and infections. Tehranzadeh et al. (1983), using Craig and Ackerman trocar needles, reported an overall diagnostic accuracy of 72% in 120 lesions.

In general the most accurate diagnoses have been obtained with malignant tumours and the least accurate with infections. Biopsy of the spine seems to be more accurate than biopsy of other bones. Trocar needles, particularly the Jamshidi, seem to obtain the best specimens.

Thus percutaneous needle biopsy of bone lesions is an alternative to open surgical biopsy. The technique will diagnose malignant tumours with an accuracy of 80%–90% and benign tumours and infections with a slightly lower accuracy. The serious morbidity is low (0.03%) and the procedure can often be carried out under local anaesthesia.

Aspiration from Other Sites

Fluoroscopically guided needle aspiration has been used to detect malignant disease in the liver and pancreas, but ultrasound guidance is more satisfactory in these situations. The main exceptions occur when opacification of the duct system by transhepatic cholangiogram or endoscopic retrograde cholangiopancreatography demonstrates a localised abnormality from which a sample of tissue can be obtained by percutaneous aspiration.

Fluoroscopy has also been used to obtain tissue from para-aortic and iliac lymph nodes shown to be abnormal on lymphography.

Percutaneous Drainage Procedures

Biliary Tract

Malignant obstruction of the biliary tract may be temporarily relieved by percutaneous insertion of a drainage catheter above the obstruction (external drainage), or by passing an endoprosthesis through the obstruction (internal drainage). Combined internal and external drainage is sometimes used as an interim measure prior to inserting the prosthesis, and is occasionally used for long-term drainage. These procedures are essentially palliative and aim to render the patient fit for surgery or to relieve the distressing symptoms of biliary obstruction.

Technique and Complications

The technique has been well described and illustrated by Dooley et al. (1981). A transhepatic cholangiogram is carried out to demonstrate the site of obstruction. The right lateral approach should be tried initially, using a 22G Chiba needle which is angled upwards through one of the lower rib interspaces into the right lobe of the liver. Contrast medium is injected during withdrawal and a bile duct is usually entered after a few passes. The injection is continued until the whole of the biliary tree above the obstruction has been opacified. This can take 20–30 minutes if the system contains viscous bile.

If the obstruction is situated in the right hepatic duct or common bile duct, a right lateral approach is used for drainage. A dilated intrahepatic duct in the right lobe is chosen for puncture and a sheathed needle (usually FG5) is passed percutaneously through the same rib space as the Chiba needle into the dilated duct. Lateral screening is an advantage at this stage, but it is usually possible to enter a dilated duct with single-plane screening. When the duct has been entered the stillette is withdrawn and a guide wire (0.035 or 0.038 inches) is passed through the sheath into the dilated biliary tree as far as the obstruction, or through it if possible. The tract through the skin and liver is dilated to FG7 or FG8 and the catheter of the same size, or one size smaller, is passed over the guide wire into the biliary tree.

Dilating the tract can kink the guide wire in the peritoneal space, and this can be a major problem, particularly in the presence of ascites. The dilators should be screened frequently to check that the wire is not bending in the peritoneal space and if a bend develops the dilator should be withdrawn, the original sheath passed and the flexible wire replaced with a Lunderquist wire. This wire has to be used cautiously as it can damage the biliary tree if it kinks at the junction between the rigid and flexible parts.

External drainage can readily be established by passing a self-retaining FG6 or FG7 pigtail catheter over the wire, which is then withdrawn.

Obstruction of the left hepatic duct may require an anterior approach for the transhepatic cholangiogram and will certainly require an anterior approach for drainage. This is technically more difficult than a right lateral approach as the left hepatic duct is usually punctured at a sharp angle close to the hilum and as it may be impossible to screen the needle and guide wire during manipulation because the operator's hands cannot be kept out of the field. The technique of passing the guide wire, dilating the tract and inserting the drainage catheter is similar to that used in draining the right hepatic duct.

External biliary drainage has few complications, the principal one being cholangitis.

Before establishing *internal drainage* the guide wire has to be passed through the obstruction into the duodenum. This difficult manoeuvre can sometimes be facilitated by passing an arterial catheter with a curved tip, or by using a torque control guide wire (Dooley et al. 1984). If the obstruction cannot be negotiated, a second attempt may be successful after a few days of external drainage. When the guide wire has been passed into the duodenum a Ring drainage catheter with side holes above and below the obstruction may be left *in situ* for a few days to provide combined external and internal drainage, before inserting the endopros-thesis.

The tract through the skin, liver parenchyma and obstructed segment has to be dilated, usually to 12FG, before inserting the endoprosthesis. This can be done with dilators, balloon angioplasty catheters or a combination of the two, and is best carried out over a Lunderquist wire. Once the tract has been dilated the endoprosthesis is passed over the wire and advanced with a "pusher" until its lower end is in the second or third part of the duodenum. The pusher and the guide wire are withdrawn, leaving the endoprosthesis in place (Fig. 5.3).

A variety of prostheses are available. All have side holes and end holes and most are 12FG. The Lunderquist–Owman endoprosthesis (William Cook) has a flange at its upper end to stabilise its position (Fig. 5.4) and the newer Miller prosthesis (William Cook) is stabilised by a mushroom configuration at both ends. The Carey–Coons prosthesis (Fig. 5.3c) (Meditech) is a tapered Teflon tube which is easier to insert than most other prostheses of a similar diameter, but it seems to be less stable. Haq and Fond (1985) used thinner double pigtail catheters which are readily inserted under local anaesthesia.

A combined oral and transhepatic approach was recently described and this may allow a larger gauge prosthesis to be passed in the future (Kerlan et al. 1984).

The procedure is often carried out under local anaesthesia by experienced operators, but the less experienced find general anaesthesia an advantage. Broad-spectrum antibiotics should be administered, starting 24 hours before the procedure and continuing for at least 5 days afterwards.

Percutaneous biliary drainage has been combined with iridium wire implantation in patients with hilar cholangiocarcinoma. The mean survival of a group of patients thus treated was 16.8 months compared with an expected survival of 8.5 months (Karani et al. 1985).

Complications are common, the most serious being biliary peritonitis, migration of the prosthesis, cholangitis, pneumonia and renal failure. Coons and Carey (1983) had two deaths within 30 days of inserting 71 prostheses; Dooley et al. (1984) had two deaths following attempted insertion of an endoprothesis in 62 patients. Mueller et al. (1985) reported serious morbidity or mortality in 17% (19/113) of their series and Neff et al. (1983) reported a mortality of 28% (13/46) within 30 days of the procedure. The morbidity and mortality following attempted drainage are often due to progression of the underlying disease and not necessarily to the procedure.

Results

Dooley et al. (1984) reported technical success in 77% (40/52) of attempted insertions of an endoprosthesis and satisfactory drainage in 53% (28/52) of patients with malignant obstruction. They commented that the treatment of intrahepatic or hilar obstruction was less successful than the treatment of extrahepatic obstruction. Mueller et al. (1985) reported technical success in 83% (94/113) of their series, with satisfactory drainage in 55% (62/113) of 113 patients with biliary obstruction (109 malignant, 4 benign).

The long-term results of insertion of an endoprosthesis depend upon the prosthesis remaining patent and *in situ*. Ring and Kerlan (1984) stated that most correctly placed 12FG endoprostheses remained open for at least 6 months, and they pointed out that this is longer than the expected survival of most patients

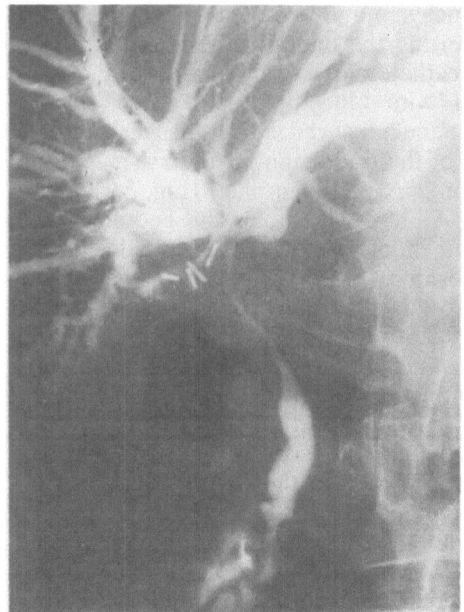
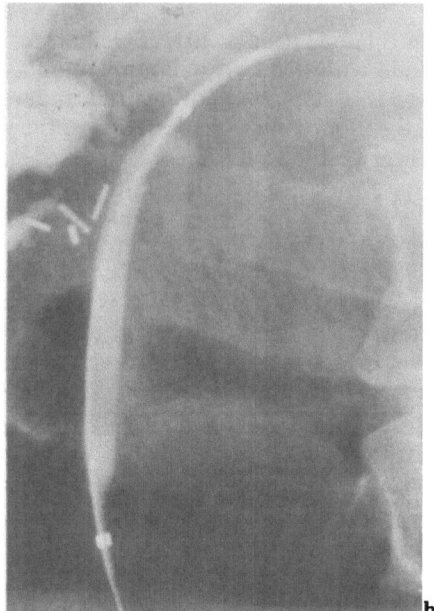
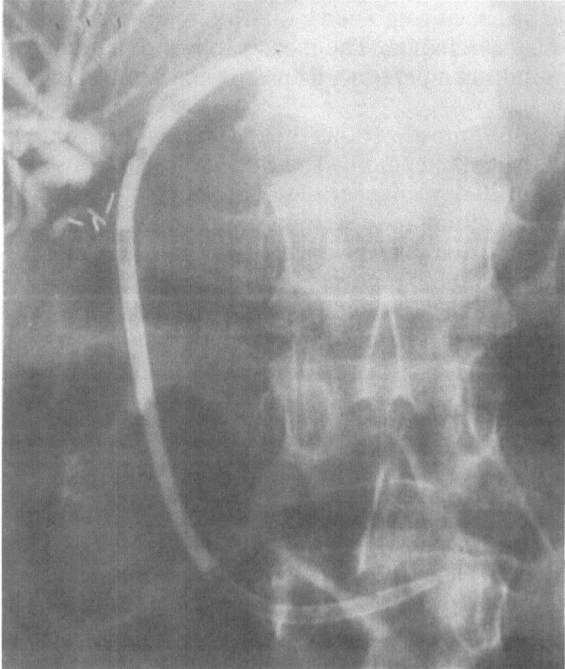

Fig. 5.3.a Percutaneous cholangiogram showing severe narrowing of the left and common hepatic ducts, with complete obstruction of the right hepatic duct in a patient with cholangiocarcinoma. The metallic clips were placed at a previous drainage operation. **b** Inflated balloon angioplasty catheter in the narrowed duct over a Lunderquist wire. **c** Carey–Coons prosthesis passing from the left hepatic duct into the second part of the duodenum. The right hepatic duct is still occluded.

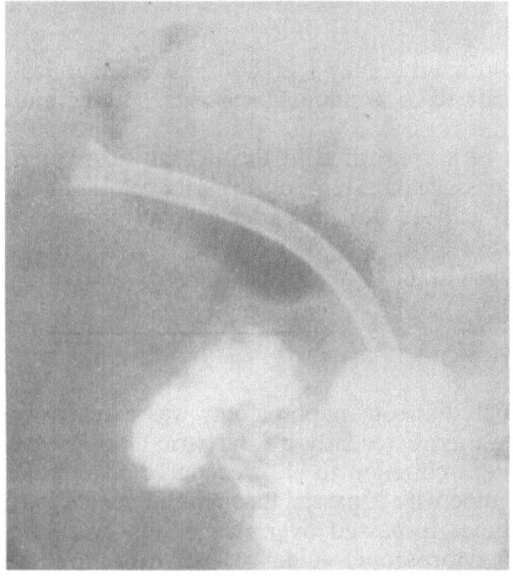

Fig. 5.4. Lunderquist–Owman endoprosthesis after percutaneous insertion through a common bile duct obstructed by pancreatic carcinoma. The upper end of the flanged prosthesis is situated in the right hepatic duct, which is dilated and partly outlined with air. The lower end of the prosthesis is obscured by contrast medium in the intestine. (Courtesy of Dr. R. Dick, The Royal Free Hospital, London.)

with malignant biliary obstruction. However, patients with cholangiocarcinoma can live for much longer as the tumour grows so slowly, and there have been cases in which an endoprosthesis has remained patent for several years (J. D. Irving pers. comm.).

A blocked prosthesis can sometimes be unblocked by passing a guide wire or dilator through the lumen (Teplick et al. 1985), or removed by passing an angioplasty catheter into the upper end, inflating the balloon and withdrawing the prosthesis (Coons and Carey 1983). However, it is more common to insert a second prosthesis alongside the first (Irving 1981).

Although pre-operative drainage of an obstructed biliary tree is usually followed by substantial biochemical improvement, the therapeutic benefit is uncertain. Gobien et al. (1984) and Dooley et al. (1986) found that the procedure reduced the morbidity of subsequent surgery, but the overall morbidity was not significantly reduced, as the drainage procedure itself carried complications, particularly cholangitis.

In conclusion, malignant obstruction of the biliary tree can be temporarily relieved in 50%–80% of patients by insertion of an endoprosthesis, but the procedure has a high morbidity and an early mortality of 3%–5%. The therapeutic value of external biliary drainage prior to surgery is uncertain owing to the increased risk of cholangitis. Iridium wire combined with internal drainage can improve the survival of patients with obstruction due to cholangiocarcinoma.

Percutaneous Renal Drainage

Percutaneous nephrostomy of an obstructed kidney is an alternative to surgical nephrostomy. The procedure is carried out under local anaesthesia and complications are extremely rare.

Percutaneous antegrade insertion of a ureteral stent through an obstructed ureter is an alternative to retrograde passage of a stent, or surgical exploration of the ureter. The procedure is usually carried out under local anaesthesia and serious complications are rare.

Technique and Complications

The long-established procedure of percutaneous nephrostomy was extensively reviewed by Stables et al. (1978) and more recently by Barbaric (1984). The details vary, but there are certain steps common to all procedures. The renal pelvis is punctured from the loin, a guide wire is passed through the needle into the pelvis and a self-retaining catheter is passed over the guide wire. The procedure may be carried out with fluoroscopic guidance, but ultrasound is usually preferred, particularly if the collecting system is dilated or renal function seriously impaired.

The patient is placed in the prone or prone-oblique position, with the affected side elevated. The ribs are identified by palpation, fluoroscopy or ultrasound and a puncture site between the ribs or below the twelfth rib infiltrated with local anaesthetic. The more lateral the puncture site the more comfortable it will be for the patient to lie supine with the drain in position. The needle is advanced from the skin to the renal capsule where more local anaesthetic is injected. The needle is then passed through the renal capsule and parenchyma into the pelvis. It is technically easier to puncture a lower than a middle calyx and this is quite satisfactory if the aim of the procedure is drainage, but if antegrade passage of a stent is contemplated, a middle calyx should be punctured.

It is usual to puncture the pelvi-calyceal system with a sheathed needle and to confirm the position of the needle by aspiration, urine having a distinctive straw colour. However, the technique is not reliable if there is blood in the pelvi-calyceal system, as may happen after a few unsuccessful passes of the needle. In these cases a J-shaped guide wire should be gently advanced through the sheath. If the tip is in the pelvi-calyceal system, the wire will pass easily and will be seen to coil within the renal pelvis on fluoroscopy. It is seldom difficult to enter a dilated collecting system, but problems are common with undilated systems.

The position of the needle may be checked by the injection of contrast medium, but if the needle is outside the collecting system contrast will pass into the renal substance, or into the peri-renal space, making subsequent fluoroscopy difficult.

For short-term drainage a pigtail catheter (FG7, FG8 or FG9) is satisfactory and can usually be passed into the renal pelvis without difficulty if the tract has been dilated to one FG size larger than the drainage catheter. The catheter sometimes coils at the level of the renal capsule and in such cases the flexible guide wire should be replaced with a Lunderquist wire before passing the self-retaining catheter.

Long-term external drainage requires a larger catheter (usually 12FG or 14FG). The tract is enlarged with a series of dilators or a balloon angioplasty catheter and it is often helpful to dilate the tract to one FG size larger than the catheter before passing it. There are a variety of catheters, but the 14FG Malecot self-retaining catheter is probably the most widely used and should provide satisfactory drainage for weeks or months, provided it is flushed at intervals of a few days. Dilating the tract and inserting the larger catheter can be painful and the patient may require a narcotic analgesic in addition to local anaesthesia.

Antegrade insertion of a double pigtail ureteral stent is a more recent development and can replace retrograde stent insertion. The renal pelvis is punctured and catheterised percutaneously, preferably through a middle calyx. A guide wire is passed into the renal pelvis and down the ureter as far as the obstruction, or through it if possible. Directing the guide wire from the pelvis into the ureter can be tricky, but can usually be accomplished with a curved arterial catheter. Anatomical abnormalities, such as pelvi-ureteric narrowing or horseshoe kidney, can make this manoeuvre impossible, however.

If the guide wire is held up at the site of obstruction, a straight catheter (FG7 usually) should be passed over the guide wire as far as the stricture and a straight guide wire pushed through the catheter and, if possible, through the stricture. If this manoeuvre fails, a slightly larger catheter (FG8) can be tried, as it takes a slightly larger guide wire (0.045 inches). Once the stricture has been negotiated the guide wire and catheter are advanced to the bladder. A tortuous or kinked ureter can usually be negotiated with a J wire and the catheter should follow the wire.

The stent should be as wide as possible as the wider stents are less likely to occlude. An FG8, FG9 or FG10 stent is desirable, but FG7 or even FG6 or FG5 may be used if the stricture cannot be sufficiently dilated. Angioplasty balloons have been used with some success to dilate benign and malignant strictures (Glanz et al. 1983; Banner and Pollack 1984). The length of the ureter should be measured from the guide wire and the length of the stent should allow the upper and lower pigtails to form without leaving a length of catheter in the bladder or renal pelvis. Before passing the stent it is often wise to replace the flexible guide wire with a Lunderquist wire, particularly if the flexible wire has shown any sign of bending in the renal pelvis (Mitty et al. 1983).

Another technique (Mitty 1984) is to pass the flexible antegrade wire out through the urethra so that both ends may be controlled.

The tract through the skin and obstruction should be dilated to one FG size larger than the stent before it is passed over the guide wire and down the ureter. When the lower pigtail forms in the bladder, the guide wire and pusher are withdrawn, allowing the upper coil to form in the renal pelvis (Fig. 5.5).

Combined external and internal drainage can be used to manage ureteric leaks at the site of surgical anastomosis, and the ureter will usually heal without developing a stricture.

Serious complications of percutaneous nephrostomy, ureteric catheterisation or stent insertion are rare. Although haemorrhage into the renal pelvis is common, it is rarely serious. Traumatic perforations of the renal pelvis or ureter can occur, but heal rapidly if internal or external drainage is satisfactorily established.

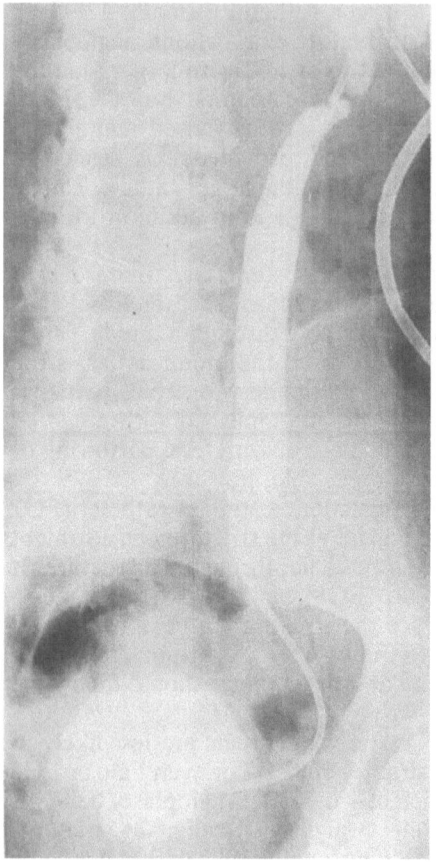

Fig. 5.5. Double pigtail catheter providing internal drainage of a left ureter obstructed by carcinoma of the cervix. The pusher is still in position and was removed a few minutes later. The 14G nephrostomy catheter had become dislodged after draining satisfactorily for some weeks.

Results

Bigongiara et al. (1979) attempted antegrade stent insertion through 14 ureteral strictures, most of which were malignant, and were successful on 8 occasions. Mitty et al. (1983) described 24 successful antegrade stent insertions for a variety of lesions. In most cases the aim of the procedure was temporary drainage prior to surgery, but in one patient the stent functioned satisfactorily for 8 months and, in another patient, 6 months.

In summary, percutaneous nephrostomy under local anaesthesia has a high success rate and few complications. It is readily carried out as an emergency procedure under ultrasound or fluoroscopic guidance. Percutaneous insertion of a double pigtail ureteral stent under local anaesthesia can be used as a pre-operative or palliative procedure for benign or malignant ureteric obstruction. The procedure is usually successful and has few serious complications.

Oesophageal Dilatation

Malignant strictures of the oesophagus have been successfully dilated with angioplasty balloon catheters (Dawson et al. 1984; Starck et al. 1984). Although the procedure can be carried out under local anaesthesia and is usually successful, there is a risk of perforation, and malignant strictures tend to recur soon after dilatation. The insertion of an oesophageal tube is occasionally undertaken by radiologists (J. D. Irving pers. comm.) and gives more prolonged palliation. The radiological appearances of two commonly used tubes, and the complications of the technique, have been described by Lipinski et al. (1982).

Therapeutic Arterial Embolisation

Arterial embolisation is an alternative to surgical ligation and has been used to control the symptoms of malignant tumours, particularly those situated in the abdomen and pelvis. The procedure is carried out under local anaesthesia and the morbidity is low.

Table 5.1. Embolisation materials

Physical
Absorbable
Blood clot
Gel foam
Non-absorbable
Fat and muscle tissue
Polyvinyl alcohol fragments (Ivalon)
Plastic spheres
Metallic spheres
Steel coils
Balloons
Cyanoacrylate cement
Silicone rubber

Chemical
Ethanol (ethyl alcohol)
Ethanolamine

A wide variety of materials have been used (Table 5.1) and the length of the list indicates that none is entirely satisfactory. Particulate materials block the arterial tree at a level which depends upon the size of the particle, whereas liquid material, such as ethanol and cyanoacrylate, probably reaches the arterioles or even the capillary bed. When the flow of blood is stopped or severely reduced, thrombus usually extends through the arterial tree, increasing the length of the block and turning partial occlusion into complete occlusion. Although this seems desirable, it means that the block produced may be largely due to thrombus and not to the embolisation material itself. Thrombus can be quite rapidly resorbed by normal physiological processes and this may account for the short-lived therapeutic benefit of some embolisation procedures.

The proximal end of the occlusion can easily be checked on the post-embolisation arteriogram and it is usually assumed that the process extends as far as the capillary bed. Radio-opaque embolisation materials are becoming more widely used and should make it possible to distinguish between obstruction due to the embolic material itself and obstruction due to thrombosis.

Liver Embolisation

Complete or partial embolisation of the hepatic artery has been widely used to control pain arising from primary or secondary tumours and to control the endocrine effects of metastatic hormone-secreting tumours in the liver. The therapeutic effect depends on the fact that malignant tumours which appear vascular on arteriography are much more dependent on the arterial blood supply than normal liver parenchyma, so that a sudden reduction in the arterial supply to the liver will produce extensive cell death within the tumour while leaving the normal parenchymal liver cells relatively unscathed (Chuang and Wallace 1981).

Technique and Complications

The patient should receive broad-spectrum antibiotics, starting 24 hours prior to embolisation and continuing for 7–10 days afterwards. An abdominal arteriogram is carried out to detect the origin of the hepatic artery or arteries. The common hepatic artery usually arises from the coeliac axis, but in about 20% of patients the right hepatic artery has a separate origin from the superior mesenteric and in a very small proportion of patients the left hepatic shares an origin with the left gastric artery. The hepatic artery (or arteries) should be selectively catheterised and the hepatic circulation demonstrated during the arterial, capillary and venous phases to check the vascularity of the tumour or tumours.

A patent portal vein must be demonstrated before arterial embolisation is carried out, as an occluded portal vein is an absolute contraindication to the procedure. The vein usually opacifies on delayed films taken 15–30 seconds after injecting 50 ml of contrast medium into the superior mesenteric artery, but in patients with portal hypertension and splenomegaly it may only show after injection into the splenic artery. Occasionally simultaneous injection into the superior mesenteric and splenic arteries may be required. Conventional photographic subtraction may demonstrate a portal vein which did not show on the arteriogram films, particularly if the vein lies over the spine. Digital subtraction should be used, if it is available, as it is quicker and requires less contrast medium. It has been suggested that the portal vein can be severely narrowed or occluded by extrinsic pressure from a hepatic tumour and that limited arterial embolisation in these patients will shrink the tumour and restore flow through the portal vein, but the conventional wisdom is that arterial embolisation should not be carried out unless the portal vein is clearly patent.

Hepatic embolisation requires selective catheterisation of the common hepatic artery, or of the right and left hepatic arteries if they have separate origins. This can usually be achieved using a sidewinder catheter with a pre-formed loop. In difficult cases it may be helpful to use a steerable system, or to approach the coeliac axis from the left axillary artery. The same technique can be applied to the right hepatic artery if it has a separate origin.

Fragments of gel foam are commonly used to achieve palliation (Fig. 5.6), as the material is readily available and easy to use, but the arterial occlusion is

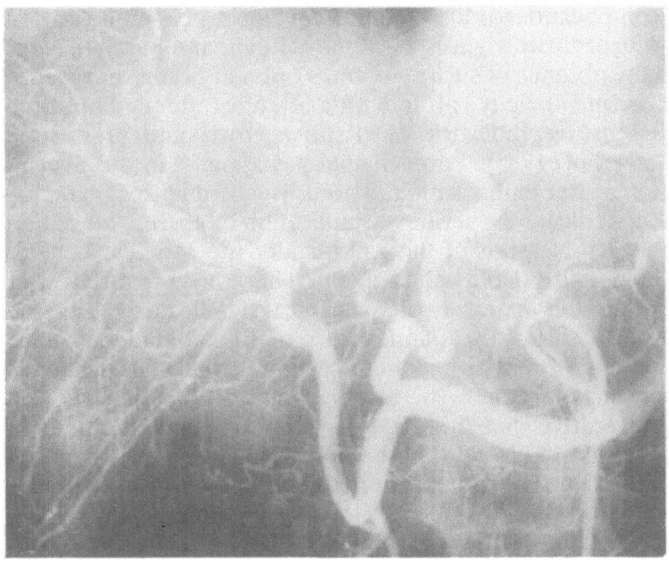

a

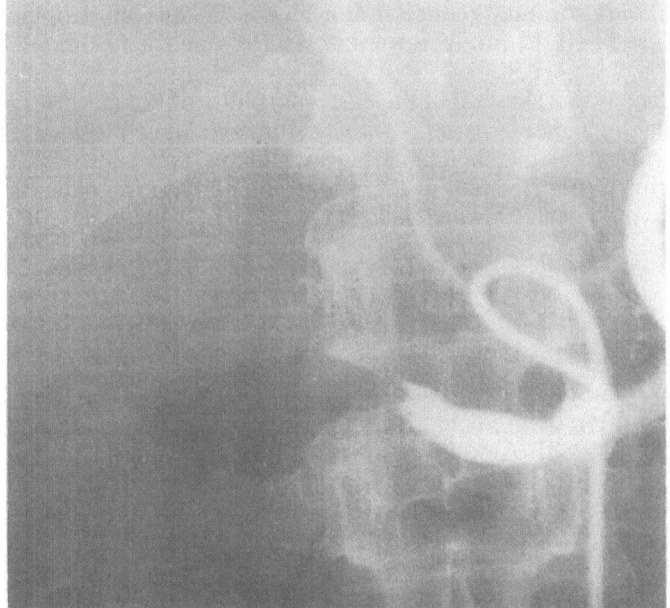

b

Fig. 5.6. Before **a** and after **b** embolisation of the common hepatic artery with gel foam and thrombin in a 64-year-old male with the carcinoid syndrome. He remained well for 10 months, when he developed intestinal obstruction from local tumour spread.

temporary and lasts only weeks or months. More permanent materials, such as fragments of dura mater or polyvinyl alcohol sponge, are preferable if the aim is long-term palliation of hormone-secreting metastases. Coils have been used, but suffer from the disadvantage that the liver may revascularise through small collateral vessels, which can be difficult or impossible to catheterise and embolise if the symptoms recur and a second embolisation is attempted.

The procedure has complications. Most patients develop a post-embolisation syndrome of pyrexia, leucocytosis, right hypochondrial pain and paralytic ileus for a few days. Indeed the absence of such symptoms often indicates an absence of tumour necrosis. A rise in C-reactive protein for a few days after embolisation seems to be a fairly sensitive indicator of tissue necrosis and of a good therapeutic result (Hind et al. 1985). Parenchymal gas appears in the liver in about one third of patients after embolisation. This is usually due to gas coming out of solution, but it can indicate the serious complication of abscess formation (Henessy and Allison 1983). Necrosis of the gall bladder (de Jode et al. 1976) and emphysematous cholecystitis (Coldwell et al. 1985) have been reported after hepatic artery embolisation, but are rarely of any clinical significance. Takayasu et al. (1985) reported on the histological appearance of 10 gall bladders which were removed in the course of partial hepatic resection 3 weeks after hepatic embolisation which had included the cystic artery. Nine gall bladders showed changes of necrotising ulcerative cholecystitis, typical of ischaemia, but none of these patients had required laparotomy. These findings suggest that necrosis of the gall bladder after hepatic artery embolisation is common but rarely serious.

Acute liver failure resulting in early death does occur after hepatic artery embolisation and, like abscess formation, seems to be more likely if liver function is grossly abnormal and if the hepatic artery is totally occluded by the procedure. Partial embolisation may reduce the incidence of this catastrophic complication, but is less likely to produce tumour necrosis and a favourable therapeutic result.

There is some evidence which shows that the early morbidity of hepatic artery embolisation is significantly higher in patients with a serum alkaline phosphatase in excess of 45 King Armstrong units than in patients with more normal levels. It is our practice at Charing Cross Hospital to exclude from embolisation patients with such elevated enzyme levels (Powell-Tuck et al. 1984).

Results

The response of liver tumours to embolisation depends largely upon their vascularity, and this can often be predicted from the arteriogram films (Chuang and Wallace 1981; Allison 1983). Among the primary liver tumours hepatoma (Yamada et al. 1983) and the much rarer sarcoma are usually vascular and respond well to embolisation, whereas cholangiocarcinomas, which are almost invariably avascular, do not respond. Metastatic tumours arising from the stomach, pancreas, colon etc. usually respond if they appear vascular or hypervascular on arteriography, but the avascular deposits do not. Metastases from the kidney are usually hypervascular, but are rarely confined to the liver and are rarely symptomatic. Some rare metastatic sarcomas are highly vascular and respond favourably to embolisation.

Metastatic hormone-secreting tumours are usually highly vascular and the results of arterial embolisation can be quite dramatic. Most patients with the carcinoid syndrome get complete or substantial relief of symptoms (Melia et al. 1982; Maton et al. 1983; Odurny and Birch 1985; Mitty et al. 1985). The procedure can be repeated if the symptoms recur and some patients have been kept reasonably symptom-free for several years by multiple embolisations. Hepatic artery embolisation usually relieves the symptoms of metastatic tumours producing gastrin or ACTH (Allison 1983; Carrasco et al. 1983).

Embolisation is usually followed by shrinkage of the tumour or tumours and this probably contributes to pain relief. However, there is no convincing evidence that the procedure prolongs life. Most patients with hepatoma or metastatic carcinoma survive for less than a year afterwards, but patients with hormone-secreting metastases may live for several years and are often helped by second and subsequent embolisation procedures.

In conclusion, there is little doubt that hepatic artery embolisation can improve the quality of life of some patients with malignant disease by relieving pain and by reducing or abolishing the endocrine effects of hormone-secreting metastases. Serious complications should be rare, if liver function is not grossly disturbed.

Kidney Embolisation

Renal artery embolisation has been used to devascularise renal carcinoma prior to nephrectomy and to relieve the symptoms of pain and haematuria arising from unresectable carcinoma.

Technique and Complications

An intravenous urogram and an ultrasound examination should be carried out to demonstrate the position and size of the mass before arteriography is undertaken. Following an abdominal arteriogram, the renal artery or arteries of the affected kidney are selectively catheterised to establish the presence of a pathological circulation. The decision to embolise pre-operatively is almost invariably made on the basis of the arteriographic findings and the previous examinations, as it is very rare to have histological proof of malignancy at this stage. An extensive pathological circulation is good evidence of malignancy if angiomyolipoma can be excluded. Lesions containing small areas of hypervascularity are almost invariably malignant and should be embolised, but totally avascular lesions should not, although avascular renal cell carcinomas can occur.

A wide range of embolisation materials have been used, including detachable balloons (White et al. 1979), balloon catheters (Mee 1982), absorbable gelatin sponge and coils (Wallace et al. 1981), polyvinyl alcohol fragments (Chuang et al. 1981), ethanol (Wells et al. 1983) and cyanoacrylate cement. Short-acting materials such as absorbable gelatin sponge and thrombin are adequate for pre-operative devascularisation of a tumour, provided the main stem of the renal artery is totally occluded (McIvor et al. 1984), but more permanent materials such as coils, balloons, cement or ethanol should be used if the intention is prolonged occlusion and long-term palliation.

Renal artery embolisation carries complications. Most patients develop a post-embolisation syndrome of fever, nausea and loin pain. Reflux of embolic material from partially or totally occluded renal arteries has resulted in spinal cord infarction, ischaemic changes in the small intestine, buttock claudication and ischaemic changes in the foot (Kaisary et al. 1982). Renal abscess and tubular necrosis have also been reported (Goldstein et al. 1976).

Results

The main indications for renal artery embolisation in malignant disease are persistent pain or haemorrhage from unresectable renal carcinoma. There are several reports and all show that the procedure has a low morbidity and a high incidence of therapeutic success (Ekelund et al. 1979; Macerlean et al. 1980). Our experience at Charing Cross Hospital has been encouraging, even with avascular tumours. The procedure does, of course, destroy the function of the affected kidney, but in these patients it is an alternative to surgical nephrectomy (Fig. 5.7).

There is an extensive literature about pre-operative embolisation of renal cell carcinoma, but the value of the procedure is questionable. There is little doubt that embolisation reduces the vascularity of tumours and makes nephrectomy easier, particularly if the tumour is large and vascular (Guilani et al. 1981; Wallace et al. 1981; Mee 1982). However, the more important question of its effect on patient survival has not yet been answered.

Swanson et al. (1983) reported complete or partial regression of metastases, mostly pulmonary, in 28% (28/100) of patients who received a prolonged course of medroxyprogesterone acetate after embolisation and nephrectomy, and

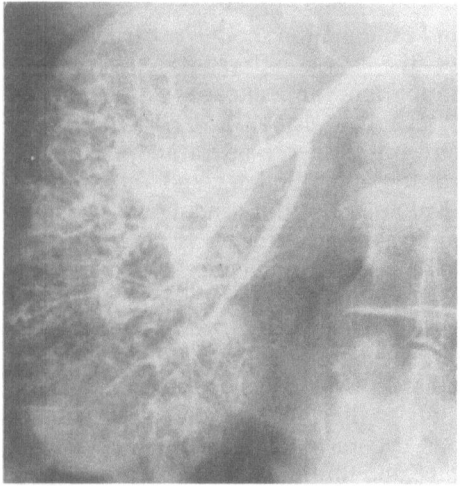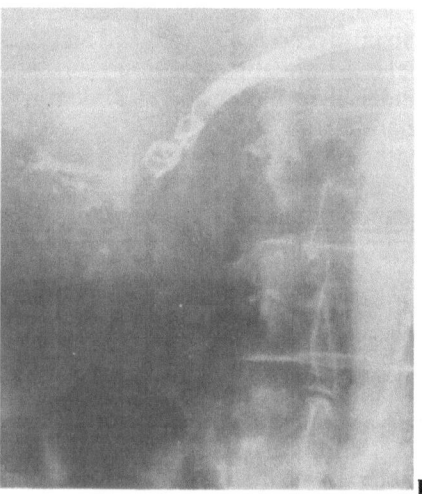

a   b

Fig. 5.7. Before **a** and after **b** embolisation of the right renal artery with gel foam and coils. The patient, a 76-year-old female, had persistent haematuria from renal carcinoma and bone metastases which had been well controlled by radiotherapy. The haematuria stopped after the embolisation and the patient remained symptom-free for some months.

found some evidence of prolonged survival compared with historical controls. There have been a few other accounts of pulmonary metastases regressing after embolisation and nephrectomy (Mohr and Whitesel 1979; Kaisary et al. 1984) but these reports do not establish the value of embolisation, as metastases from renal carcinoma occasionally regress after nephrectomy alone. Fairlamb (1981) collected 57 such cases from the literature.

Renal carcinoma is highly immunogenic; de Kernion et al. (1979) found that 94% (70/75) of patients with the tumour had circulating complement-fixing antibodies and that the level of the titre fell when the tumour was removed. The idea that embolisation might stimulate the production of tumour antibodies and cause regression of metastases is attractive, but is far from proved. Although Wallace et al. (1981) found an increase in "general immunocompetence" after embolisation and nephrectomy, these results have not been repeated elsewhere (Kaisary et al. 1984). A controlled trial is clearly desirable and is already under way at the Bristol Royal Infirmary (Jeans 1984). However, it will be some years before the effect of embolisation on metastatic disease and patient survival become clear, as the course of metastatic renal carcinoma is so unpredictable.

In conclusion, renal artery embolisation can usually be relied upon to control pain or haemorrhage arising from renal carcinoma, and the procedure is an alternative to surgical nephrectomy in these cases. The technique has also been used to reduce the vascularity of renal carcinoma prior to nephrectomy. Although it may make nephrectomy easier, particularly if the tumour is large and vascular, there is no evidence that it prolongs survival.

Bladder and Pelvic Embolisation

Embolisation of the internal iliac arteries is an alternative to surgical ligation and will usually control haemorrhage arising from malignant disease in the bladder or female genital tract.

Technique and Complications

The internal iliac artery may be catheterised from the femoral artery on the same or opposite side, using a catheter with a pre-formed loop, or from the left axillary artery, using a catheter with a slight distal curve. Although the axillary artery can be difficult to puncture and poses difficult surgical problems if damaged or thrombosed, it is an attractive approach to the internal iliac arteries: the operator's hands are well away from the field of interest and the same FG7 catheter can usually be passed into the anterior divisions of both internal iliac arteries. We have carried out over 100 axillary artery catheterisations at Charing Cross Hospital during the last few years with no serious complications.

Short-acting embolisation materials such as gelatin sponge are generally used to control haemorrhage, and seem to be as effective as more permanent materials.

Embolisation should be limited to the anterior divisions of the internal iliac arteries if possible (Fig. 5.8), as occlusion of the posterior division often results in severe gluteal pain for a day or two and persistent buttock claudication has

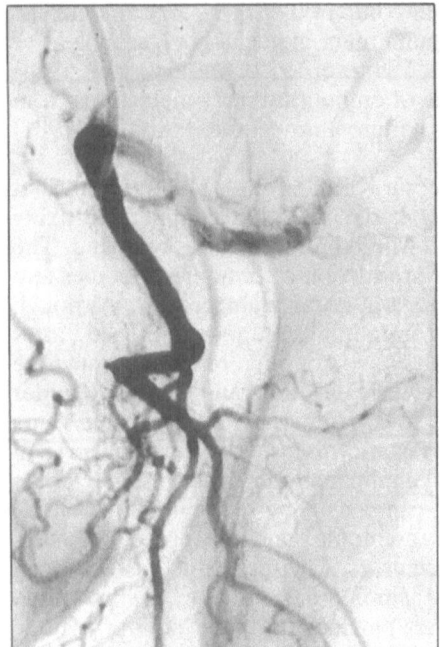
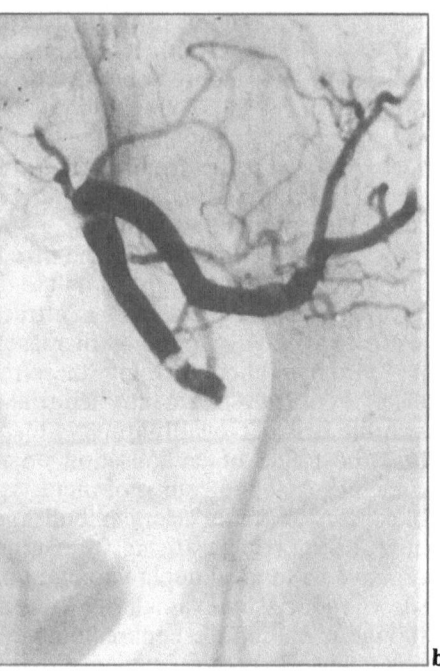

a   b

Fig. 5.8. Before **a** and after **b** embolisation of the anterior division of the left internal iliac artery with fragments of gel foam. The patient was a 67-year-old male with severe haematuria from an invading carcinoma of the sigmoid colon. The anterior division of the right internal iliac artery was occluded at the same time and the haematuria was controlled for nearly a year.

been reported. However, embolisation of the posterior division is sometimes unavoidable as arteries supplying the bladder may arise from the main stem of the internal iliac artery, or even from its posterior division.

The most serious complication of internal iliac artery embolisation is a neurological defect which can affect one or both lower limbs (Carmignani et al. 1980; Hare and Holland 1983). This is probably due to sciatic nerve damage caused by occluding the arteria comitans nervi ischiadicis, a branch of the anterior division of the internal iliac artery.

Necrosis or gangrene of the bladder is frequently mentioned as a complication of the procedure (Bullock and Whitaker 1985)—usually accompanied by a reference to the case of a sky diver who sustained severe pelvic injuries when his parachute failed to open, and who developed necrosis of the bladder after embolisation of one internal iliac artery. The same case seems to have been reported twice (Braf and Koontz 1977; Hietala 1978) and both reports mention that there was widespread pelvic vein thrombosis at the time of embolisation. It seems likely that the pelvic circulation was already compromised at the time of embolisation and that this contributed to bladder necrosis. There are now over 100 cases of internal iliac artery embolisation in the literature and this case seems to be the only example of extensive soft tissue necrosis, so the complication must be rare.

Results

Embolisation of the internal iliac arteries will usually control severe haemorrhage from an unresectable carcinoma which has arisen in the bladder itself, or invaded the bladder from an adjacent organ. A review of the literature (McIvor et al. 1982) found a success rate of over 90%. Although haematuria from a tumour which is localised to one side of the bladder can be controlled by unilateral embolisation (Kobayashi et al. 1980), it is necessary to occlude the anterior divisions of both internal iliac arteries if the tumour is extensive (Carmignani et al. 1980) or if the patient has received radiotherapy, as haemorrhage in these cases may be due to post-irradiation telangiectasis. The procedure seems to be more effective than surgical ligation, probably because it occludes the small arteries within the tumour and bladder wall and not just the main feeding vessel.

Embolisation of the internal iliac arteries has also been used to control severe haemorrhage arising from carcinoma of the rectum or uterus, and the results are favourable.

Lung Embolisation

Embolisation of the bronchial arteries has been used to control massive haemoptysis in patients who are poor candidates for surgery. Most reports describe haemorrhage from chronic inflammatory lung disease, but there are a few cases of haemorrhage from bronchial carcinoma being successfully controlled by embolisation (Remy et al. 1977; Vujic et al. 1982; O'Halpin et al. 1984).

In patients with bilateral lung disease, bronchoscopy should be carried out prior to embolisation to identify when possible the side of bleeding. Selective catheterisation of the bronchial arteries can be difficult, as the arteries are small and the anatomy is variable. In 90% the lung is supplied by one or two bronchial arteries which arise directly from the aorta at, or below, the level of the carina, but in the remaining 10% a bronchial artery arises from an intercostal artery, usually at another level. Embolisation should not be carried out unless a pathological circulation is demonstrated.

There are several reports of permanent damage to the spinal cord with resultant paraplegia following embolisation, and the risk of this complication should restrict the procedure to patients with life-threatening haemorrhage. Paraplegia can follow embolisation even when no communication with the spinal arteries has been demonstrated on arteriography (Vujic et al. 1982). White and Lundell (1984) have suggested that particulate materials such as fragments of gel foam or polyvinyl alcohol sponge should be used in preference to liquid embolisation materials, as the particles will impact in moderate-sized arteries and will not travel on into the very small arteries which supply the spinal cord.

Bone Embolisation

Embolisation has been used to devascularise malignant bone tumours prior to surgery and to control pain from unresectable primary and secondary tumours

(Keller et al. 1983). The technique has also been used as a primary or sole treatment for benign bone tumours where radical resection would result in severe disfigurement, and the results are encouraging, particularly with aneurysmal bone cysts in the pelvis (Wallace et al. 1979; Murphy et al. 1982; Keller et al. 1983).

Transluminal Angioplasty

Percutaneous transluminal angioplasty seems to have a role in managing arterial or venous narrowing after radiotherapy. The pathology of this rare complication is uncertain, the most likely cause being perivascular fibrosis or endothelial proliferation, but accelerated development of atheroma is also a possibility. Angioplasty has been successfully used to dilate post-radiotherapy arterial stenosis of the iliac artery (Saddekni et al. 1980), the femoral artery (Guthaner and Schmitz 1982) and the renal artery (Minton et al. 1986).

Conclusion

Interventional radiology provides a new dimension in the management of some patients with cancer. Some of the conditions for which such techniques are possible have been discussed. There is little doubt that with further experience, other conditions and techniques will be defined that will expand the range of possibilities.

References

Allison DJ (1983) Intervential radiology. In: Steiner RE (ed) Recent advances in radiology and medical imaging, vol 7. Churchill Livingstone, Edinburgh, pp 139–170
Allison DJ, Hemingway AP (1981) Percutaneous needle biopsy of the lung. Br Med J 282: 875–878
Ayala AG, Zornosa J (1983) Primary bone tumours: percutaneous needle biopsy. Radiologic-pathologic study of 222 biopsies. Radiology 149: 675–679
Banner MP, Pollack HM (1984) Dilatation of ureteral stenosis: techniques and experience in 44 patients. AJR 143: 789–793
Barbaric ZL (1984) Percutaneous nephrostomy for urinary tract obstruction. AJR 143: 803–809
Berquist TH, Bailey PB, Cortese DA, Miller WE (1980) Transthoracic needle biopsy: accuracy and complications in relation to location and type of lesion. Mayo Clin Proc 55: 475–481
Bigongiara LR, Lee KR, Moffat RE, Mebust WK, Foret J, Weigel J (1979) Percutaneous ureteral stent placement for stricture management and internal urinary drainage. AJR 133: 865–868
Braf ZF, Koontz WW (1977) Gangrene of bladder: complication of hypogastric artery embolisation. Urology 9: 670–671
Bullock N, Whitaker RM (1985) Massive bladder haemorrhage. Br Med J 291: 1522–1523
Carmignani G, Belgrano E, Puppo P, Chichero A, Giuliani L (1980) Transcatheter embolisation of the hypogastric arteries in cases of bladder haemorrhage from advanced pelvic cancers: follow-up in 9 cases. J Urol 124: 196–200
Carrasco CH, Chuang VP, Wallace S (1983) Apudomas, metastatic to the liver. Treatment by hepatic artery embolisation. Radiology 149: 79–83

Chin WS, Yee IST (1978) Percutaneous aspiration biopsy of malignant lung lesions using the Chiba needle: an initial experience. Clin Radiol 29: 617–619

Chuang VP, Wallace S (1981) Hepatic artery embolisation in the treatment of hepatic neoplasms. Radiology 140: 51–58

Chuang VP, Soo CS, Wallace S (1981) Ivalon embolisation in abdominal neoplasms. AJR 136: 729–733

Coldwell DM, Hottenstein DW, Ricci JA, Wengert PA (1985) Emphysematous cholecystitis as a complication of hepatic arterial embolisation. Cardiovasc Intervent Radiol 8: 36–38

Coons HG, Carey PH (1983) Large bore long biliary endoprosthesis (biliary stents) for improved drainage. Radiology 148: 89–94

Dawson SL, Mueller PR, Ferrucci JT et al. (1984) Severe oesophageal strictures: indications for balloon catheter dilatation. Radiology 153: 631–635

de Jode LR, Nicholls RJ, Wright PL (1976) Ischaemic necrosis of the gallbladder following hepatic artery embolisation. Br J Surg 63: 621–623

de Kernion JB, Ramming KP, Gupta RK (1979) The detection and clinical significance of antibodies to tumour associated antigens in patients with renal carcinoma. J Urol 122: 300–305

de Santos LA, Murray JA, Ayala AG (1979) The value of percutaneous needle biopsy in the management of primary bone tumours. Cancer 43: 735–744

Dick R, Heard BE, Hinson KFW, Kerr IH, Pearson MC (1974) Aspiration needle biopsy of thoracic lesions: an assessment of 227 biopsies. Br J Dis Chest 68: 86–94

Dooley JS, Dick R, Irving D, Sherlock S (1981) Relief of bile duct obstruction by the percutaneous transhepatic insertion of an endoprosthesis. Clin Radiol 32: 163–172

Dooley JS, Dick R, George P, Kirk RM, Hobbs KEF, Sherlock S (1984) Percutaneous transhepatic endoprosthesis for bile duct obstruction: complications and results. Gastroenterology 86: 905–909

Dooley JS, Dick R, George P, Kirk RM, Hobbs KEF, Sherlock S (1986) An evaluation of the results of percutaneous external bile drainage in patients with obstructive jaundice. Gastroenterology (in press)

Ekelund L, Mansson W, Olsson AM, Stigsson L (1979) Palliative embolisation of arterial renal tumour supply: results in 10 cases. Acta Radiol [Diagn] (Stockh) 20: 323–336

Fairlamb DJ (1981) Spontaneous regression of metastases of renal cancer: a report of 2 cases, including the first recorded regression following irradiation of a dominant metastasis and review of the world literature. Cancer 47: 2102–2106

Flower CDR, Verney GI (1979) Percutaneous needle biopsy of thoracic lesions: an evaluation of 300 biopsies. Clin Radiol 30: 215–218

Frable WJ (1982) Needle aspiration biopsy of pulmonary tumours. Semin Resp Med 4: 161–168

Glanz S, Gordon DH, Butt K, Rubin B, Hong J, Sclafani SJA (1983) Percutaneous transrenal balloon dilatation of the ureter. Radiology 149: 101–104

Gobien RP, Stanley JH, Soucek CD, Anderson MC, Vujic I, Gobien BS (1984) Routine pre-operative biliary drainage: effect on management of obstructive jaundice. Radiology 152: 353–356

Goldstein HM, Wallace S, Anderson JM, Bree RL, Gianturco C (1976) Transcatheter occlusion of abdominal tumours. Radiology 120: 539–545

Greenman RL, Goodall PT, King D (1975) Lung biopsy in immunocompromised hosts. Am J Med 59: 488–496

Guilani L, Carmignani G, Belgrano E, Puppo P, Quattrini S (1981) Usefulness of pre-operative transcatheter embolisation in kidney tumours. Urology 17: 431–434

Guthaner DF, Schmitz L (1982) Percutaneous transluminal angioplasty of radiation induced arterial stenosis. Radiology 144: 77–78

Haq N, Fong PLC (1985) Percutaneous transhepatic internal drainage, using polyurethane double pigtail endoprosthesis. Clin Radiol 36: 57–59

Hare WSC, Holland CJ (1983) Paresis following internal iliac artery embolisation. Radiology 146: 47–51

Harrison BDW, Thorpe RS, Kitchner PG, McCann BG, Pilling JR (1984) Percutaneous tru-cut biopsy in the diagnosis of localised pulmonary lesions. Thorax 39: 493–499

Hennessy OF, Allison DJ (1983) Intrahepatic gas following embolisation. Br J Radiol 56: 348

Hietala S (1978) Urinary bladder necrosis following selective embolisation of the internal iliac artery. Acta Radiol [Diagn] (Stockh) 19: 316–320

Hind CRK, Thomas AMK, Pepys MB, Allison DJ (1985) Serum C-reactive protein response to therapeutic embolisation: possible role in management. Clin Radiol 36: 179–183

Irving JD (1981) Interventional radiology: relief of biliary obstruction. Br J Hosp Med 26: 329–338

Jamshidi K, Swaim WR (1971) Bone marrow biopsy with unaltered architecture: a new biopsy device. J Lab Clin Med 77: 335–342

Jeans WD (1984) Embolisation of renal carcinoma. Clin Radiol 35: 335

Kaisary AV, McIvor J, Williams G (1982) Conservative management of unintentional distal embolisation following intravascular occlusive therapy. Br J Surg 69: 422

Kaisary AV, Williams G, Riddle PR (1984) The role of pre-operative embolisation in renal cell carcinoma. J Urol 131: 641–646

Karani J, Fletcher M, Brinkley D, Dawson JL, Williams R, Nunnerley H (1985) Internal biliary drainage and local radiotherapy with Iridium-192 wire in treatment of hilar cholangiocarcinoma. Clin Radiol 36: 603–606

Keller FS, Rosch J, Bird CB (1983) Percutaneous embolisation of bony pelvic neoplasms with tissue adhesive. Radiology 147: 21–27

Kerlan RK, Ring EJ, Pogany AC, Jeffrey RB (1984) Biliary endoprosthesis: insertion using a combined per oral–transhepatic method. Radiology 150: 828–830

Kobayashi T, Kusano S, Matsubayashi T, Uchida T (1980) Selective embolisation of the vesical artery in the management of massive bladder haemorrhage. J Urol 121: 30–36

Lipinski JK, Conway SS, Kottler RE, Werner DI (1982) The radiology of oesophageal tubes for malignant strictures. Clin Radiol 33: 435–459

Macerlean DP, Owens AP, Bryan PJ (1980) Hypernephroma embolisation: is it worthwhile? Clin Radiol 31: 297–300

McIvor J, Williams G, Southcote RCC (1982) Control of severe vesical haemorrhage by therapeutic embolisation. Clin Radiol 33: 561–567

McIvor J, Kaisary AV, Williams G, Grant RW (1984) Tumour infarction after pre-operative embolisation of renal carcinoma. Clin Radiol 35: 59–64

Maclarnon JC (1982) Biopsy of the spine using a needle with a rigid guide wire. Clin Radiol 33: 189–192

Maton PN, Camilleri M, Griffin G, Allison DJ, Hodgson HJF, Chadwick VS (1983) Role of hepatic arterial embolisation in the carcinoid syndrome. Br Med J 287: 932–935

Mee AD (1982) Prognosis after radical nephrectomy for carcinoma: the influence of pre-operative arterial balloon occlusion. Br J Urol 54: 201–203

Melia WM, Nunnerly HB, Johnson PJ, Williams R (1982) Use of arterial devascularisation and cytotoxic drugs in 30 patients with the carcinoid syndrome. Br J Cancer 46: 331–339

Minton MJ, McIvor J, Cappuccio FP, MacGregor GA, Newlands ES (1986) Renovascular hypertension following radiotherapy and chemotherapy treated by transluminal angioplasty. Clin Radiol (in press)

Mitty HA (1984) Ureteral stenting facilitated by antegrade transurethral passage of guide wire. AJR 142: 831–832

Mitty HA, Train JS, Dan SJ (1983) Antegrade ureteral stenting in the management of fistulas, strictures and calculi. Radiology 149: 433–438

Mitty HA, Warner RRP, Newman LH, Train JS, Parnes IH (1985) Control of carcinoid syndrome with hepatic artery embolisation. Radiology 155: 623–626

Mohr SJ, Whitesel JA (1979) Spontaneous regression of renal cell carcinoma metastases after embolisation of primary tumour and subsequent nephrectomy. Urology 14: 5–8

Mueller PR, Ferrucci JT, Teplick SK et al. (1985) Biliary stent endoprosthesis: analysis of complication in 113 patients. Radiology 156: 637–639

Murphy WA, Destouet JM, Gilula LA (1981) Percutaneous skeletal biopsy: a procedure for radiologists—results, review and recommendations. Radiology 139: 545–549

Murphy WA, Strecker WB, Schoenecker PL (1982) Transcatheter embolisation therapy of an ischial aneurysmal bone cyst. J Bone Joint Surg [Br] 64: 166–168

Neff RA, Fankuchen EI, Cooperman AM, Helmrich ZV, Martin EC (1983) The radiological management of malignant biliary obstruction. Clin Radiol 34: 143–146

Odurny A, Birch SJ (1985) Hepatic arterial embolisation in patients with metastatic carcinoid tumours. Clin Radiol 36: 597–602

O'Halpin D, Legge D, Macerlean DP (1984) Therapeutic arterial embolisation: report of five years experience. Clin Radiol 35: 85–93

Payne CR, Stovin PGI, Barker V, McVittie S, Stark JE (1979) Diagnostic accuracy of cytology and biopsy in primary bronchial carcinoma. Thorax 34: 294–299

Powell-Tuck J, McIvor J, Reynolds KW, Murray Lyon IM (1984) Prediction of early death after therapeutic hepatic artery embolisation. Br Med J 288: 1257–1259

Remy J, Arnauld A, Fardon H, Girard R, Voisin C (1977) Treatment of haemoptysis by embolisation of bronchial arteries. Radiology 122: 33

Ring EJ, Kerlan RK (1984) Interventional biliary radiology. AJR 142: 31–34

Saddekni S, Sniderman KW, Hilton S, Sos TA (1980) Percutaneous transluminal angioplasty of non-atherosclerotic lesions. AJR 135: 975–982

Shaltot A, Mitchell PA, Betts JA, Darby AJ, Gishen P (1982) Jamshidi needle biopsy of bone lesions. Clin Radiol 33: 193–196

Sinner WN (1976) Complication of percutaneous thransthoracic needle aspiration biopsy. Acta Radiol [Diagn] (Stockh) 17: 813–827

Sinner WN, Zajicek J (1976) Implantation metastases after percutaneous transthoracic needle aspiration biopsy. Acta Radiol [Diagn] (Stockh) 17: 473–480

Stables DP, Ginsberg NJ, Johnson ML (1978) Percutaneous nephrostomy: a series and review of the literature. AJR 130: 75–82

Starck E, Paolucci V, Herzer M, Crummy AB (1984) Esophageal stenosis: treatment with balloon catheters. Radiology 153: 637–640

Stoker DJ, Kissin CM (1985) Percutaneous vertebral biopsy: a review of 135 cases. Clin Radiol 36: 569–577

Swanson DA, Johnson DE, von Eschenbach AC, Chuang VP, Wallace S (1983) Angio-infarction plus nephrectomy for metastatic renal cell carcinoma: an update. J Urol 130: 449–452

Takayasu K, Moriyama N, Muramatsu Y et al. (1985) Gall bladder infarction after hepatic artery embolisation. AJR 144: 135–138

Tehranzadeh J, Freiberger RH, Ghelman B (1983) Closed skeletal needle biopsy: review of 120 cases. AJR 140: 113–115

Teplick SK, Haskin PM, Pavlides CA, Goldstein RC (1985) Management of obstructed biliary endoprosthesis. Cardiovasc Intervent Radiol 8: 164–167

Thornbury JR, Burke DP, Naylor BN (1981) Transthoracic needle aspiration biopsy. Accuracy of cytological typing of malignant neoplasms. AJR 136: 719–724

Vujic I, Pyle R, Hungerford GD, Griffin CN (1982) Angiography and therapeutic blockade in the control of haemoptysis. The importance of non-bronchial systemic arteries. Radiology 143: 19–23

Wallace S, Granmayeh M, de Santos LA (1979) Arterial occlusion of pelvic bone tumours. Cancer 43: 322–328

Wallace S, Chuang VP, Swanson D et al. (1981) Embolisation of renal carcinoma: experience with 100 patients. Radiology 138: 563–570

Wells IP, Hammonds JC, Franklin K (1983) Embolisation of hypernephromas: a simple technique using ethanol. Clin Radiol 34: 689–692

Westcott JL (1981) Percutaneous needle aspiration of hilar and mediastinal masses. Radiology 141: 323–329

White RI, Lundell C (1984) Prevention of complications during embolotherapy of the lung. Ann Radiol 27: 310–315

White RI, Kaufman SL, Barth KH, de Caprio V, Strandbert JD (1979) Embolotherapy with detachable silicone balloons. Radiology 131: 619–627

Wolinsky H, Lischner MW (1969) Needle track implantation of tumour after percutaneous lung biopsy. Ann Intern Med 71: 359–362

Yamada R, Sato M, Kawabata M, Nakatsuka H, Nakamura K, Takashima S (1983) Hepatic artery embolisation in 120 patients with unresectable hepatoma. Radiology 148: 397–401

Zavala DC, Schoell JE (1981) Ultrathin needle aspiration of the lung in infections and malignant disease. Am Rev Resp Dis 123: 125–131

6 Computerised Tomography

Adrian K. Dixon

Introduction

Ever since the initial development of cranial computerised tomography (CT) by Hounsfield (1973), it has been anticipated that this technique would make a substantial impact on the diagnosis, staging, treatment and follow-up of various malignancies. When whole-body CT machines became available in the mid 1970s, this hope started to be fulfilled—despite the fact that the images obtained by these early models were somewhat primitive compared with the high-resolution images produced by modern scanners. Now that such modern scanners are quite widely available within the UK, a rational outline of some of the uses of body CT in oncological practice can be considered. A few technical and procedural points will be considered first and then some of the clinical problems in which CT has a role will be discussed.

Technical Considerations

The Machine

There is still considerable controversy about the optimal design of a CT scanner. Some manufacturers favour a rotating gas-filled detector system, others prefer a rotating scintillation detector system, while yet others use a static array of detectors distributed around the traverse of the tube. Each has some advantages and disadvantages and these do not greatly affect the quality of the resulting image. Much, however, depends on the design of the X-ray tube and its cooling system. A tube failure renders the CT scanner out of action for longer than the scheduled down time for servicing, with resulting inconvenience to all. A tube with poor heat capacity and a limited cooling system may result in interruptions in the examination procedure with a deleterious effect on patient throughput. The machine may not provide full rapid-sequence facilities, which are very useful for assessing vascular aspects of various tumours (e.g. renal vein involvement in renal carcinoma). The computing aspects of the machines also vary considerably; those machines which allow fast image reconstruction and recall have certain advantages as regards patient throughput. However, apart from these differences, most modern machines have fairly similar technical characteristics and yield images of approximately comparable quality.

The Patient

The first requirement of the patient is that he or she should be able to lie flat. For studies involving the chest and abdomen, he or she should also be able to suspend respiration for the duration of each slice (nowadays 5 seconds or less).

For abdominal examinations it is essential that some system of opacification of the small bowel is used. This usually involves drinking dilute oral contrast medium (iodinated compounds or even dilute barium) an hour or so before, and again immediately before, the study. This allows differentiation between small bowel loops and lesions of soft tissue density which otherwise can have similar CT appearances. For pelvic examinations it is helpful to opacify the rectosigmoid colon by giving similar dilute contrast medium per rectum. This is, of course, impossible in patients who have had abdomino-perineal surgery for rectal carcinoma; here even more rigorous preparation with oral contrast medium is essential.

It is worth remembering that CT will give much better images in obese patients than emaciated ones. This is because CT relies heavily on the negative attenuation of fat to provide contrast with the soft tissue density of most lesions. In those patients with little intra-abdominal fat subtle lymph node enlargement may be difficult to interpret. The slender young female is an especially difficult customer; women have only half as much intra-abdominal fat as men (Dixon 1983). Fewer than 1 in 2000 patients are so obese that they will not fit through the gantry aperture!

The thin patient who is unable to suspend respiration on command is thus a less than easy subject for body CT. Most children fall into this category and so CT in the paediatric group poses some particular problems both in procedural technique and in interpretation (Berger et al. 1981). Some sedation is needed, but it is often surprising what can be achieved with calm and reassuring explanation. Before CT is considered in this group it is always worth considering whether the necessary information could be obtained from ultrasound (see Chapter 8), which is so ideally suited to the thin, and mobile, patient.

The Examination

Many studies in oncology follow a routine, such as staging bronchial carcinoma, and the examination can be performed using an established radiographic protocol. Clearly some compromise about slice thickness and table movement increments must be adopted for each clinical problem. If contiguous thin slices are used for each examination, then correspondingly fewer patients can be studied in a working day. However, whatever protocol is adopted, it is essential that a radiologist assesses the examination as it proceeds and alters the protocol as appropriate. For example if, in a patient with bronchial carcinoma, low-attenuation lesions within the hepatic parenchyma consistent with metastases are seen, possible mediastinal involvement becomes less relevant. However if all other sites are clear, an equivocal 1.5 cm diameter nodal structure in the mediastinum is of crucial concern with regard to possible surgical cure; here the radiologist must use every manoeuvre to confirm or disprove the presence of a node by using magnification and enhancement techniques.

Opinion is varied as to the use of intravenous contrast medium and the timing of its administration. For possible intracranial or juxtacranial lesions many workers routinely give intravenous contrast medium before starting the study, as lesions affecting the blood–brain barrier will usually become more obvious. For cervical work some would leave an infusion of contrast medium running during the study to allow optimal differentiation of nodes from vessels. In the chest and upper abdomen an approach of withholding contrast medium at the outset can be justified, reserving its use for bolus rapid-sequence enhancement techniques to identify vessels and vascular characteristics of tumours as appropriate. Such rapid-sequence techniques are particularly important for staging studies of bronchial neoplasia where vascular structures such as the left atrium and pulmonary vessels can simulate subcarinal and hilar nodes respectively. Some lesions within a solid organ (e.g. liver) may only be identified after intravenous contrast medium; a full dynamic series after a bolus injection provides the best chance of seeing such a lesion (Moss et al. 1982). For studies of the pelvis it is useful to have the ureters and bladder delineated by contrast medium; only a small intravenous dose (c. 5–6g iodine) is needed for this purpose—indeed larger doses can lead to artefacts from the resulting dense bladder.

It is important to realise that a CT study undertaken to assist with radiotherapy treatment planning is a rather different procedure from a diagnostic study. In the diagnostic study the examination is arranged to give the best diagnostic images, using suspended respiration, full bowel opacification, arms above head to avoid artefacts, magnification techniques, and other manoeuvres if required. In the study aimed purely at assisting treatment planning, with subsequent computer-generated treatment schemes, the patient is positioned in the precise position in which radiotherapy will be administered; normal breathing will continue during as long a time of data acquisition as possible, to simulate radiotherapeutic conditions. Finally the images should not be magnified, as the whole point of the study is to relate the target area to the outline of the torso and a known reference point on the skin. In many situations this will necessitate a full initial diagnostic CT study to stage the lesion followed by a further study (which can often be quite abbreviated) to assist in planning.

Interpretation

Even assuming the radiologist has closely checked each CT image during the procedure, the detailed interpretation of the data must be carried out at leisure when all the images have been processed into hard copy suitable for viewing on an X-ray viewing box. The radiologist must also have the electronic data available on a viewing console at this stage. This dual need comes about because of the vast amount of data available for further analysis, only a proportion of which is retained on the hard copy films generally made for viewing. For example a series of abdominal films in a patient with lymphoma is generally displayed at a relatively wide window of approximately 500 Hounsfield units (HU) around a soft tissue density setting (*c.* +45 HU). However this setting would not be ideal for demonstrating subtle changes of bone infiltration, which would be better seen using a wider window (*c.* 1000 HU) and a much higher level (*c.* +500 HU) (Fig. 6.1). Similarly, subtle areas of diminished attenuation within the hepatic parenchyma and lesions in the lung bases may only be evident with careful viewing on the monitor; further hard copy images should be made as appropriate to display any significant lesions.

Abnormalities can only be demonstrated by CT either if the normal anatomy is recognisably distorted (e.g. abnormal lymph nodes) or if the attenuation of a normal structure is altered by disease (before, during or after intravenous enhancement). In oncology it is usually the abnormal anatomy which is most helpful. The primary lesion may be recognised as a mass of soft tissue density displacing normal structures; its relation with, or extension into, adjacent organs can be assessed. Lymph nodes are generally regarded to be abnormal when their diameter is over 1.5 cm, although inflammatory nodes can easily attain this size. Nodes of 2 cm, in the presence of a known malignancy, can be assumed with a high degree of confidence to be due to infiltration (Sagel 1982). In certain sites, such as the retrocrural area, smaller nodes than this are worrying (Callen et al. 1978) (see Fig. 6.5c). Even when the anatomy is definitely abnormal and the patient is known to have a malignancy it must be remembered that other conditions may be responsible for the abnormality. Lymph node enlargement could be due to coexistent granulomatous disease, and abnormal structures could be due to congenital anomalies (especially venous: Royal and Callen 1979) or even normal variants (Nightingale and Dixon 1984). The radiologist must be constantly aware of these possibilities.

The lack of tissue specificity is one great drawback of CT. The CT attenuation coefficient (number) does not often help. Although it is quite reliable at distinguishing between lesions of fatty composition, fluid-filled structures (−10 to +20 HU) and lesions of soft tissue density (20+ HU and usually *c.* 40 HU), problems still occur. The low attenuation (*c.* 10 HU) of some solid nodal deposits in testicular teratoma provides an example; this is particularly common following treatment, when decreasing attenuation provides some measure of the chemotherapeutic effect (Husband et al. 1982). Occasionally the distribution of disease provides clues as to the aetiology (Fig. 6.2). But for absolute certainty of the nature of an abnormal anatomical structure biopsy is necessary, and this type of radiologically guided interventional procedure is becoming increasingly common (see Fig. 6.6).

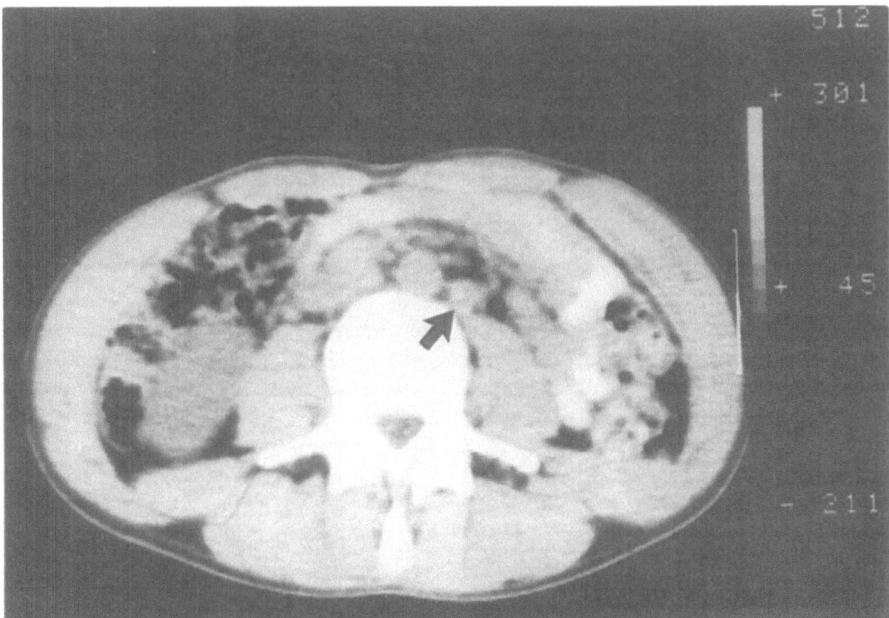

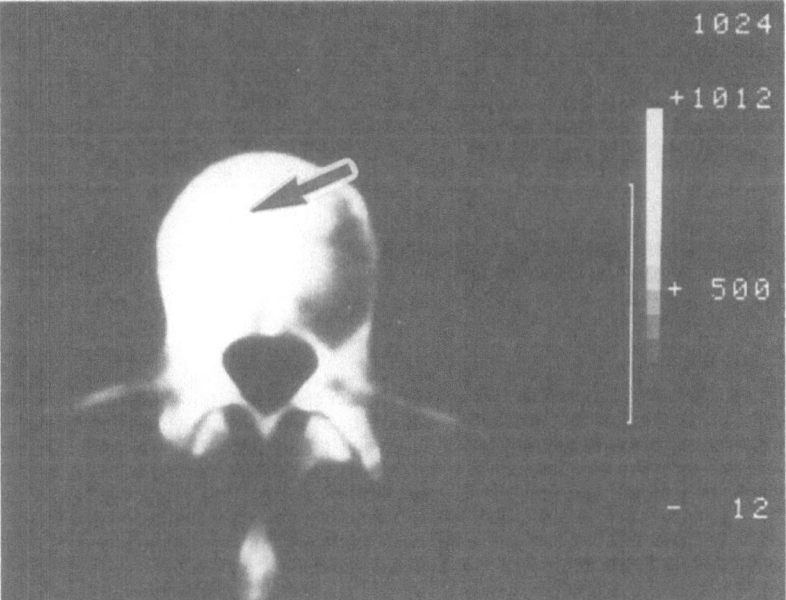

Fig. 6.1.a,b. A 22-year-old patient complaining of malaise and back pain. Chest X-ray showed extensive mediastinal and hilar lymphadenopathy. **a** Abdominal image shown at window width 512 HU and level +45 HU. A 1.5 cm diameter left para-aortic node is illustrated (*arrow*). There were many other enlarged nodes in the para-aortic chain. No bone detail was seen at this setting. **b** The same image as **a** but expanded and shown at a wider window (1024 HU) and a much higher level (+500 HU). Extensive bone involvement of the right half of the vertebra is now clearly seen (*arrow*). Hodgkin's lymphoma was diagnosed on bone marrow aspirate.

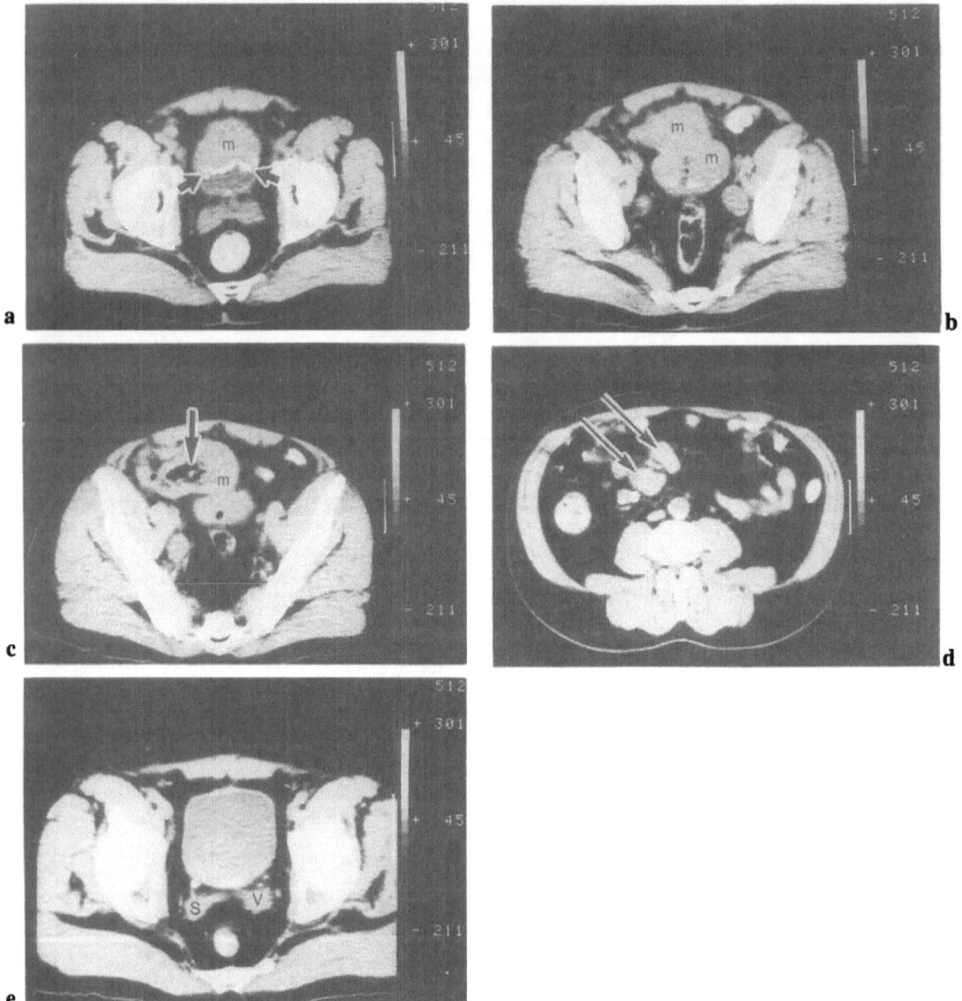

Fig. 6.2.a–e. A 57-year-old male referred for staging of bladder carcinoma. Initial CT (**a–d**) showed an extensive soft tissue mass (m) within the bladder, with surface calcium encrustation (*arrows* in **a**), and extension through the dome of the bladder (**b**) to involve a loop of small bowel (**c**). Note the thickened bowel wall around central air in the lumen (*arrow* in **c**). More cranially (**d**) enlarged mesenteric nodes were demonstrated (*arrows*). Because of the pattern of the extent of disease the possibility of a lymphoma was raised. This latter diagnosis was subsequently confirmed on histological review. **e**   Normal bladder following chemotherapy. All sites of involvement had regressed. Note normal fat between bladder and seminal vesicles (sv).

Radiation Dose

The radiation dose received by a patient during CT is usually not much of a problem for patients with a known malignancy. However, for those where CT is used to diagnose, maybe treat (via percutaneous drainage) and then follow up a condition such as a liver abscess, several CT studies may be needed over a short period and the radiation dose becomes more worrying. Similarly a young patient with a curable malignant lesion may undergo numerous CT studies during the years of follow-up.

With a typical modern machine (e.g. Siemens Somatom 2) the radiation dose is 12.5 mGy (1.25 rad) for a single slice using 125 kV and 230 mAs. For more detailed work using 460 mAs per slice, the skin dose would be doubled. Clearly the surface dose per centimetre of the body will depend upon the number of slices per centimetre. Discontinuous thick (8 mm) slices will lead to a lower dose per centimetre than contiguous/overlapping thin slices. A series of thin contiguous slices at high exposure rates, such as used for lumbar spine studies, could lead to a surface dose of around 50 mGy (5 rad) (Claussen and Lochner 1985). As the dose is highest at or just under the skin, it follows that superficial structures are potentially most at risk. The radiation dose to the eyes should be considered when sequential cranial CT studies are needed, though this is less of a problem with more modern machines; the early rotate/translate machines caused especial problems here.

Cost

Cost has always been a controversial part of CT on account of the fact that this relatively expensive technique emerged at a time of economic recession when the costs of health care generally were being closely scrutinised. It is likely that no other diagnostic technique has been subjected to such stringent evaluation (*Lancet* editorial 1984). However the cost of a CT machine (ranging from £200 000 to £600 000) now compares quite favourably with that of equipment used for other accepted radiological techniques (angiography, fluoroscopy). In many centres, CT was initially funded independently from the main X-ray department; accordingly precise costing data are available. In the unit at Addenbrooke's Hospital in Cambridge, which is used exclusively for body CT studies, the overall cost per patient is around £75. This sum allows for the initial purchase cost and all running costs (consumables, power, staffing and service contracts). A mixture of cranial and body examinations would allow a higher patient throughput and an even lower overall cost per patient. Of course this cost is an extra cost to the imaging department if the CT unit is developed as an additional facility. However when a CT unit is installed so that it replaces existing radiological equipment such as an outdated and underused fluoroscopic room, then there is little extra cost to the imaging department. Furthermore it is likely that some of the extra cost can be recouped by a reduction in the use of other tests such as lymphography (Dixon 1985) and in the time for which patients are hospitalised (Dixon et al. 1981a).

Clinical Problems

Testicular Tumours

The use of CT in the modern management of testicular tumours can be held up as one of the banners of the success of the technique. Many centres are coming to depend more and more on the CT findings and foregoing much lymphography which hitherto had been the mainstay of radiological staging. The one test can assess both the lungs and the abdomen, albeit at some cost. Such a study will require slices at 1 cm intervals through the chest where very small lesions are being sought; in the abdomen, where only lesions over 1 cm diameter are of much significance, slightly wider increments are usually chosen in the interests of economy and increased patient throughput.

The characteristic peripheral, sharply defined lung nodule of soft tissue density in a young patient born and bred in the UK can usually be assumed to be due to a metastasis (see Fig. 6.8c). However if the lesion is very small and single, or if the site is unusual, or if there are other features which do not fit, such as lack of elevation of levels of biochemical markers, then slight caution should be exercised before labelling the patient as having stage IV disease. A benign granuloma could be responsible, although this is relatively unlikely in this age group and is also less of a problem in this country than in some parts of the world (Edwards and Kelsey Fry 1982); furthermore such granulomata are usually calcified. A small pleural tag or another benign variant could be simulating a lesion. A fibrotic process could be present and in some situations metastases can be simulated; this can be a particular problem in the follow-up of patients following bleomycin therapy, although the characteristic peripheral rind-like appearance of this iatrogenic condition is now becoming well recognised (Bellamy et al. 1985; Rimmer et al. 1985). However these problems rarely arise at the time of the staging examination.

When there is concern about a possible lesion at chest CT, a repeat limited study (maybe just five cuts) through the possible lesion, after a short interval of perhaps 3 weeks, may resolve the dilemma. A small lung metastasis should be noticeably larger after such an interval. Such a policy may also be needed in other cancers where the development of a solitary lung nodule is critical to management; osteogenic sarcoma provides an example, although here many workers would proceed straightaway to a thoracotomy and removal of the supposed solitary lesion. It is humiliating that when such surgery is performed there are quite frequently several small nodular deposits present, over and above the one which had been demonstrated by CT. These are often discoid and arranged in a plaque-like fashion in an immediately sub-pleural situation so as to be virtually impossible to detect on the axial CT image. Thus there is an increasing tendency for clinicians to believe abnormal CT lung findings in patients with testicular teratoma as indicative of metastases and proceed with suitable chemotherapy forthwith. There is good evidence that CT is more sensitive than whole-lung tomography for the detection of lung nodules in this condition (Husband et al. 1979) and most hospitals have discontinued this latter technique.

Before considering the abdominal findings in patients with testicular lesions, the history of the development of abdominal CT will be briefly considered. Even with second-generation CT equipment (e.g. 5005 EMI model) it was quickly shown that enlarged para-aortic nodes could be reliably demonstrated, and in diseases such as the lymphomas, where detailed comparisons of lymphographic and CT findings were made, CT emerged favourably (Best et al. 1978; Earl et al. 1980). The obvious advantage of CT in demonstrating other areas besides the para-aortic chain was also appreciated; the liver, the spleen, the hepatic portal region, the mesenteric nodal region and the retrocrural nodal chains can all be assessed. The extensive literature describing anatomical variants which can simulate disease then emerged (Callen et al. 1978; Royal and Callen 1979; Nightingale and Dixon 1984). Now that radiologists are aware of these problems, and are armed with much more sophisticated equipment than was initially available, the results of CT should be that much better. However fewer and fewer patients with lymphoma are being subjected to full staging laparotomies and thus the detailed node by node comparisons may never again be undertaken.

Testicular lesions share with lymphoma the useful characteristic of tending to cause lymph node expansion, rather than mere replacement, as nodal involvement progresses. Thus the initial CT results of abdominal studies in patients with testicular teratoma were similarly very encouraging and there is every reason to believe that there may have been improvement recently with better equipment (Lee et al. 1979; Husband et al. 1980; Lien et al. 1983b). However in the United States, where surgical para-aortic lymphadenectomy is still widely practised, neither the results obtained by CT or lymphography, nor the two tests combined, are considered sufficiently reliable to forego staging procedures (Rowland et al. 1982). In this country extensive para-aortic nodal surgery has never been widely adopted, partly because of anxiety about potential complications (Kedia et al. 1975). Hence there is considerable reliance on radiological and biochemical parameters in the UK. Although lymphography may occasionally show nodal involvement, by architectural change within nodes of normal size which could be called normal at CT, this yield is low (Lien et al. 1983a). For these reasons many centres have discontinued or are in the process of reducing the use of lymphography in patients with testicular teratoma (Lien et al. 1983a; Marincek et al. 1983; Dixon 1985). This does presuppose that CT is sufficiently widely available to allow early review of those patients with equivocal or normal CT who are placed under surveillance, many of whom have tumour within para-aortic nodes of normal size. The diseased nodes increase in

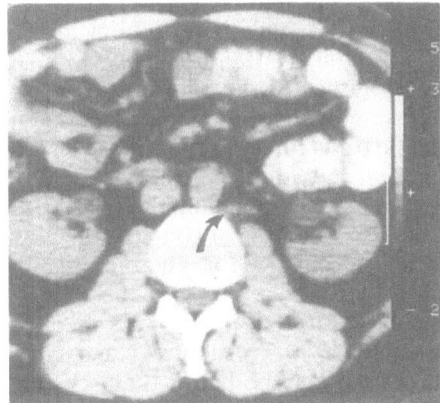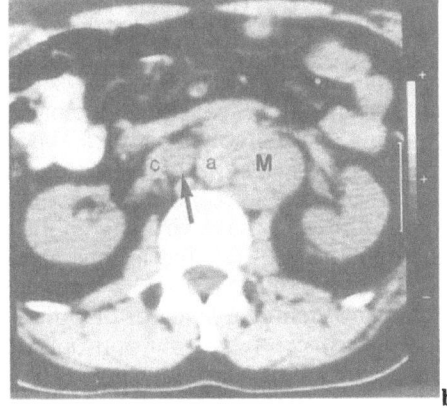

a   b

Fig. 6.3.a Staging CT in a patient with left-sided testicular teratoma and a suspicious node in the left para-aortic region (*arrow*). At this size interpretation should be guarded. **b** Eleven weeks later there is a huge left-sided para-aortic mass (M) with an additional 1.6 cm diameter node (*arrow*) between the inferior vena cava (c) and aorta (a) indicating crossover. (Reproduced with permission from Dixon et al. 1986.)

size at an alarming rate (Fig. 6.3) and early review at 4–6 weeks is recommended. This was one area where the lymphogram had some advantages; the one follow-up plain abdominal radiograph might show sufficient change to convert a node of equivocal interpretation to one with a definitely abnormal appearance (Macdonald et al. 1968). However the limitations of post-lymphogram plain abdominal radiographs in the longer term have been exposed by CT (Lee et al. 1980).

Such reliance on the radiological findings, especially in those patients with normal biochemical tumour markers, does mean that the CT procedure and the subsequent reporting must be performed with the utmost care. Again most difficulties will occur in the thin patient with little retroperitoneal fat; scrupulous attention to bowel opacification is essential. Knowledge of the normal distribution of early metastatic lymphatic spread may help reduce both false positive and false negative interpretations. Early nodal involvement tends to be ipsilateral: in the anterior inter-aorticocaval nodes for tumours of the right testicle; in the upper left para-aortic nodes for left-sided lesions (Donohue et al. 1982; Dixon et al. 1986).

Carcinoma of the Uterine Cervix

An area where CT is generally regarded to be less rewarding than in the preceding example is carcinoma of the cervix. The reasons for this difference are manifold. First the nature of cervical cancer means that involved nodes are often of normal size and such nodes will inevitably be undetectable at CT; indeed they are often not recognised to be involved at surgery or on macroscopic grounds at post-mortem, where there is a 20% error rate compared with histological examination (Henriksen 1949). Secondly it is much easier at CT to identify and interpret normal and abnormal nodes in the para-aortic chain than in the pelvic chains which are the most important sites for early spread of cervical cancer. In the para-aortic region the plane of the axial slice is at right angles to a constant vascular anatomy; in the pelvis the plane of the CT slice is tangential to the lymphatic chains, which pursue a rather variable course around a slighly variable vascular anatomy. The scene is set for some difficulties in interpretation. A further difficulty is caused by the patient; as stated above, the female abdomen contains considerably less intra-abdominal fat than that of the male (Dixon 1983). This seems to be a particular problem in the younger female, who is a likely candidate for cervical cancer; even a seemingly quite plump patient of this age and sex may have virtually no intra-abdominal fat. It is of course largely by the contrast with fat that lesions of soft tissue density such as enlarged lymph nodes or tumour extension can be recognised by CT.

Having identified some of the inherent problems for CT in the assessment of cervical cancer it is now appropriate to evaluate the results. As a staging procedure CT is probably as good as, and overall may be better than, clinical assessment (Photopulus et al. 1979; Kilcheski et al. 1981; Walsh and Gopelrud 1981), although precise comparisons are difficult because full surgical staging is rarely performed (Kademian and Bosch 1977). CT's weakest area, however, is in the distinction between stage Ib and IIb lesions—a distinction that involves a large potential difference in management.

The FIGO (International Federation of Obstetricians and Gynaecologists) classification does not take account of nodal involvement and thus some centres manage their patients on the basis of clinical findings with no investigations apart from chest X-ray and intravenous urogram. However many workers consider that evaluation of the presence and extent of nodal involvement allows a more logical decision as to the use of surgery or radiotherapy. Lymphography has long been used in this context and, despite the limitation that bipedal lymphography does not fill much of the internal iliac chains, has had considerable success (Douglas et al. 1972). So far the accuracy of CT for pelvic nodal involvement has not quite matched that of lymphography (Ginaldi et al. 1981), although a detailed comparison using the most modern equipment is awaited. In the para-aortic region CT performs better, for the reasons outlined above, with positive and negative predictive values of 80% and 92% respectively and an overall accuracy of 89% (Whitley et al. 1982). Fine needle cytological aspiration of abnormal or equivocal nodes can be used to confirm either lymphographic or CT findings.

Despite the slightly disappointing results of CT in the interpretation of pelvic nodes it is of interest that there is an increasing use of CT in the staging of patients with carcinoma of the cervix, both in centres which did and in those that

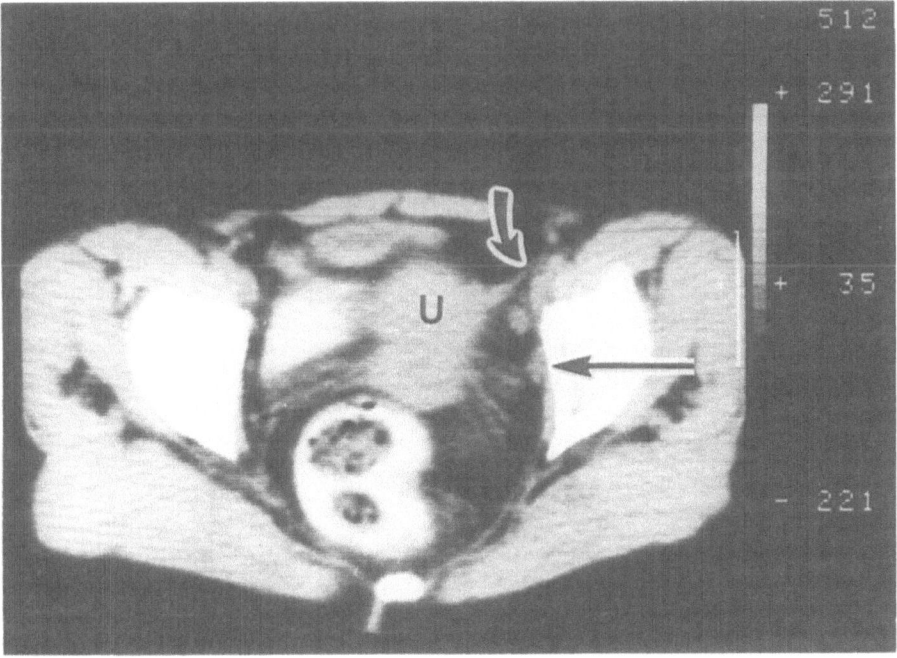

Fig. 6.4. A 59-year-old female with clinical stage III carcinoma of the cervix. The uterus (u) and round ligament (*curved arrow*) anterior to cervix proper are shown. The cervix has a slightly irregular border and there are numerous strands of soft tissue material within both parametria (left more than right) compatible with infiltration. There is no convincing CT evidence of a confluent mass of soft tissue density extending to the pelvic sidewall, but there is a 1.2 cm diameter node present in the left obturator chain (*straight arrow*).

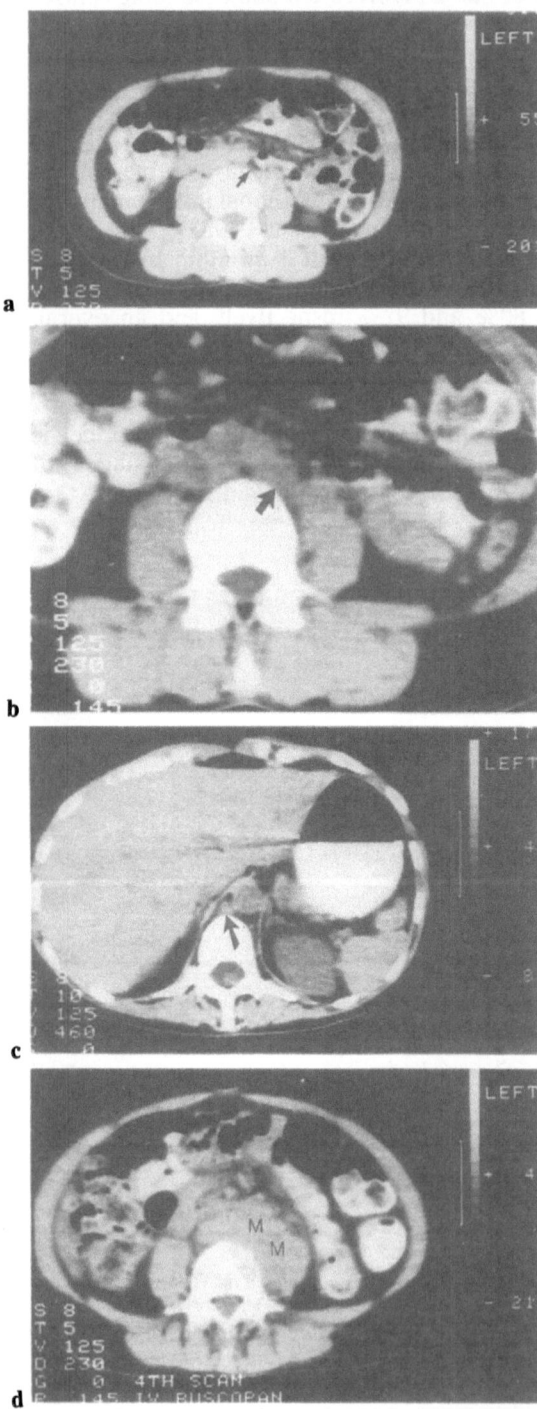

Fig. 6.5

did not use lymphography in the past. CT gives useful confirmation of the clinical stage in 65% of patients and will suggest upstaging in 19% and downstaging in 16% (Walsh and Gopelrud 1981). It can show intraperitoneal, rectal and bladder involvement in stage IV lesions. It is quite reliable at demonstrating sidewall extension by virtue of obliteration of the pelvic fat plane and all but the earliest of hydronephroses will be clearly evident. CT is slightly less reliable at demonstrating the irregular border of the cervix or the subtle parametrial infiltration of an early IIb lesion and it is still worse at demonstrating the presence and extent of vaginal extension. For these reasons it will always be used as an adjunct to clinical evaluation. However the same test can give useful information about pelvic nodes (Fig. 6.4) and quite accurate information about para-aortic nodes. Local treatment policies will determine which patients will benefit most from CT.

If the role of CT in the staging of primary cervical cancer varies from centre to centre there is little controversy about its usefulness in those patients with possible recurrence of malignancy. Here the one test can show both kidneys, the para-aortic and pelvic nodes as well as the pelvic structures. Sadly the nodal masses at this stage can be quite large, and may show bone involvement (Fig. 6.5). In the pelvis the tissue planes are often poorly defined following radiotherapy which causes a characteristic rind of material of soft tissue density around the perirectal fat (Doubleday and Bernadino 1980). However this tends to be symmetrical and any area of concern can be biopsied with a fine needle, which should allow differentiation between post-radiation fibrosis and recurrence.

Bladder

Cystoscopy remains essential for the diagnosis and histological grading of urothelial bladder neoplasms. The cystoscopic and histological findings can also assess the extent of muscular invasion. However cystoscopy cannot assess possible extension into the perivesical fat or the status of adjacent organs and lymph nodes. By virtue of its negative attenuation value, the perivesical fat is well demonstrated by CT. Although infiltration at microscopic level will not be recognised, more advanced infiltration will be evident by blurring of these fat planes or even by a soft tissue mass which may extend into adjacent structures. The angle between the posterior aspect of the bladder and the anterior aspect of

---

Fig. 6.5.a–d. a Initial CT in a patient who presented with clinical stage IIb carcinoma of the cervix. A normal left para-aortic region (*arrow*) is shown. Note the normal fat planes, with contrast medium and gas in an adjacent bowel loop. **b** Eighteen months later the patient is now complaining of back pain. Note that material of soft tissue density now occupies the gap between the aorta and left psoas (*arrow*) with features highly suggestive of para-aortic involvement, even though no discrete node over 1 cm in diameter is visible. The image could have been improved with better bowel preparation and an antiperistaltic agent. Aspiration biopsy could have been performed for confirmation. **c** An 8 mm diameter node in the right retrocrural region (*arrow*) has also developed over this period. Nodes of this size at this site should be regarded as abnormal. **d** Four months later there is now a huge para-aortic mass (M) with associated bone destruction. Hydronephrosis is evident on more cranial slices.

the seminal vesicles is normally well demarcated by fat (see Fig. 6.2e) (an overdistended rectum may cause approximation of these structures). Thus if this fat plane is lost, the extension of the neoplasm into the seminal vesicles is probable. Sadly there is no fat plane between the bladder and the prostate and therefore prostatic extension of tumour is difficult to recognise. The fact that the prostate is often quite bulky further contributes to the problem. So too does the inherent difficulty for axial CT in demonstrating tumour extension in the sagittal and coronal planes. To avoid this difficulty some workers (e.g. van Waes and Zonneveld 1982) advocate direct coronal CT. This is just possible for the pelvis using machines with spacious apertures provided the patient has adequate hip flexion. However many potential candidates for this technique are quite elderly and it has not been widely adopted; magnetic resonance imaging has clear advantages here. Nevertheless CT is a useful adjunct in staging (Kellett et al. 1980) and has an overall accuracy in recognising perivesical and seminal vesicle involvement of about 75% (Lee and Balfe 1982).

With respect to lymph nodes, the same overriding problem pertains as has been discussed for other tumours, namely CT's inability to recognise tumour within normal-sized nodes. However enlarged nodes should be recognised whether these are in the external or internal iliac chain. Few centres routinely performed lymphography in the pre-CT era and few workers now perform CT purely for nodal data as the accuracy is no better than that of lymphography. But the nodes should be carefully assessed as well as the pelvic organs. This ability to assess the bladder, the bladder wall, the perivesical space, the adjacent organs *and* the nodes makes CT a powerful technique.

Many patients will be treated on the basis of cystoscopic/clinical findings alone. However where there is uncertainty as to the appropriate treatment, CT can be helpful. In those patients who are to receive radiotherapy, a CT study for planning purposes will assist the design of suitable treatment fields.

A final role for CT in carcinoma of the bladder is in those patients who relapse following radiotherapy. In some a salvage cystectomy may be beneficial. However, enlarged pelvic or para-aortic nodes would strongly suggest dissemination; this could be confirmed if necessary by fine needle aspiration biopsy. Definite evidence of extension into adjacent structures would also be a contraindication to cystectomy. The sign of poorly defined fat planes is less useful in this situation as radiotherapy itself can cause this appearance (Doubleday and Bernadino 1980).

Bronchogenic Cancer

CT has become quite an important technique in the diagnosis of carcinoma of the bronchus. Occasionally it may reveal a small lesion in a patient presenting with either haemoptysis, clubbing or inappropriate endocrine secretion even when the chest X-ray is entirely normal and the results of bronchoscopy negative. But much more common is the patient with an equivocal mass at the hilum or elsewhere on the chest X-ray in whom CT may be used to determine whether the mass is real or apparent (e.g. prominent pulmonary artery). CT can not only establish the presence of additional material of soft tissue density but should also provide an indication as to the best method of obtaining a biopsy (bronchoscopic, percutaneous or via mediastinoscopy).

However it is in the staging of tissue-proven bronchial carcinoma that CT has come to play a major role (Rhea et al. 1981; Baron et al. 1982)—even if some controversy remains (Glazer et al. 1984; Libshitz and McKenna 1984; Brion et al. 1985). CT can accurately delineate the site of the primary lesion. In some instances the primary tumour can be seen extending into the mediastinal fat, encasing mediastinal vessels or causing adjacent bony destruction (rib or vertebra). Most surgeons regard such signs as reliable indicators of inoperability. It is important to realise that a lesion shown by CT merely to abut an important structure such as the aorta may well still be operable if there is no infiltration of the structure concerned. Even a lesion abutting the pleura and evoking pleural thickening or a small effusion may not have caused true invasion.

Although CT can prove or disprove the presence of enlarged hilar nodes secondary to a more peripheral lesion, the presence of such hilar nodes would merely alter the proposed need for a lobectomy to a pneumonectomy. It is the presence or absence of mediastinal nodes which is so important for the determination of operability. And in patients of the age at which cancer of the lung most frequently occurs, in whom the mediastinum is normally largely composed of vessels and fat (Dixon et al. 1981b), CT is a very good technique for demonstrating the size of mediastinal nodes. However CT cannot always predict whether the nodes contain tumour or not. Most workers (e.g. Sagel 1982) consider that nodes of diameter 2 cm or more in a patient with a known primary bronchogenic carcinoma can be assumed to contain tumour; but this is not invariable (Brion et al. 1985). Nodes between 1 and 2 cm in diameter are considered indeterminate; they may be large due to tumour infiltration, long-standing granulomatous disease or an inflammatory response to the effects of the tumour. Brion et al. (1985) have shown that in this setting 72% of involved nodes will be over 1 cm in diameter. Apart from demonstrating such a node, CT provides a very accurate map that allows appropriate biopsy. Mediastinoscopy allows biopsy of pretracheal nodes, anterior subcarinal nodes and nodes anterior to the right main bronchus. But mediastinoscopy cannot evaluate the anterior mediastinum or the aorticopulmonic space. Percutaneous aspiration may be possible for large nodes at such sites, but more often mediastinotomy or even thoracotomy is the final arbiter. If CT shows no node over 5 mm in diameter, mediastinoscopy is very likely to be unrewarding (Brion et al. 1985) and the surgeon should proceed directly to thoracotomy—although many centres use a larger nodal size for this decision (e.g. Glazer et al. 1984: 1.0–1.5 cm).

Because of the propensity of bronchial tumours to spread to the adrenals, assessment of the upper abdomen is an essential part of the staging procedure. Although it is relatively unusual for adrenal metastases to occur without other evidence of spread, the demonstration of an adrenal lesion considerably increases the confidence of the radiologist in his diagnosis when mediastinal nodes are of indeterminate size (1–2 cm in diameter). A unilateral adrenal lesion in the absence of other evidence of spread should be viewed with caution; an incidental adrenal adenoma is quite a common serendipitous finding. Fine needle aspiration may resolve the problem and provide definite evidence of dissemination (Fig. 6.6). Because of the frequency of adrenal involvement, some workers (Pagini 1983) have advocated CT-guided fine needle aspiration of normal adrenals in the work-up for bronchial cancer, but few centres in the UK have adopted this approach. Bilateral adrenal enlargement can be fairly safely assumed to be due to metastatic disease in the presence of a known primary tumour, although the possibility of ACTH production by the tumour should be considered.

By extending slices into the upper abdomen, the hepatic parenchyma can also be evaluated for metastatic deposits. Although the liver can also be assessed by ultrasound or scintigraphy, such tests can probably be dispensed with if CT is performed. Some workers include cranial CT as part of the staging procedure, but others (e.g. Poon et al. 1982) would argue that the relatively low detection rate of cerebral metastases (5% for small cell carcinoma) would mitigate against its routine use.

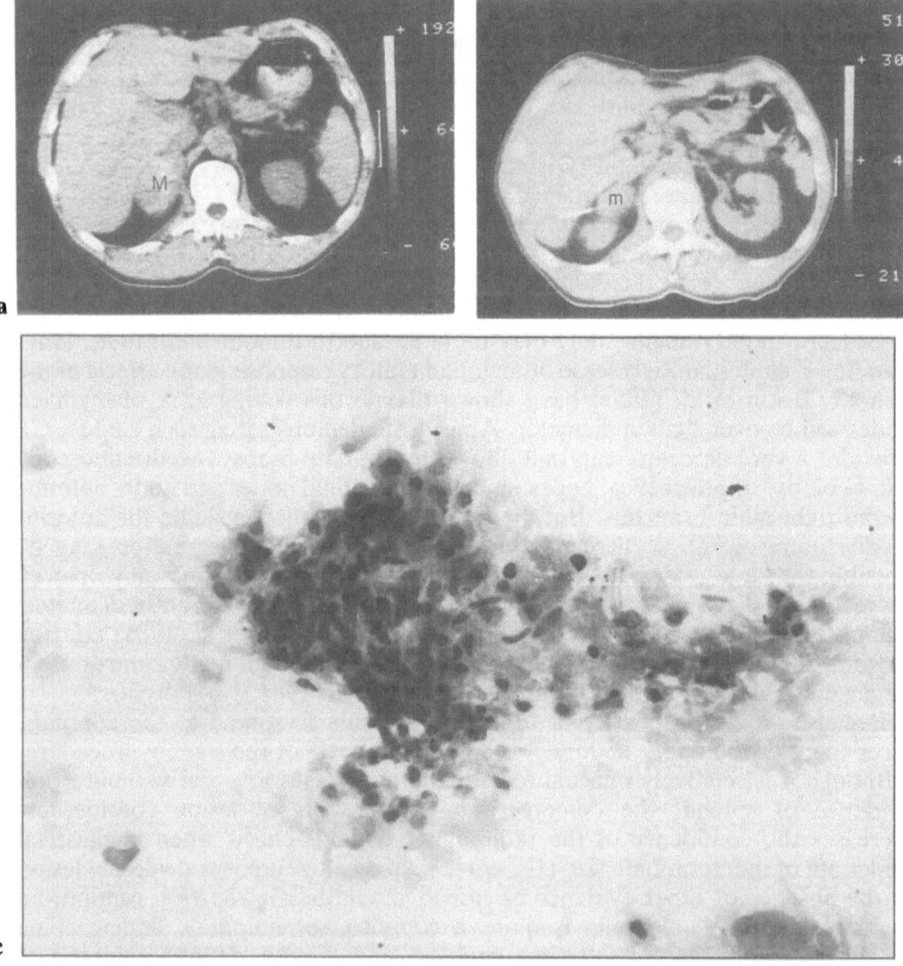

Fig. 6.6.a,b.   A 58-year-old male with biopsy-proven squamous cell carcinoma in the left upper lobe bronchus. CT of the mediastinum showed no definite contraindication to surgical resection. **a**   A large right adrenal mass (M). This was subsequently biopsied under CT control. **b**   A section of the needle leading to the mass (only the more caudal portion is seen; m on this slice). **c**   The malignant squamous cells obtained by adrenal aspirate, which matched the cells found in the initial fibreoptic biopsy (Papanicolau stain, ×128).

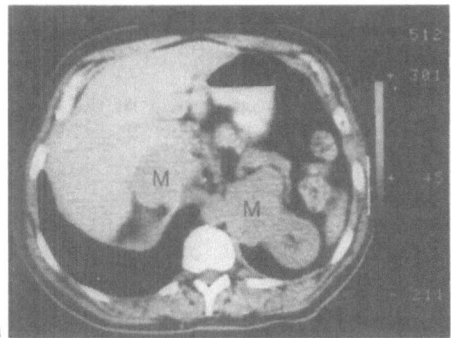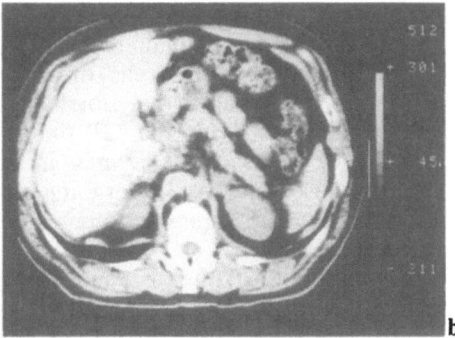

a   b

Fig. 6.7.a,b. A middle-aged male with small cell lung carcinoma. **a** CT scans show massive adrenal metastases at presentation (M, M). **b** Three months later, after chemotherapy, the adrenals have almost returned to normal size; they did not extend more cranially at this stage. This improvement has been maintained (1 year after presentation).

One management problem arises from the fact that carcinoma of the bronchus is a very common disease; if every patient in the community who developed such a lesion were to have CT, then the workload of many CT units would be heavily oversubscribed. Carcinoma of the bronchus (all histological types, all types of CT requests) accounts for well over 10% of the workload of the body CT unit in Addenbrooke's Hospital. So the first question that must be asked is whether the patient is suitable for surgical treatment. Many patients are unsuitable in terms of age, general clinical condition or lung function tests and thus do not need CT for the purposes of surgical evaluation. Some patients have clear evidence on the chest X-ray of bone destruction or mediastinal widening which again would mitigate against surgery. However some of these patients may be referred for radiotherapy. As CT can greatly assist therapy treatment planning (Emmai et al. 1978; Prasad et al. 1981) there may well be a good case for examining these patients by CT after all. CT seems to have little to offer the patient who develops a small irregular peripheral lung lesion but has an otherwise normal chest X-ray; mediastinal nodes are unlikely to be involved and thoracotomy is probably the quickest and safest method of sorting out such a problem. Patients with small cell carcinoma are not usually referred for surgery; however knowledge of the extent of metastatic disease is of importance as a base-line before starting chemotherapy, and here again the use of CT is probably justifiable. Such small cell lesions seem to have an even greater propensity than other bronchial lesions to spread to the adrenals (Fig. 6.7).

Tumours of the Musculoskeletal System

CT has many advantageous features when compared with other techniques of imaging tumours of the musculoskeletal system. In particular the simultaneous appreciation of bone and soft tissue structures is especially valuable (Genant et al. 1980).

In patients with osteogenic sarcoma, CT can accurately delineate the extent of the primary lesion (de Santos et al. 1979). Such lesions often have a much larger soft tissue component and more extensive intramedullary spread (Fig. 6.8) than is appreciated from the plain radiographs. Inevitably there are some problems in interpretation. Not all areas of osteopaenia are due to bone destruction. Furthermore oedema or haemorrhage may lead to over-estimation of the soft tissue component. But the CT findings can certainly influence the site and approach of the biopsy. They may influence the nature of the definitive surgery and, in those patients undergoing pre-operative chemotherapy, they allow determination of tumour volume before, during and after various drug regimens.

The ability of CT to detect small lung metastases means that it is an essential part of the staging procedure. There is currently considerable enthusiasm for surgical resection of lung metastases, provided these do not number more than a handful. However, as mentioned in the section on testicular teratoma, the thoracic surgeon often finds many more metastases than were seen at CT. For this reason it seems worth while to repeat the thoracic CT immediately before proposed thoracotomy, as additional metastases may have developed during the intervening period making surgery a less attractive proposition. Alternatively,

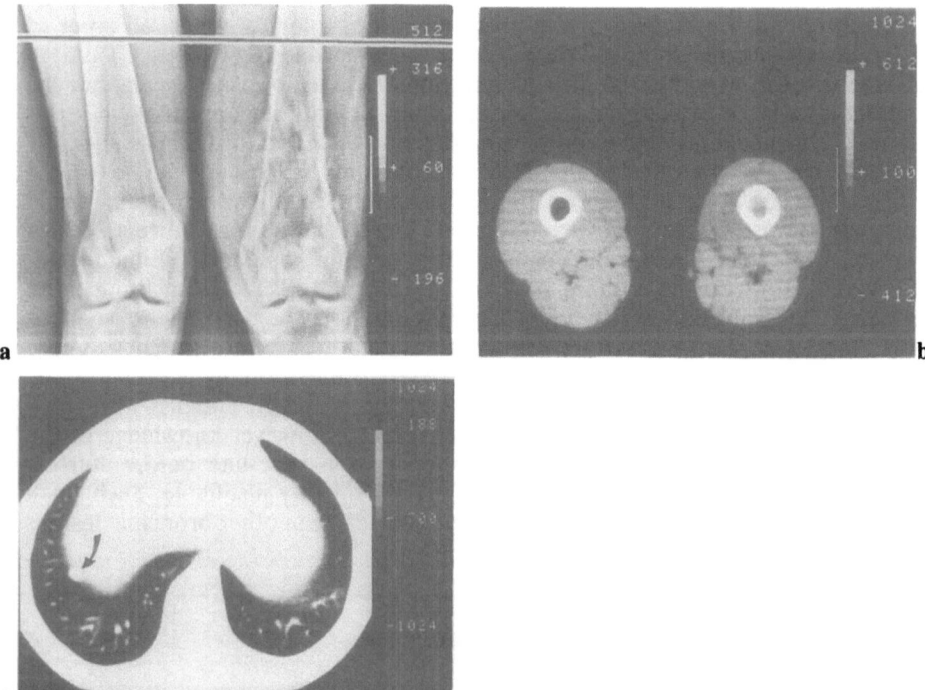

Fig. 6.8.a–c A 19-year-old male with osteogenic sarcoma of the left lower femur. **a** Scanogram film taken as an initial localising procedure. **b** Infiltration of tumour extending more proximally in the left medullary canal than anticipated. This should be compared with the normal fat-filled right medullary canal. This image was obtained at the level of the horizontal line in **a. c** Despite treatment a lung metastasis (*arrow*) developed in the right lower lobe 1 year later. This lesion was hard to see on the chest X-ray due to its proximity to the right hemidiaphragm.

the absence of new metastases during this period is an encouraging sign which should make the proposed thoracotomy all the more rewarding.

In Ewing's sarcoma CT is again helpful in demonstrating the soft tissue component of the tumour, and here knowledge of the precise site of the tumour bulk may influence the radiation field. Again assessment of the lungs is essential. These patients tend to be younger and full general anaesthesia may be needed for accurate thoracic assessment.

In tumours arising from the soft tissues (e.g. fibrosarcoma), the chief use of CT is to define the precise anatomical extent of the lesion in the hope that complete surgical excision can be effected with minimal residual loss of function. In the adult patient there is usually adequate adipose tissue to distinguish the planes of cleavage between the various muscle groups. By comparing the abnormal limb/site with the contralateral side, a good appreciation of the anatomy can be gained. In some children and very emaciated adults, recognition of the fat planes may be difficult.

Summary

Now that modern computerised tomography facilities are becoming more widely available and many of the initial diagnostic pitfalls are understood, many oncologists are increasingly coming to rely on CT data. In most centres this has resulted in a decrease in referrals for lymphography and other invasive radiological procedures. The use of the CT image as a road-map to allow accurate radiotherapy planning and placement of biopsy needles is a further advance. The continued need for biopsy highlights the major limitation of the technique: whilst CT provides exquisite anatomical information, its ability to differentiate between benign and malignant processes is limited.

References

Baron RL, Levitt RG, Sagel SS, White MJ, Roper CL, Marbarger JP (1982) Computed tomography in the preoperative evaluation of bronchogenic carcinoma. Radiology 145: 727–732
Bellamy EA, Husband JE, Blaquiere RM, Law MR (1985) Bleomycin-related lung damage: CT evidence. Radiology 156: 155–158
Berger PE, Kuhn JP, Brusehaber J (1981) Techniques for computer tomography in infants and children. Radiol Clin North Am 19: 399–408
Best JJK, Blackledge G, Forbes WStC et al. (1978) Computed tomography of abdomen in staging and clinical management of lymphoma. Br Med J ii: 1675–1677
Brion JP, Depauw L, Kuhn G et al. (1985) Role of computed tomography and mediastinoscopy in preoperative staging of lung carcinoma. J Comput Assist Tomogr 9: 480–484
Callen PW, Filly RA, Korobkin M (1978) Computed tomography of the diaphragmatic crura. Radiology 26: 413–416
Claussen C, Lochner B (1985) Dynamic computed tomography. Springer-Verlag, Berlin Heidelberg New York, pp 11–12
de Santos LA, Bernadino ME, Murray JA (1979) Computed tomography in the evaluation of osteosarcoma: experience with 25 cases. AJR 132: 535–540
Dixon AK (1983) Abdominal fat assessed by computed tomography: sex difference in distribution. Clin Radiol 34: 189–191

Dixon AK (1985) The current practice of lymphography: a survey in the age of computed tomography. Clin Radiol 36: 287–290

Dixon AK, Fry IK, Kingham JGC, McLean AM, White FE (1981a) Computed tomography in patients with an abdominal mass. Lancet I: 1199–1201

Dixon AK, Hilton CJ, Williams GT (1981b) Computed tomography and histological correlation of the thymic remnant. Clin Radiol 32: 255–257

Dixon AK, Ellis M, Sikora K (1986) Computed tomography in testicular tumours: distribution of abdominal lymphadenopathy. Clin Radiol (in press)

Donohue JP, Zachary JM, Maynard BR (1982) Distribution of nodal metastases in nonseminomatous testis cancer. J Urol 128: 315–320

Doubleday LC, Bernadino ME (1980) CT findings in the peri-rectal area following radiation therapy. J Comput Assist Tomogr 4: 634–638

Douglas B, Macdonald JS, Baker JW (1972) Lymphography in carcinoma of the uterus. Clin Radiol 23: 286–294

Earl HM, Sutcliffe SBJ, Kelsey Fry I et al. (1980) Computerised tomographic (CT) abdominal scanning in Hodgkin's disease. Clin Radiol 31: 149–153

Edwards SE, Kelsey Fry I (1982) Prevalence of lung nodules on computed tomography of patients without known malignant disease. Br J Radiol 55: 715–716

Emmai B, Melo A, Carter BL, Munzenrider JE, Piro AJ (1978) Value of computed tomography in radiotherapy of lung cancer. AJR 131: 63–67

Genant HK, Wilson JS, Bovill EG, Brunelle FO, Murray RO, Rodrigo JJ (1980) Computed tomography of the musculoskeletal system. J Bone Joint Surg [Am] 62: 1088–1101

Ginaldi S, Wallace S, Jing B-S, Bernadino ME (1981) Carcinoma of the cervix: lymphangiography and computed tomography. AJR 136: 1087–1091

Glazer GM, Orringer MB, Gross BH, Quint LE (1984) The mediastinum in non-small cell lung cancer: CT–surgical correlation. AJR 142: 1101–1105

Henriksen E (1949) The lymphatic spread of carcinoma of the cervix and body of the uterus. Am J Obstet Gynecol 58: 924–942

Hounsfield GN (1973) Computerized transverse axial scanning (tomography). I. Description of system. Br J Radiol 46: 1016–1022

Husband JE, Peckham MJ, Macdonald JS, Hendry WF (1979) The role of computed tomography in the management of testicular teratoma. Clin Radiol 30: 243–252

Husband JE, Peckham MJ, Macdonald JS (1980) The role of abdominal computed tomography in the management of testicular tumours. Comput Tomogr 4: 1–16

Husband JE, Hawkes DJ, Peckham MJ (1982) CT estimations of mean attenuation values and volume in testicular tumours. Radiology 144: 553–558

Kademian MT, Bosch A (1977) Staging laparotomy and survival in carcinoma of the uterine cervix. Acta Radiol [Ther] (Stockh) 16: 314–324

Kedia KR, Markland C, Fraley EE (1975) Sexual function following high retroperitoneal lymphadenectomy. J Urol 114: 237–239

Kellett MJ, Oliver RTD, Husband JE, Fry IK (1980) Computed tomography as an adjunct to bimanual examination for staging bladder tumours. Br J Urol 52: 101–106

Kilcheski TS, Arger PH, Mulhern CB, Coleman BG, Kressel HY, Mikuta JI (1981) Role of computed tomography in the presurgical evaluation of carcinoma of the cervix. J Comput Assist Tomogr 5: 379–383

Lancet editorial (1984) Body computed tomography: wanted or needed? Lancet II: 961–962

Lee JKT, Balfe DM (1982) The pelvis. In: Lee JKT, Sagel SS, Stanley RJ (eds) Computed body tomography. Raven Press, New York, pp 393–413

Lee JKT, McClennan BL, Stanley RJ, Sagel SS (1979) Computed tomography in the staging of testicular neoplasms. Radiology 130: 387–390

Lee JKT, Stanley RJ, Sagel SS, Melson GL, Koehler RE (1980) Limitations of the post-lymphangiogram plain abdominal radiograph as an indicator of recurrent lymphoma: comparison to computed tomography. Radiology 134: 155–158

Libshitz HI, McKenna RJ (1984) Mediastinal lymph node size in lung cancer. AJR 143: 715–718

Lien HH, Fossa SD, Ous S, Stenwig AE (1983a) Lymphography in retroperitoneal metastases in non-seminoma testicular tumour patients with a normal CT scan. Acta Radiol [Diagn] (Stockh) 24: 319–322

Lien HH, Kolbenstvedt A, Talle K, Fossa SD, Klepp O, Ous S (1983b) Comparison of computed tomography, lymphography, and phlebography in 200 consecutive patients with regard to retroperitoneal metastases from testicular teratoma. Radiology 146: 129–132

Macdonald JS, Laugier A, Schlienger M (1968) Observations on the growth of tumours in lymph nodes changing from normal to abnormal while remaining opacified after lymphography. Clin Radiol 19: 120–127

Marincek B, Brutschin P, Triller J, Fuchs WA (1983) Lymphography and computed tomography in staging nonseminomatous testicular cancer: limited detection of early stage metastatic disease. Urol Radiol 5: 243–246

Moss AA, Dean PB, Goldberg HJ (1982) Dynamic CT of hepatic masses with intravenous and intraarterial contrast material. AJR 138: 847–852

Nightingale RC, Dixon AK (1984) Crural change with respiration: a potential mimic of disease. Br J Radiol 57: 101–102

Pagini JJ (1983) Normal adrenal glands in small cell lung carcinoma: CT-guided biopsy. AJR 140: 949–951

Photopulus GJ, McCartney WH, Walton LA, Staab EV (1979) Computerized tomography applied to gynaecological oncology. Am J Obstet Gynecol 135: 381–383

Poon PY, Feld R, Evans WK, Ege G, Yeoh JL, McLoughlin ML (1982) Computed tomography of the brain, liver, and upper abdomen in the staging of small cell carcinoma. J Comput Assist Tomogr 6: 963–965

Prasad S, Pilepich MV, Perez CA (1981) Contribution of CT to quantitative radiation therapy planning. AJR 136: 123–128

Rhea HH, Shevland JE, House AJS (1981) Accuracy of computed tomographic scanning in assessment of the mediastinum in bronchial carcinoma. J Thorac Cardiovasc Surg 81: 825–829

Rimmer MJ, Dixon AK, Flower CDR, Sikora K (1985) Bleomycin lung: computed tomographic observations. Br J Radiol 58: 1041–1045

Rowland RG, Weisman D, Williams SD, Einhorn LH, Klatte EC, Donohue JP (1982) Accuracy of preoperative staging in Stages A and B nonseminomatous germ cell testis tumours. J Urol 127: 718–720

Royal SA, Callen PW (1979) CT evaluation of anomalies of the inferior vena cava and left renal vein. AJR 132: 759–763

Sagel SS (1982) Lung, pleura, pericardium and chest wall. In: Lee JKT, Sagel SS, Stanley RJ (eds) Computed body tomography. Raven Press, New York, p 110

van Waes PFGM, Zonneveld FW (1982) Direct coronal body computed tomography. J Comput Assist Tomogr 6: 58–66

Walsh JWS, Gopelrud DR (1981) Prospective comparison between clinical and CT staging in primary cervical carcinoma. AJR 137: 997–1003

Whitley NO, Brenner DE, Francis A et al. (1982) CT evaluation of carcinoma of the cervix. Radiology 142: 439–446

7 Magnetic Resonance Imaging in Oncology

R. J. Johnson, J. P. R. Jenkins and I. Isherwood

Introduction

Nuclear magnetic resonance (NMR) employs radio-frequency radiation in the presence of a static magnetic field to produce signals from naturally occurring nuclei in biological tissue. The information in magnetic resonance imaging (MRI) can be derived from these signals in any orthogonal plane. Hydrogen is the most abundant of such nuclei, occurring naturally in water and lipid, and can be detected at relatively low magnetic field strength (0.04 tesla (T) upwards). The MR signal from hydrogen depends not only on the *proton density* and the T_1 and T_2 *relaxation times* of those protons following radio-frequency disturbance, but also on the timing parameters of the radio-frequency pulse sequences employed. Image contrast depends on the interaction between all these factors; not simply as in X-ray computed tomography (CT) on the properties of the tissue itself. Therefore an understanding of both the imaging process and the pathology under investigation is essential in the proper use of MRI.

Approach to Tissue Characterisation

Tissue characterisation by MRI can be approached in a variety of ways: through measurement of *proton density*, *relaxation times*, blood flow, chemical shift or the use of paramagnetic tracers. In Manchester we have attempted quantitative characterisation by determination of the three signal parameters: *proton density*, and the T_1 and T_2 *relaxation times*. The difficulty is to ensure the independence of *proton density* and *relaxation times*. In vitro experiments can be undertaken using radio-frequency pulse sequences with long repetition times. This is not practical in clinical imaging where limited time is available. It is difficult for patients to remain stationary in the instrument for periods exceeding 1 hour and therefore pulse sequences with shorter repetition times than can be used in vitro have to be employed. This time constraint also means that only a limited number of regions of interest can be studied (Isherwood et al. 1986).

The important physical factors to consider in the measurement of T_1 and T_2 *relaxation times* from MR images include the acquisition of multiple data points to plot exponential decay, the consistency of slice profile, the use of a suitable algorithm to take into account the interaction between signal intensity and the signal parameters and finally the optimisation of any spatial variation within the image. Details of our methodology have been described elsewhere (Hickey et al. 1986). Multiple data points are used to minimise error and improve reproducibility. Data from seven *Total Saturation Recovery* (TSR) (Waterton et al. 1984) and six *Spin Echo* (SE) *sequences* are used to calculate T_1 and T_2 *relaxation times* and the *proton density* using an iterative least squares technique. Data acquisition time to collect these 13 images for a single section in each patient has been approximately 50 minutes. Pulse sequences have been designed in which the slice profile is independent of repetition time (Hickey et al. 1986). Inappropriate sequences can result in a slice profile changing from a Gaussian to a bi-modal shape by shortening the repetition time (Bryant et al. 1984).

The equation employed for T_1 calculations from *Saturation Recovery* data is:

$$I = M_\infty e^{-2\tau/T_2} [1 - e^{-TR/T_1}]$$

and that for the estimation of T_2 is:

$$I = M_\infty [1 - 2e^{-(TR-\tau)/T_1} + e^{-TR/T_1}] e^{-2\tau/T_2}$$

where I is signal intensity, M_∞ is *proton density*, TR is the repetition time of the pulse sequence used, and $2\tau = TE$ where TE is the echo delay time in the *Spin Echo sequences* used.

The accuracy of T_1 estimations in studies in vitro is, as discussed earlier, dependent upon a very long repetition time. Since time is clearly restricted in clinical studies, appropriate corrections must be applied to compensate for the necessarily shorter TR values. The steps to achieve this correction have been described elsewhere (Isherwood et al. 1986; Hickey et al. 1986). The least squares regression line is then calculated for data obtained from a series of scans with TR varied. For the T_2 estimations TR is fixed and TE is varied in the *Spin Echo sequences* employed.

This method has been used in a series of clinical and experimental studies on a Picker superconducting whole-body imaging system operating at 0.26 T and 10.98 mHz (Jenkins et al. 1985a, b, 1987; Johnson et al. 1987). The results obtained suggest that the method is robust and reproducible. It is important, however, to recognise that a measured parameter will vary with the imaging instrument's field strength and the pulse sequences employed. Reproducibility in longitudinal clinical studies depends upon these factors remaining constant.

Described below are various clinical studies we have undertaken in patients with cancer. Some of these studies involve the use of the tissue characterisation methods described above; in others we have looked at the role of MR as an imaging technique for staging cancer. The studies related to pelvic malignancy are described first. Sections on carcinoma of the pancreas and musculoskeletal tumours follow.

Carcinoma of the Rectum

Staging

As an imaging technique MRI is often compared with CT, and the pelvis is one anatomical region where it has potential advantages over CT. The display of pelvic anatomy is well suited for study by MRI due to the absence of motion artefact. There is a high intrinsic contrast between pelvic fat, urine in the bladder, air and faeces in the rectum and the pelvic soft tissues which MRI with its superior contrast resolution should be able to exploit and thereby improve the staging of pelvic malignancies. The ability to scan directly in the coronal and sagittal planes in addition to the transverse axial plane is another advantage. It

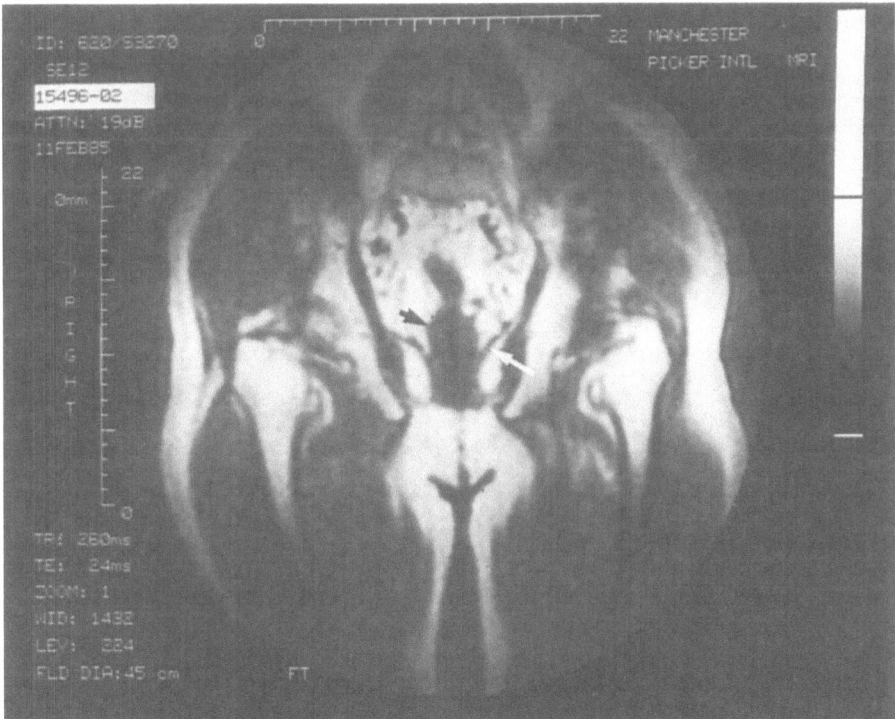

Fig. 7.1. Coronal MR scan (*Spin Echo sequence*; TR = 260 ms, TE = 24 ms (SE = 260/24)) through a normal pelvis illustrating the relationship of the rectum (*black arrow*) to the pelvic floor (*white arrow*).

allows better identification and delineation of tumour spread to adjacent structures and to the pelvic floor and perineum. To date there are limited published data comparing MRI with CT in the pre-operative staging of rectal carcinoma. Butch et al. (1985) compared pre-operative staging by MRI and CT with findings at surgery in 13 patients and concluded that the two techniques were equal in their ability to assess the local extent of disease. The disease itself, however, was more easily delineated by MRI. Neither technique could distinguish normal lymph nodes from those involved with tumour.

In Manchester we have compared MRI and CT in patients presenting with carcinoma of the rectum extending through the bowel wall (advanced disease) and in patients with biopsy-proven recurrent rectal carcinoma. The techniques compared favourably with each other in assessing the extent of disease, delineation of disease being easier by MRI, mainly as a result of images obtained in the coronal and sagittal planes. Such images can demonstrate the relationship of the primary tumour to the pelvic floor, which may be helpful to the surgeon in deciding operative technique, that is whether to undertake an anterior or abdominoperineal resection (Fig. 7.1). Delineation of the intraluminal extent of tumour can be difficult due to the presence of faeces, which have a varied signal intensity. If necessary the patient can be prepared prior to the MR scan with a rectal wash-out and installation of a contrast agent such as air or particulate iron oxide (magnetite) (Saini et al. 1986). Butch et al. (1985) scanned patients in the prone position with a distended bladder. However, we have not found this an advantage.

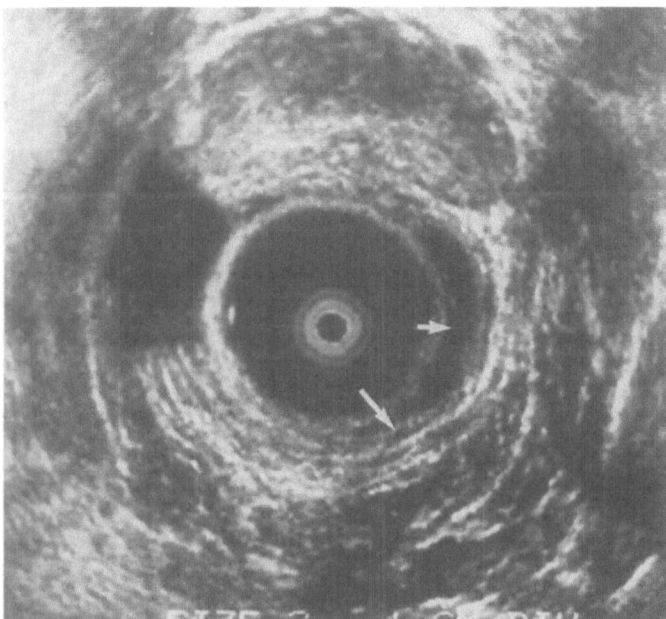

Fig. 7.2. Transrectal ultrasound illustrating a stage T1 carcinoma of the rectum (*short arrow*). The tumour has not penetrated the submucosa (*long arrow*). (Reproduced by courtesy of Mr J. Beynon, Dept. of Surgery, Bristol Royal Infirmary.)

The depth of tumour penetration into the bowel wall is a most important prognostic factor in carcinoma of the rectum. CT cannot ascertain this or identify early perirectal invasion, though it is accurate in detecting spread beyond 1–2 cm (Dixon et al. 1981; Van Waes et al. 1983; Zheng et al. 1984). There are no studies yet published documenting the ability of MRI to detect the depth of tumour penetration or early perirectal invasion. Early studies suggest that transrectal ultrasound is a technique able to do this (Beynon et al. 1986) (Fig. 7.2).

MRI therefore compares favourably with CT in assessing the local extent of disease in patients with both advanced and recurrent rectal carcinoma. Both techniques are limited in assessing the lymph node status of the patient. Neither can detect metastases in normal-sized nodes and, as with CT, MRI is unlikely to distinguish nodes enlarged by tumour deposit, reactive hyperplasia or infection.

Tissue Characterisation

One of the clinical studies we have undertaken has been an attempt to distinguish between recurrent carcinoma of the rectum and post-operative fibrosis in patients who have had either an abdomino-perineal (A–P) or an anterior resection. An aim of the study was to improve the early detection of tumour recurrence. In this cohort of patients, particularly those who have had an A–P resection, the detection of early recurrence can be difficult. CT is usually the optimal method of confirming recurrence in symptomatic patients and planning treatment (Husband et al. 1980; Lee et al. 1981; Zheng et al. 1984). However in some asymptomatic patients, or those with minimal symptoms, CT may demonstrate a soft tissue mass in the sacro-coccygeal hollow where it is impossible to differentiate between tumour recurrence and fibrosis. An open or percutaneous biopsy is then required to obtain a tissue diagnosis. A negative percutaneous biopsy (i.e. no evidence of tumour) is unreliable in excluding tumour. Biopsy obtained at second-look laparotomy is more reliable but the patient may then have been subjected to unnecessary surgery if the mass is entirely fibrotic.

Table 7.1. Tissue characterisation in carcinoma of the rectum

	No. of patients	Mean *relaxation times* ± SE	
		T_1 (ms)	T_2 (ms)
Carcinoma of the rectum	15	*832 ± 39	**68 ± 2
Fibrosis	7	*478 ± 61	**59 ± 3

* Highly significant ($P<0.001$).
** Significant ($P<0.05$).

From our initial studies we have obtained baseline data of the T_1 and T_2 values in patients with biopsy-proven carcinoma of the rectum and pelvic fibrosis. All these patients had a tumour bulk or a fibrotic mass greater than 5 cm in one diameter. The results are detailed in Table 7.1 and indicate a highly significant difference in the T_1 *relaxation times* ($P<0.001$) between fibrosis and carcinoma. Further work is in progress to determine whether these results remain valid in a larger number of patients (Johnson et al. 1987).

We have also measured *relaxation times* in a group of patients undergoing radiotherapy for recurrent carcinoma of the rectum and in patients with previously untreated carcinoma of the rectum who have had pre-operative radiotherapy. The purpose of this study was to assess the effect of radiotherapy by comparing the clinical response with changes in tumour size on the MR scan together with the measured *relaxation times*. Each patient had:
1. MRI and CT scan prior to biopsy and radiotherapy.
2. Follow-up MR scan approximately 6 weeks after radiotherapy.
3. Further MR and CT scan approximately 12 weeks after radiotherapy.
4. Further MR scans at approximately 26 and 52 weeks after radiotherapy.

Table 7.2. Magnetic resonance characteristics before and after radiotherapy in patients with carcinoma of the rectum

Visit (see text)	Mean *relaxation times* ± SE	
	T_1 (ms)	T_2 (ms)
1 ($n = 15$)	832 ± 39	68 ± 2
2 ($n = 15$)	876 ± 41	69 ± 9
3 ($n = 5$)	1118 ± 118	81 ± 8
4 ($n = 4$)	1028	84

On each occasion T_1 and T_2 *relaxation times* and *proton density* were measured using the multi-point method described above. An estimate of tumour size was made from the scan and the clinical state of the patient documented. Our initial results on 15 patients who have had more than one MR scan are detailed in Table 7.2. Five of these patients have had a third MR scan and one patient a fourth, fifth and sixth scan. These pooled data demonstrate no significant difference between the T_1 and T_2 values before and 6 weeks after radiotherapy. Whilst an analysis of variance indicates a significant difference ($P<0.02$) between the T_1 values for the first and third visit in these pooled data, no significant difference was observed for the T_2 values. Analysis of the data on individual patients, however, is encouraging. Initial results suggest a correlation between clinical response, changes in size of the tumour seen on the MR scan and the measured *relaxation times*. Details of three representative patients are given below.

A patient with recurrent carcinoma of the rectum had no improvement in his symptoms following radiotherapy. The *relaxation times* demonstrate a sequential fall over 3½ months associated with an increase in tumour bulk on the MR images (Fig. 7.3a,b).

	Visit 1 10.10.84	Visit 2 23.11.84	Visit 3 28.1.85
T_1 (ms)	1052	897	830
T_2 (ms)	76	68	65

Fig. 7.3.a,b. Sagittal SE 1000/60 images illustrating recurrent carcinoma of the rectum (a) (*white arrow*) which has increased in size over 3½ months to involve the sacrum and upper presacral regions (b) (*white arrows*). The patient has a bladder catheter *in situ* on both scans. On the initial scan the low-intensity area (*open arrow*) probably represents post-operative fibrosis.

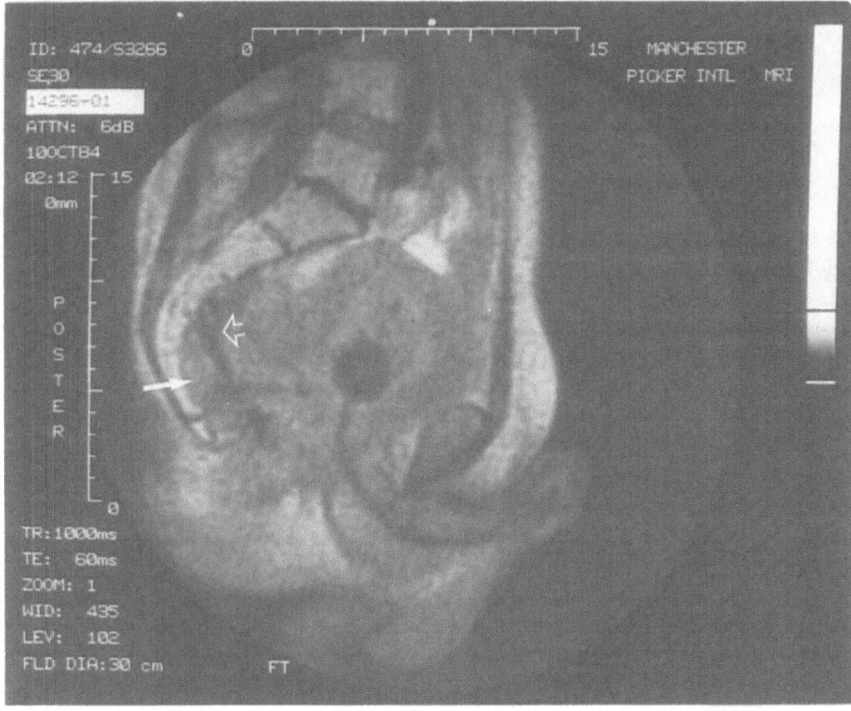

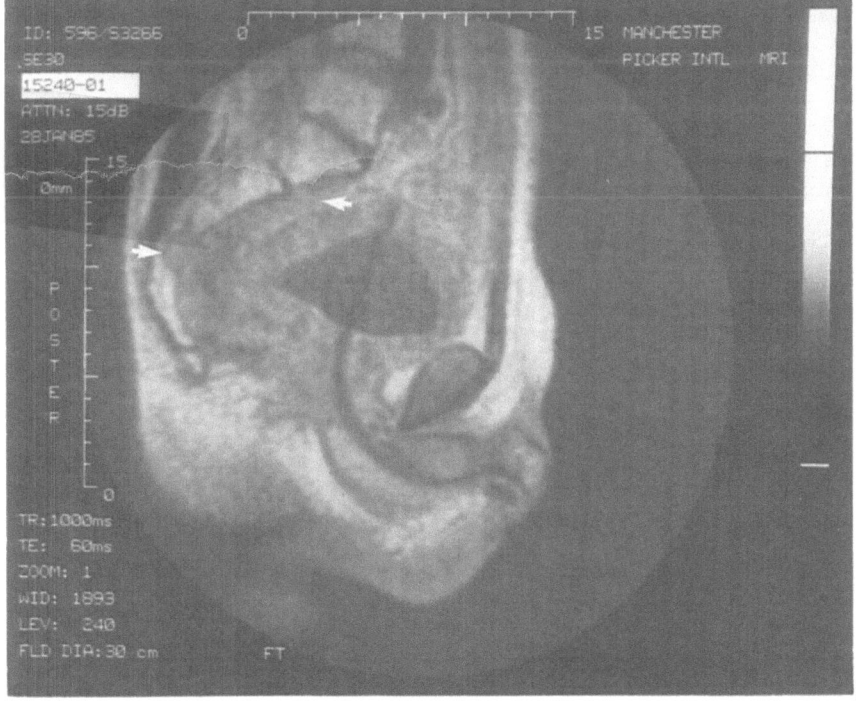

Fig. 7.3

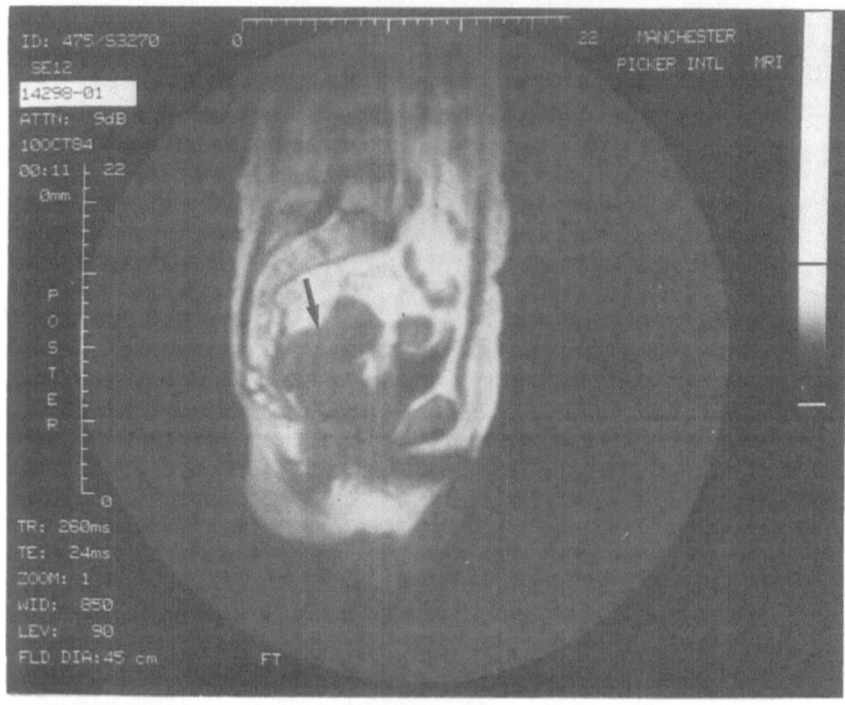

a

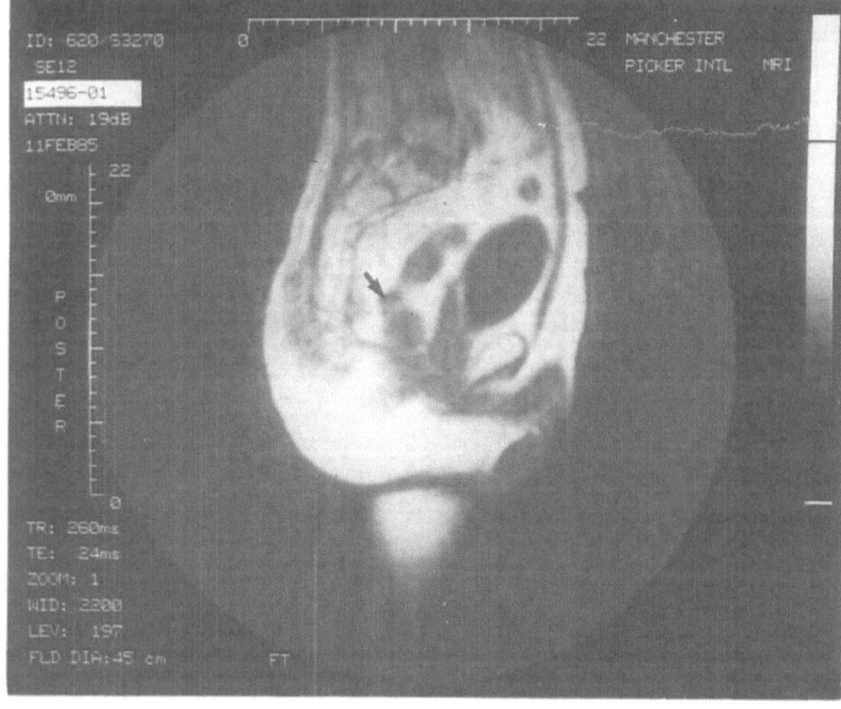

b

Fig. 7.4

A second patient with advanced, initially inoperable, carcinoma of the rectum responded to radiotherapy and was able to have an A–P resection. There was a sequential rise in the measured *relaxation times* associated with a reduction in tumour bulk, the immediately pre-operative MR scan being essentially normal (Fig. 7.4a,b). Histology of the resected specimen demonstrated a small number of viable tumour cells at the base of a small rectal ulcer.

	Visit 1 10.10.84	Visit 2 19.12.84	Visit 3 11.2.85
T_1 (ms)	606	864	1064
T_2 (ms)	64	76	83

The third patient initially had a good response to radiotherapy for his recurrent rectal tumour, with amelioration of his pelvic pain and reduction in tumour size. This was associated with a sequential rise in T_1 and T_2 values (February to July 1984). Biopsy of the residual mass at this time showed evidence of fibrosis only. A further scan in January 1985, when the patient remained well, showed a fall in the T_1 and T_2 values. The residual mass had not changed in size and a further biopsy showed evidence of fibrosis only. Five months later the patient had developed pelvic pain and repeat scan showed an increase in size of the mass with a further fall in the T_1 and T_2 values. Five months after this there had been further deterioration with obvious bulk tumour recurrence and a further fall in the T_1 and T_2 values (Fig. 7.5a–c).

	Visit 1 13.2.84	Visit 2 9.4.84	Visit 3 25.7.84	Visit 4 24.1.85	Visit 5 12.6.85	Visit 6 19.11.85
T_1 (ms)	914	930	1548	1028	1033	669
T_2 (ms)	85	94	112	84	64	65

One may conclude, therefore, that although the number of patients is small these early data suggest that a sequential rise in the measured *relaxation times* indicates a good response to radiotherapy whilst a fall is a bad prognostic sign. Of more importance, as seen in the third patient, is that a fall in the measured *relaxation times* following a sequential rise occurred before clinical evidence of recurrence or a change in tumour size on the scan. It appears that the fall in T_1 and T_2 values was the first sign of tumour recurrence which was confirmed several months later.

Fig. 7.4.a,b. Sagittal SE 260/24 images illustrating (**a**) a large, new carcinoma of the rectum (*arrow*) and (**b**) a normal appearance of the rectum (*arrow*) after radiotherapy.

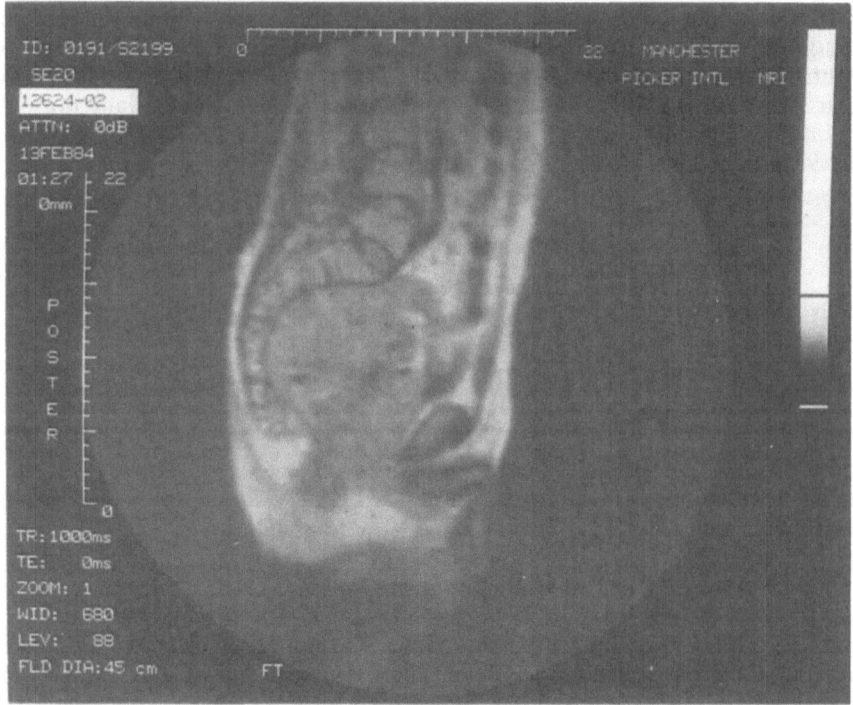

a

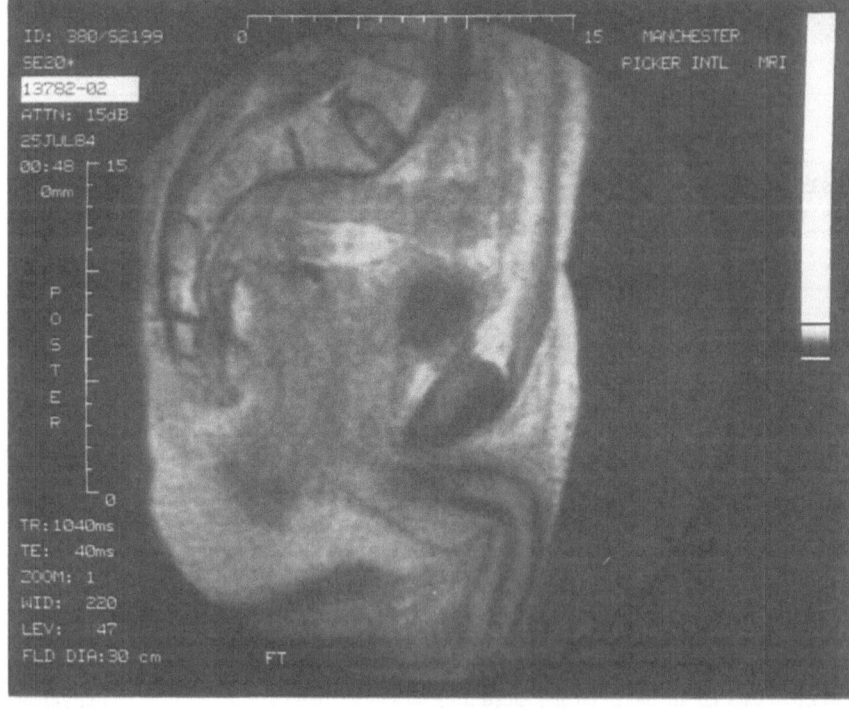

b

Fig. 7.5a,b

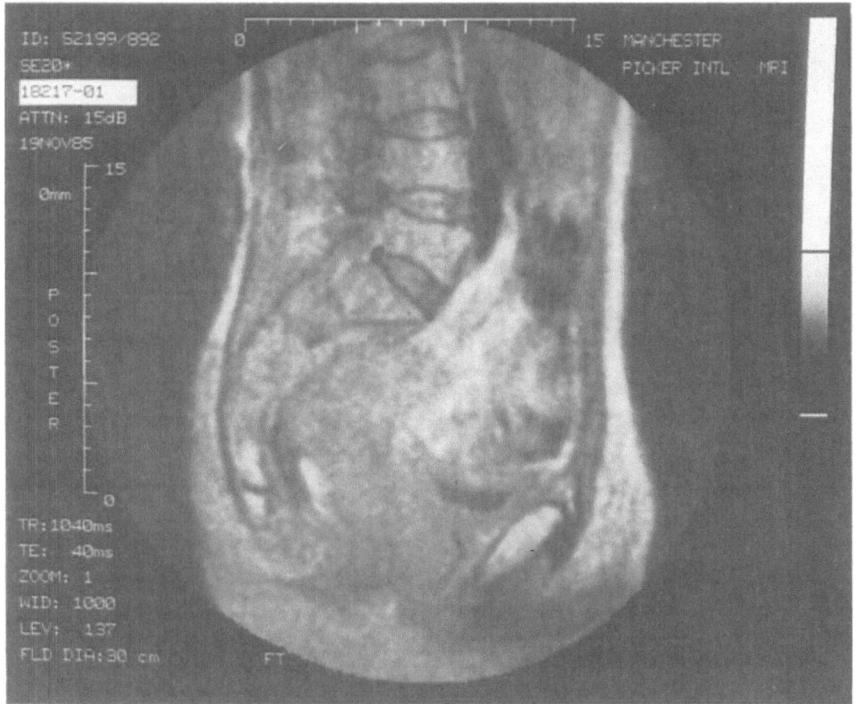

c

Fig. 7.5.a–c. Sagittal SE 1040/40 images. **a** Illustrates bulk tumour recurrence following anterior resection. **b** Illustrates reduction in size of the mass 5 months after radiotherapy. **c** Illustrates further recurrence involving the sacrum 19 months after initial treatment.

Carcinoma of the Prostate

Staging and Tissue Characterisation

As described above, the pelvic anatomy is well suited for study by MRI, its multiplanar facility (Fig. 7.6) and superior contrast resolution providing advantages over other imaging techniques. The prostate is best imaged using coronal and sagittal planes. The prostate gland and seminal vesicles can readily be separated, although they have similar signal intensities, and the rectovesical fascia can be identified posteriorly. The normal-sized urethra is not usually seen.

Further clinical studies using the tissue characterisation methods described above have been directed towards the differentiation of carcinoma of the prostate contained within the gland and benign prostatic hypertrophy (BPH). Both these conditions lead to increased T_1 and T_2 *relaxation times* and have heterogeneous signal intensities on MR images, especially when using T_2-weighted sequences. Earlier results (Bryan et al. 1983) suggested that carcinoma of the prostate and BPH could be differentiated on signal intensity alone, but this has not been substantiated (LiPuma and Bryan 1985; Poon et al. 1985).

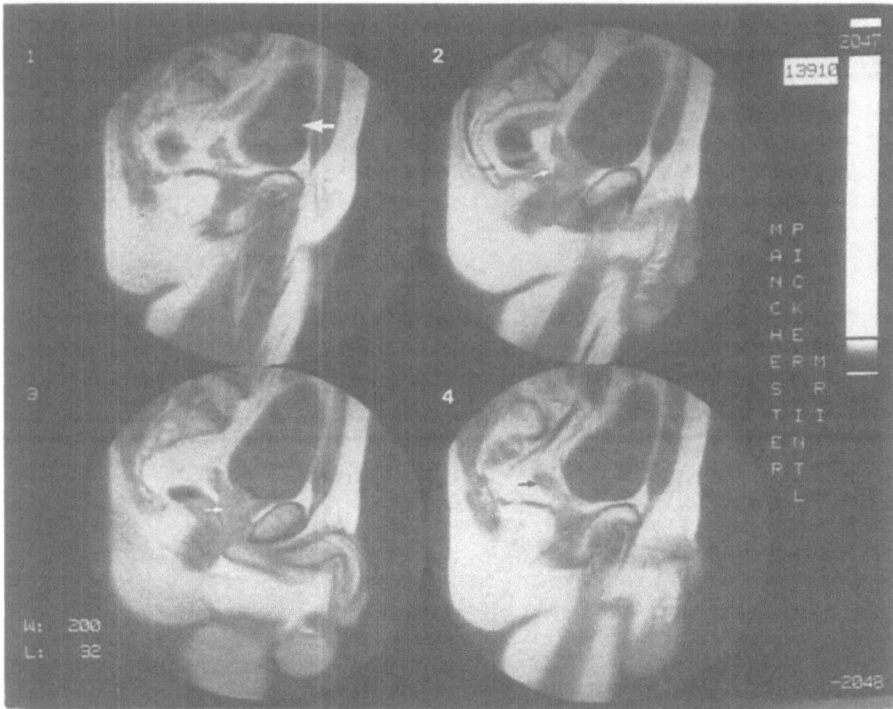

Fig. 7.6. Four multi-section sagittal SE 1840/40 images from 1 (left) to 4 (right) illustrating normal pelvic anatomy. The relevant structures are arrowed in each case. 1, bladder; 2, Denovillier's fascia; 3, prostate; 4, right seminal vesicle.

Direct spread of carcinoma of the prostate into adjacent tissues is well shown on T_1-weighted multi-section sequences because the contrast between surrounding fat and tumour tissue is increased (Fig. 7.7). Because of its superior soft tissue contrast MRI is more accurate than CT in delineating extracapsular extension of carcinoma into the seminal vesicles, bladder base and pelvic sidewalls. Bone metastases can also be demonstrated, but lymph node involvement within the normal-sized node is not detectable by MRI. Theoretically volume measurement of the prostate gland should be more accurate than with CT, indicating an important role for MRI in defining radiation treatment fields and assessing volume changes with therapy (Choyke et al. 1985; Zhu et al. 1986).

Table 7.3. Tissue characterisation in prostatic disease

	No. of patients	Mean *relaxation times* ± SE	
		T_1 (ms)	T_2 (ms)
Carcinoma of the prostate	7	843 ± 72	*63 ± 3
BPH			
Glandular stroma	10	843 ± 24	*77 ± 4
Fibrotic stroma	2	843	54

* Significant difference ($P < 0.02$).

As mentioned above no differentiation between carcinoma of the prostate and BPH can be made on signal intensity alone, but it has been noted that by measuring *relaxation times* some discrimination between the two groups can be made (Jenkins et al. 1985b). From a group of 36 patients, 19 with clinical evidence of prostatic enlargement and who subsequently underwent surgery with histological confirmation of disease were investigated by MRI with measurement of the T_1 and T_2 *relaxation times*. There were seven patients with carcinoma of the prostate and twelve with BPH. The patients in the BPH group were divided using single random sampling biopsies into those with predominantly glandular stroma and those with a predominantly fibrotic stroma. The mean T_1 and T_2 values are shown in Table 7.3. It can be seen that whilst there is no significant difference in the T_1 values between carcinoma of the prostate and the BPH groups, there is a highly significant difference between the T_2 values of carcinoma of the prostate and the BPH group with a predominantly glandular stroma. The results from this preliminary study suggest a useful role for MRI in characterising prostatic disease.

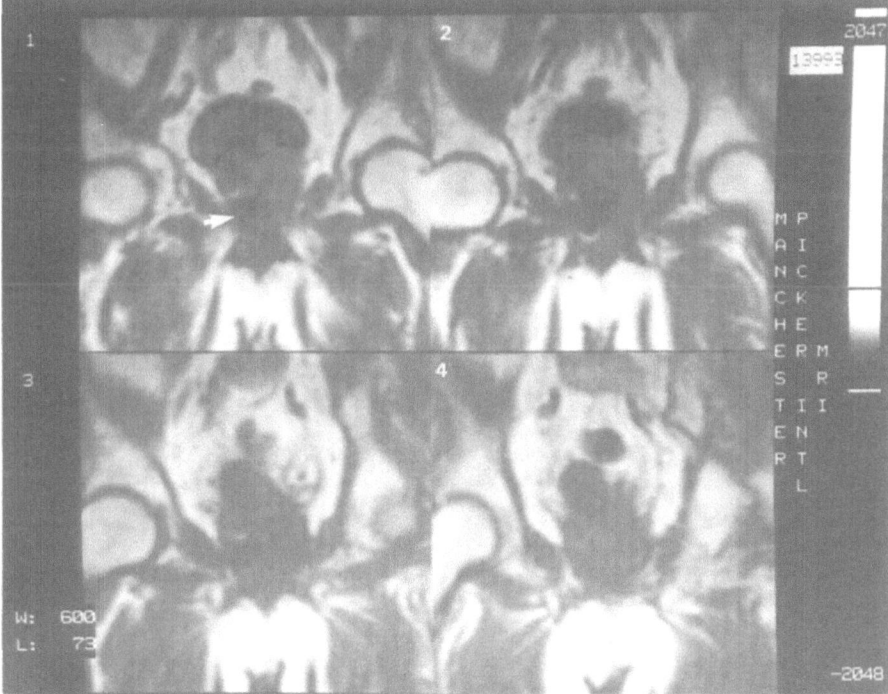

Fig. 7.7. Unconfined carcinoma of the prostrate shown on coronal multi-section *inversion recovery* (IR) 2080/500 images 1 (anterior) to 4 (posterior). A large tumour mass is infiltrating the bladder and extending laterally onto the left pelvic sidewall. The area of low signal to the right of the mid-line (*arrowed*) is a cavity containing urine remaining after a previous transvesical prostatectomy performed 13 years previously for BPH.

Carcinoma of the Bladder

The ability to identify the depth of tumour penetration into and through the bladder wall has important implications in the treatment of bladder carcinoma. The TNM system of staging bladder carcinoma is illustrated in Fig. 7.8.

In our practice T1 and T2 lesions are initially treated by endoscopic resection. Adverse factors such as poor histology, multiplicity of lesions, early recurrence and abnormal random biopsies of the bladder may necessitate the use of intravesical chemotherapy (T1 lesions only), cysto-urethrectomy or radical radiotherapy. T3a and T3b lesions are treated with radical radiotherapy, if the patient is fit, with follow-up cystoscopy. If the tumour recurs locally then a salvage cystectomy is performed if there is no evidence of major extravesical spread or metastases. T4 lesions are treated with palliative radiotherapy.

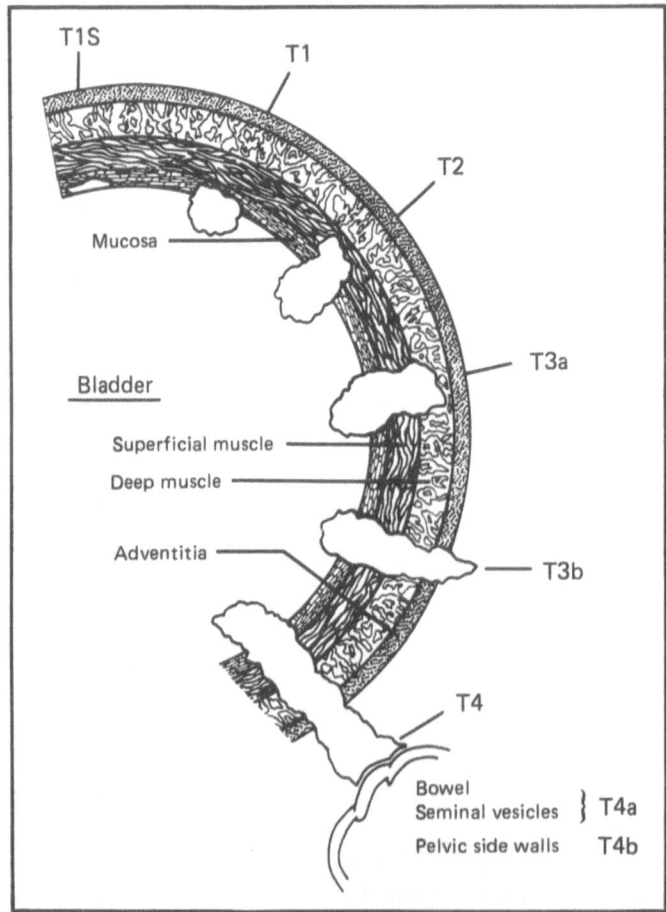

Fig. 7.8.   TNM system for staging carcinoma of the bladder. (Reproduced from Fisher et al. 1985.)

Identification of depth of tumour penetration into the bladder wall and extension beyond the wall into adjacent tissues or organs will enable appropriate treatment planning. Ideally it would be useful to the surgeon to be able to differentiate between T2 and T3a lesions. In some respects, however, the distinction between T2 and early T3a lesions is artificial as at surgery it is not possible to identify the boundary between the superficial and deep muscle layers. The important question is whether there is sufficient muscle preserved deep to the tumour to be able to hold the wall together following resection. A 3 mm thickness of muscle is thought to be adequate (R. J. Barnard pers. comm.).

The accuracy of CT in staging bladder carcinoma, as reported in the literature, ranges from 68% to 85% (Hodson et al. 1979; Frodin et al. 1980; Koss et al. 1981; Jeffrey et al. 1981). Its greatest value is in delineating accurately the extravesical extension of tumour, which helps to identify those patients who are clearly inoperable and those who may be suitable for radical cystectomy, as well as improving radiotherapy planning.

There are recognised limitations, however, in assessing the pelvic lymph nodes by CT, and the superficial lesions (T1 and T2) cannot be distinguished from each other. Early tumours, if proliferative, project into the lumen and can be associated with a normal bladder wall. Local wall thickening is sometimes due to deep muscle invasion, enabling a distinction between T2 and T3 lesions to be made. Such an interpretation, however, is unreliable. The thickening of the bladder wall may be due to muscle hypertrophy or the presence of oedema, or be the result of a T2 lesion alone. Intraluminal projections may be due to blood clot or trabeculation which cannot be distinguished from tumour by CT. Small intravesical lesions at the dome or base of the bladder can be missed entirely if images are obtained only in the transverse axial plane. More significant problems may arise if there has been transurethral resection prior to scanning. In these circumstances there may be no detectable intravesical growth, and wall thickening due to oedema can be misinterpreted as tumour invasion.

Minimal extravesical extension is recognised by loss or blurring of the perivesical fat margin. This sign is acknowledged as a potential source of error (Koss et al. 1981). The absence of fat planes between the bladder and rectum, vagina or prostate makes detection of invasion of these organs difficult. Involvement of the seminal vesicles can be recognised by the disappearance of the seminal vesicle angle (Seidelmann et al. 1978).

Initial experiences of the use of MRI in the pelvis, particularly in relation to the normal and abnormal bladder, have been reported (Hricak et al. 1983a, b; Bryan et al. 1983; Fisher et al. 1985). Fisher et al. (1985) have reported their initial results in using MR to detect and stage bladder carcinoma and in Manchester we are undertaking a study to assess its ability to detect the depth of tumour penetration into and through the bladder wall and to correlate this, where possible, with pathological staging. MRI has advantages over CT in imaging the pelvis as detailed above. Potentially it can overcome some of the problems related to the use of CT in assessing the local extent of bladder tumours. Distension of the bladder is not required and tumour is readily distinguished from blood clot and hypertrophied muscle. Multiplanar imaging enables the identification of small lesions involving the dome and base of the bladder and involvement of the prostate, vagina and rectum detected as alterations in the normal signal intensity of these structures. Assessment of lymph node status by MRI remains limited due to an inability to detect metastases in normal-sized nodes or distinguish reliably between reactive hyperplasia and metastases in nodes between 1 and 2.5 cm in diameter. Nodes larger than this are usually metastatic.

The initial observations by Fisher et al. (1985) have not enabled them to distinguish between T1 and T2 lesions, but they state that T2 lesions should be distinguished from T3a lesions that involve the entire bladder wall. They could not identify early involvement of the deep musculature. Stages T2 and T3a were readily distinguished from stage T3b and T4 lesions involving adjacent structures. Overall accuracy of staging in this reported series was 85%, although the study involved only 14 patients. To a large extent this reflects our experiences in Manchester, although tumours can be over-staged (see below).

It is important to emphasise that assessment of tumour extent depends on the use of optimal imaging planes and appropriate radio-frequency pulse sequences. Images obtained in the transverse plane usually provide adequate information on the site and extent of a tumour confined to the anterior, posterior or lateral walls. Images in the sagittal or coronal plane are necessary when tumours involve the dome or base of the bladder (Fig. 7.9). Sagittal images are required to assess involvement of the prostate, vagina or rectum and pubic symphysis. Involvement of the seminal vesicles can usually be identified on transverse axial images.

T_1-weighted images (e.g. *Spin Echo sequences* with TR = 500 ms, TE = 26 ms) delineate the intravesical component of the tumour and the perivesical extension. The signal intensity of the tumour distinguishes it readily from the

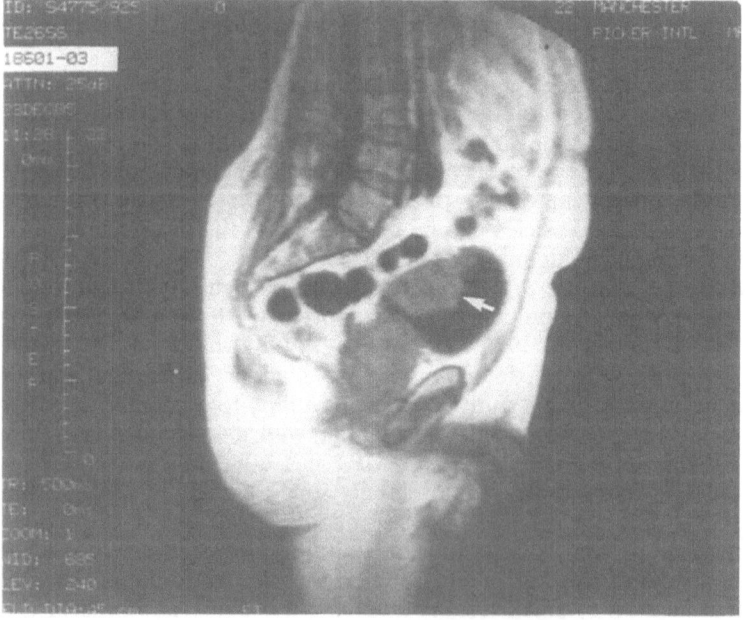

Fig. 7.9. Sagittal SE 500/26 image (T_1-weighted) illustrating a large tumour (*arrow*) involving the posterior wall and dome of the bladder. The prostate is enlarged. Note the contrast between the tumour, urine and pelvic fat.

lower signal intensity of urine and the high signal intensity of the perivesical fat (Fig. 7.9). With longer TR/TE sequences fat, urine and tumour may exhibit similar signal intensities.

Infiltration into the bladder wall is best assessed using T_2-weighted *Spin Echo sequences*. Sequences are required to optimise the contrast between the tumour, involved bladder wall and perivesical fat. A variety of sequences with varying TR and TE values may then be required. Fig. 7.10 demonstrates the appearances with varying TE values but a similar TR value. In Fig. 7.11 the TR value has been increased. These images appear at first to show tumour extending through the wall into the perivesical fat. Histology of the resected specimen, however, revealed the tumour had infiltrated deeply but not breached the wall. A fibrotic reaction adjacent to the tumour in the perivesical fat had given rise to misinterpretation of the images. Review of the images confirmed the deep penetration of the tumour and a variation in signal intensity between tumour and fibrosis. This case serves to illustrate the importance of choosing appropriate pulse sequences and the need for correlation of MR images with histology to assess accurately the role of MRI in staging carcinoma of the bladder. Other pitfalls in interpretation of the images are the presence of infection or oedema which may give rise to increases in *relaxation times* similar to those of tumour.

One may conclude that MR imaging offers potential advantages over CT in staging bladder carcinoma. Initial reports in the literature of its use in assessing the depth of tumour penetration into the bladder wall are encouraging and work in progress continues to confirm the early results and identify the role of MRI in clinical practice.

Carcinoma of the Pancreas

The pancreas represents a challenge to any imaging modality, even with the introduction of new techniques such as CT and more recently MRI (Stark et al. 1984; Haaga 1984; Clarke et al. 1985). With MRI there are a number of limitations that need to be understood when imaging the pancreas. The gland lies in the oblique plane within the retroperitoneum, making it difficult for the whole pancreas to be included in one image irrespective of the plane used. Oblique MR scanning is not yet generally available. The spatial resolution of the MR images is less than with the latest-generation CT, although MRI has a higher contrast resolution. The collection of the MR data for image production typically takes 4–8 minutes, whereas CT data is collected during suspended respiration. As a consequence there may be significant motion artefacts within the MR image, from respiratory and cardiac motion and bowel peristalsis.

The normal pancreas can be visualised as a relatively homogeneous structure on both T_1- and T_2-weighted sequences. On T_2-weighted sequences the pancreas has a similar signal intensity to the liver, but on T_1-weighted images it is slightly lower. The major vessels in close proximity to the pancreas are routinely visualised. The retroperitoneal fat is shown as high signal on both T_1- and T_2-weighted sequences and is important in separating the ventral margin of the pancreas from adjacent bowel (Fig. 7.12). Difficulty is encountered when

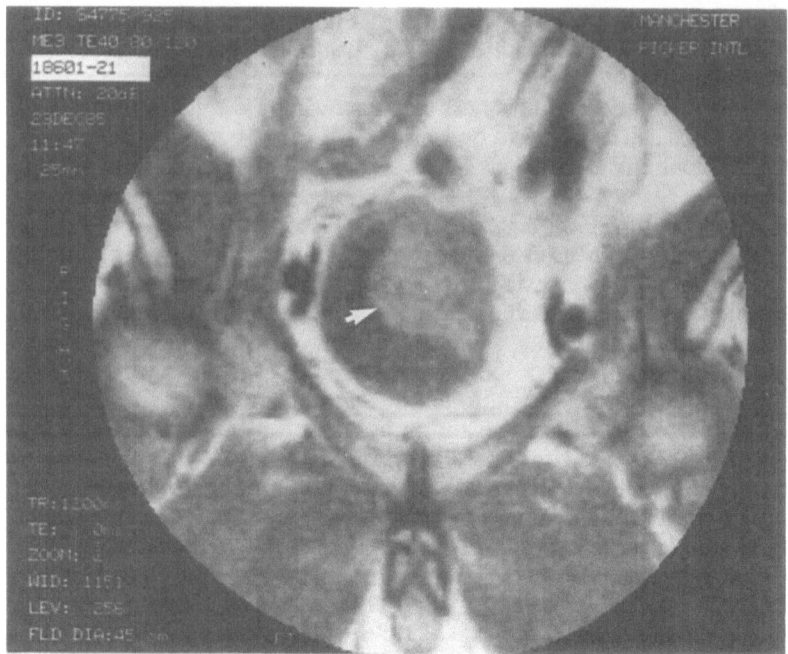

a

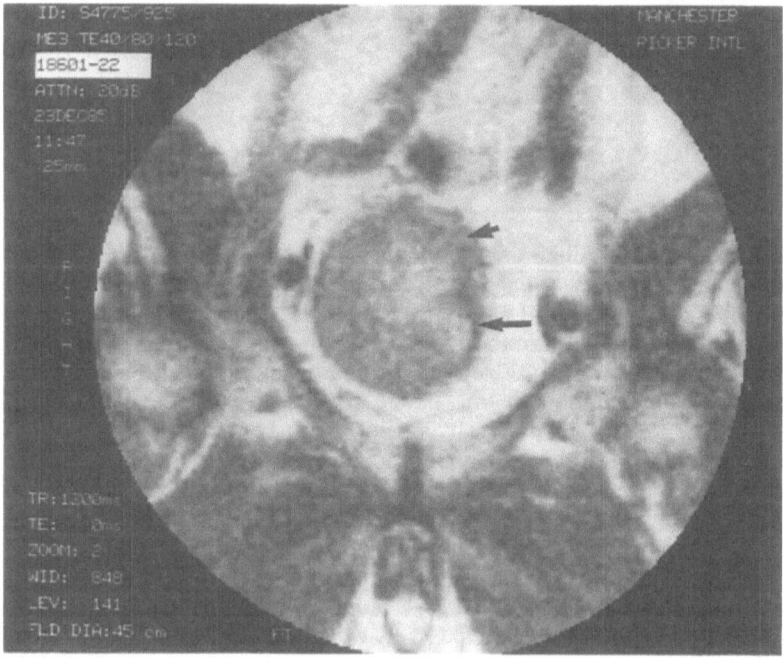

b

Fig. 7.10.a–c. T$_2$-weighted coronal SE images with a fixed TR = 1200 ms and TE = 40 (**a**), 80 (**b**) and 120 (**c**) ms. These images illustrate the alterations in signal intensity of the tumour, bladder wall, urine and perivesical fibrotic mass that occur with a varying TE. The intraluminal component of the tumour (*white arrow*) is best seen in **a**. The thickened and penetrated bladder wall (*long arrow*) and the fibrotic mass (*short arrow*) are best seen in **b** and **c**.

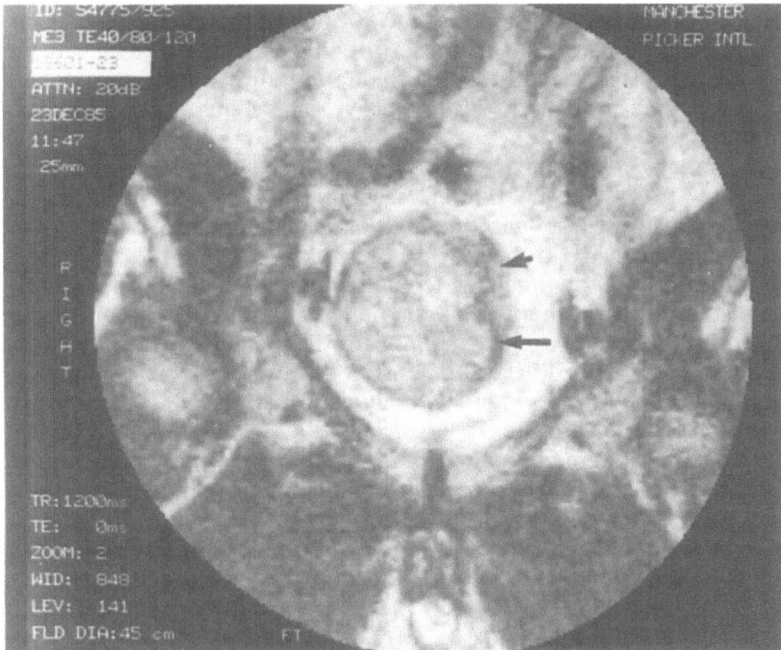

Fig. 7.10c

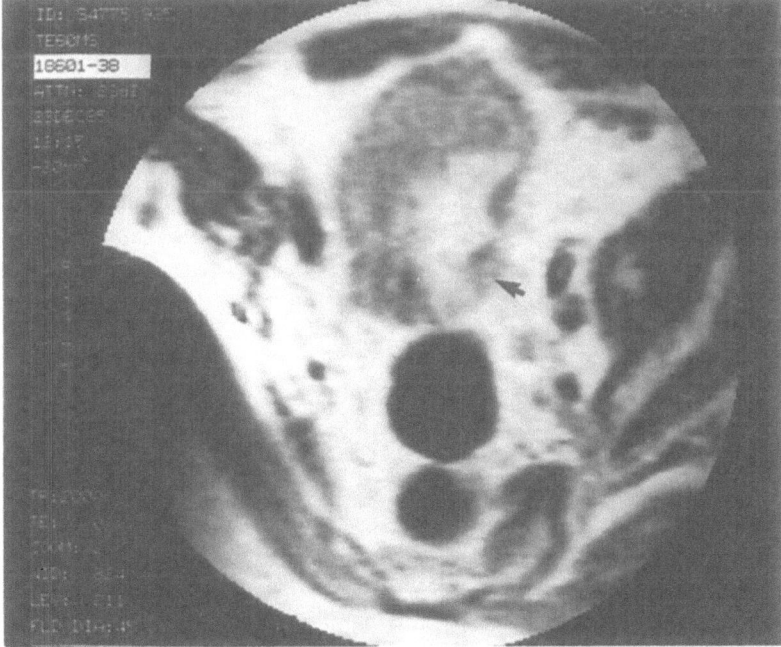

Fig. 7.11. Transverse axial SE 2000/60 image. The long TR time has improved contrast between the tumour, urine and bladder wall. The perivesical fibrotic mass (*arrow*) has a different signal intensity from that of the tumour.

retroperitoneal fat is sparse and when there is atrophy of the gland. Significant improvement in image quality and definition of the pancreas is achieved by reducing bowel peristalsis and by distending the upper bowel with gas or water. Respiratory and cardiac gating can also improve image quality but tend to increase scanning time.

Small lesions and calcification are poorly visualised when compared with images obtained by CT, but delineation of vascular structures without the need for intravenous contrast, together with the multiplanar, multi-section facility are significant advantages for MRI over CT.

The major difficulty for all imaging techniques is to distinguish between benign and malignant disease, that is between pancreatitis and carcinoma of the pancreas. The morphological criteria for demonstrating pancreatic tumours with MRI are similar to those for CT. Local extension of tumour, associated biliary obstruction and liver metastases can be demonstrated as can the patency, encasement and involvement of major vessels (Fig. 7.13). Tissue characterisation studies with measurement of *relaxation times* has not contributed significantly to the differentiation of tumour from inflammatory tissue. In a study reported in full elsewhere (Jenkins et al. 1987), 37 patients with clinical evidence of pancreatic disease were investigated by MRI and in 19 the *relaxation times* were calculated for the group of patients with chronic pancreatitis and those with

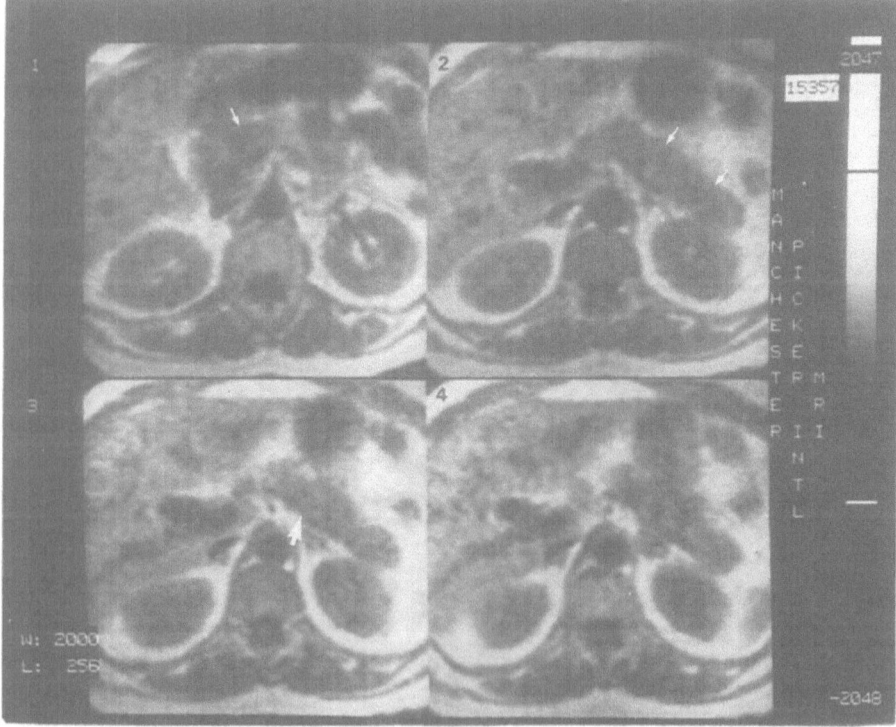

Fig. 7.12. Four transverse contiguous SE 260/24 images from 1 (inferior) to 4 (superior) through a normal pancreas (*small arrows*). The *large arrow* points to the splenic vein.

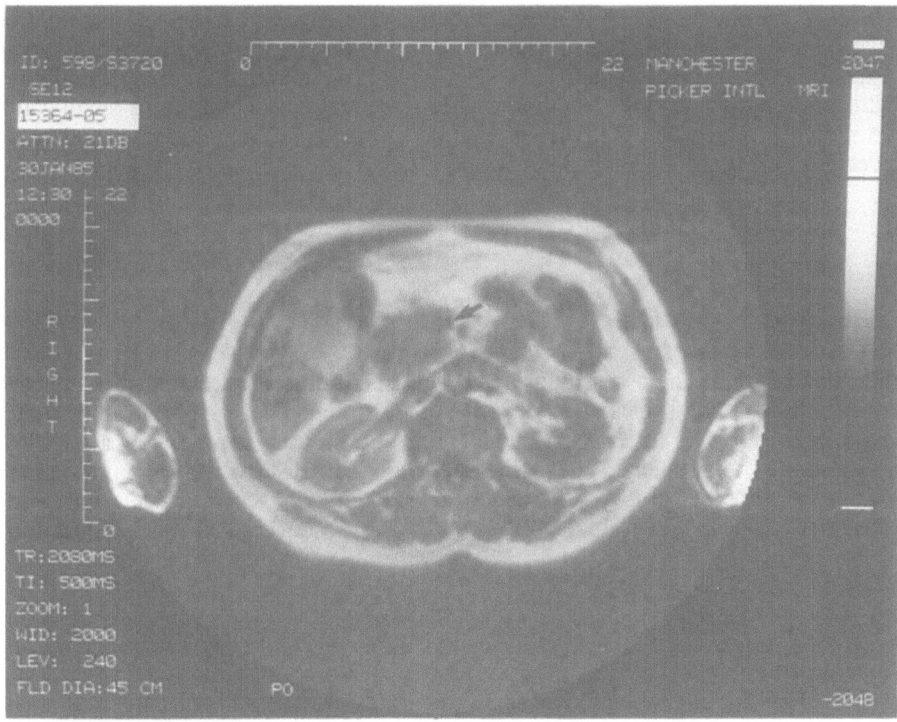

Fig. 7.13. Transverse IR 2080/500 image illustrating an enlarged uncinate process of the pancreas encasing the superior mesenteric vein (*arrow*).

carcinoma of the pancreas. In addition the T_1 and T_2 *relaxation times* for 8 normal controls were measured. The mean T_1 and T_2 values are shown in Table 7.4. These show no significant difference between the T_1 and T_2 values of the control group and patients with carcinoma of the pancreas or between patients with carcinoma of the pancreas and those with chronic pancreatitis. There is a highly significant difference in the measured T_1 values between those patients with chronic pancreatitis who exhibit calcification on CT and the control group. In addition a highly significant difference in the measured T_1 values was observed between those patients with chronic pancreatitis who show no calcification on CT and those who do.

Table 7.4. Tissue characterisation in pancreatic disease

	No. of patients	Mean *relaxation times* ± SE	
		T_1 (ms)	T_2 (ms)
Controls	8	*545 ± 38	58 ± 2
Pancreatic tumour	5	676 ± 77	65 ± 7
Chronic pancreatitis			
No calcification	6	†522 ± 59	55 ± 5
Calcification	8	*†812 ± 36	65 ± 1

*† Highly significant differences ($P<0.01$).

It may be concluded that measurements of *relaxation times* in pancreatic disease have not contributed to the differentiation of tumour from inflammatory tissue. Whilst calcification cannot be seen on an MR image, our study of patients with pancreatitis has revealed that in the presence of calcification a significant variation in pancreatic T_1 values can be observed. The reason for this is uncertain and requires further study.

Musculoskeletal Tumours

The role of MRI in the assessment and diagnosis of musculoskeletal tumours has yet to be fully defined. Even at this early stage, though, there are clear important advantages of MRI over current imaging methods (Zimmer et al. 1985; Pettersson et al. 1985a). These include high contrast resolution and tissue discrimination; the ability to image directly in the coronal, sagittal and transverse planes; the multisection facility; the absence of motion, bone and

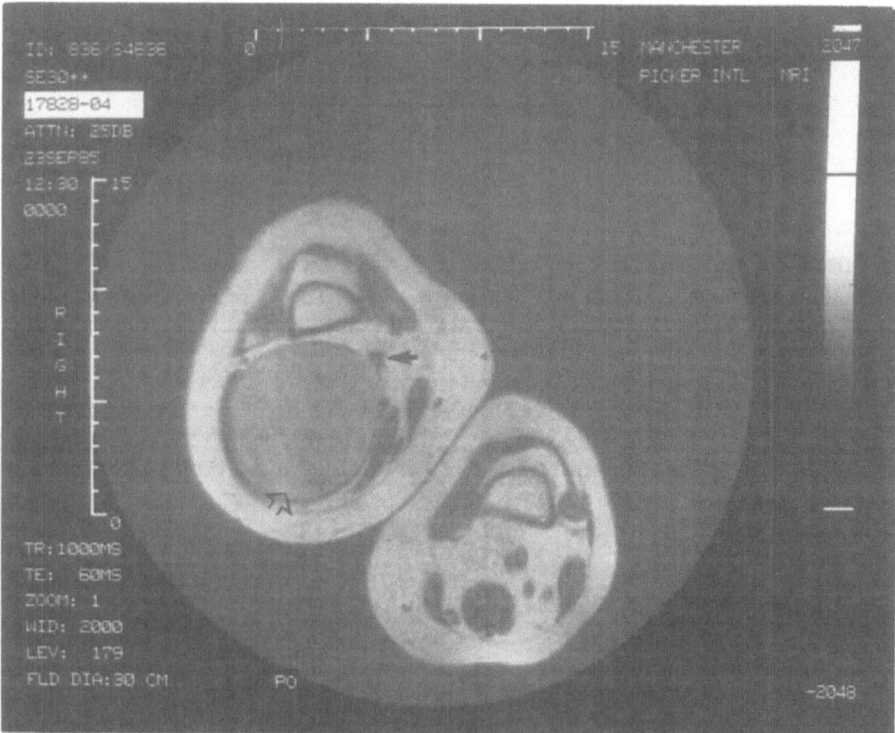

Fig. 7.14. Transverse axial SE 1000/60 image illustrating a large neurofibroma in the posterior compartment of the right lower thigh (*open arrow*). The mass is well encapsulated, and displaces and compresses the biceps femoris muscle laterally and the semimembranosus muscle medially. The popliteal neurovascular bundle is displaced but separate from the mass (*filled arrow*).

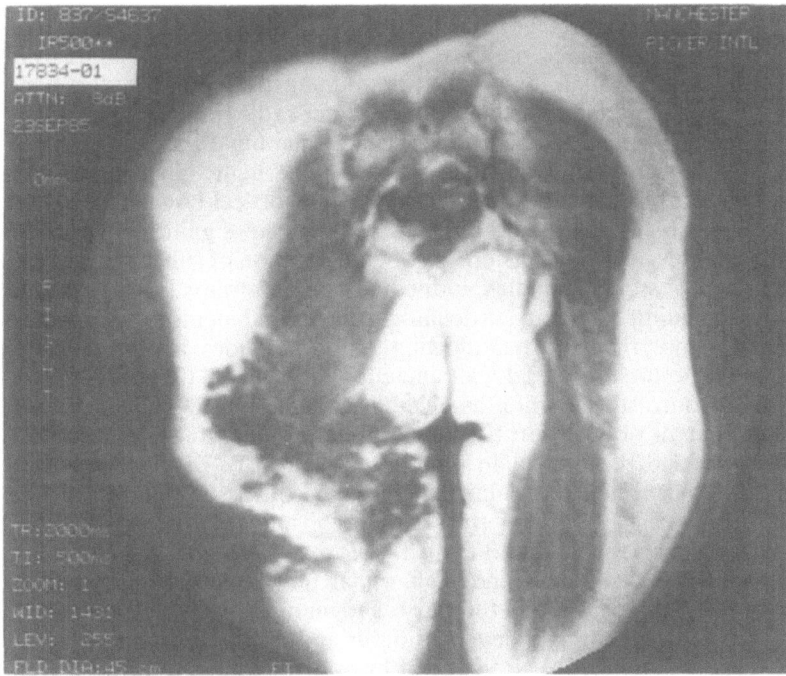

a

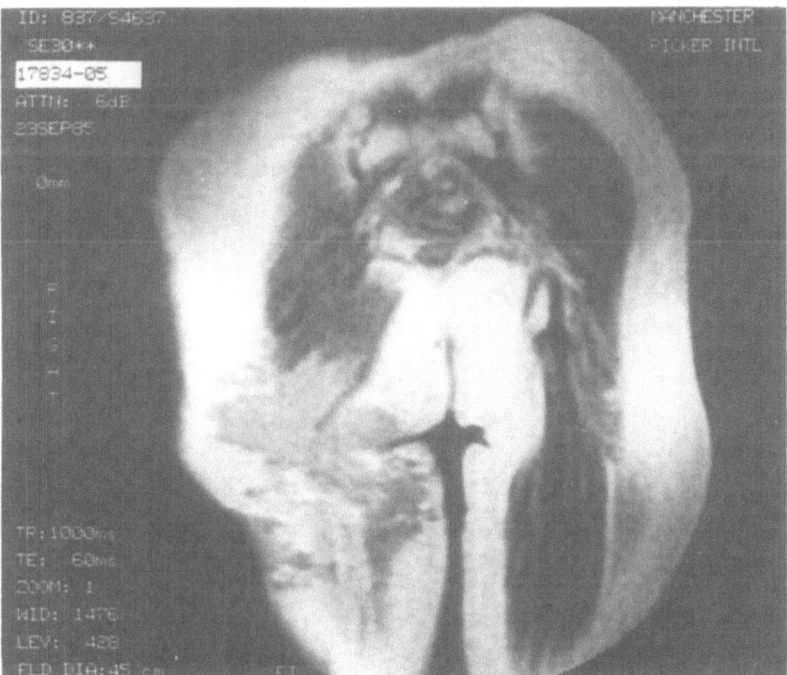

b

Fig. 7.15.a,b. A soft tissue sarcoma seen on comparative IR 2000/50 (**a**) and SE 1000/60 (**b**) coronal images through the posterior pelvis and upper thigh. There is an induration and infiltration into the subcutaneous fat (best shown in **a**: T_1-weighted image); the infiltration into the gluteus maximus muscle is more clearly illustrated in **b** (T_2-weighted image).

some metal artefacts on the image; and the use of non-ionising radiation. The main disadvantage of MRI referable to the musculoskeletal system—apart from its high cost and limited availability—is the poor demonstration of compact bone and calcium detail compared with that seen on plain radiographs and by CT.

On both T_1- and T_2-weighted sequences, cancellous bone has a high signal intensity due to the fat within the bone marrow. The high signal intensity is surrounded by a sharply defined low-intensity rim of cortical bone. A signal of intermediate intensity is obtained from muscle, with no significant variation between different muscle groups. There is good delineation of subcutaneous fat, fascial planes, neurovascular bundles, individual muscle groups (Fig. 7.14) and joint anatomy, including ligaments, articular cartilages and menisci. An absence of intraluminal signal from normal flowing blood provides a high intrinsic contrast between the lumen, vessel wall and surrounding soft tissues.

The improved contrast resolution associated with the multiplanar facility of MRI allows the extent of both soft tissue and bone tumours to be more clearly and accurately defined than on plain radiographs and CT. Displacement and involvement of adjacent neurovascular structures by soft tissue tumours can be accurately assessed (Fig. 7.14) together with involvement of adjacent bone. Most tumours have a relatively long T_1 and T_2 *relaxation time* and appear as low signal on T_1-weighted sequences and high signal on T_2-weighted sequences. Maximum contrast between fat and tumour is shown on T_1-weighted sequences (Fig. 7.15a) but the best contrast between tumour and muscle is obtained on T_2-weighted sequences (Fig. 7.15b). Regions of haemorrhage within tumour (Fig.

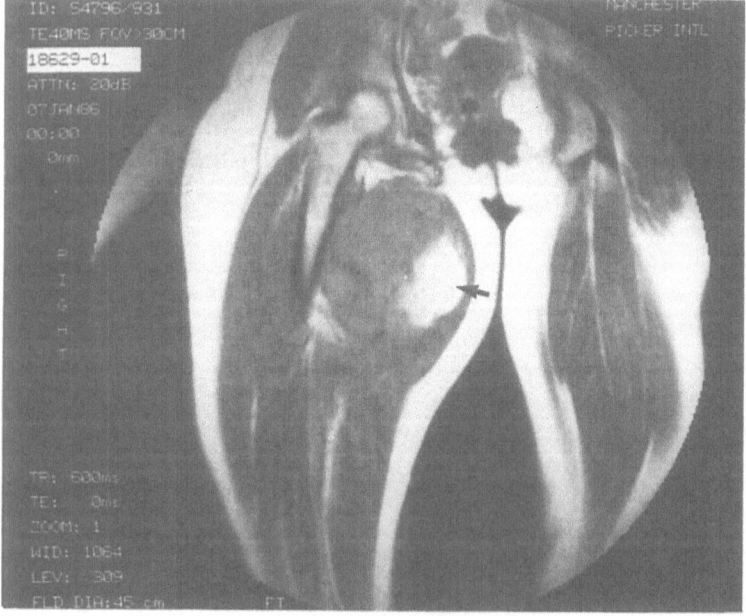

Fig. 7.16. A soft tissue sarcoma involving the adductor muscles of the upper thigh shown in coronal section on a T_1-weighted (SE 600/40) image. There is an area of high signal within the tumour mass medially (*arrow*) that is consistent with haemorrhage.

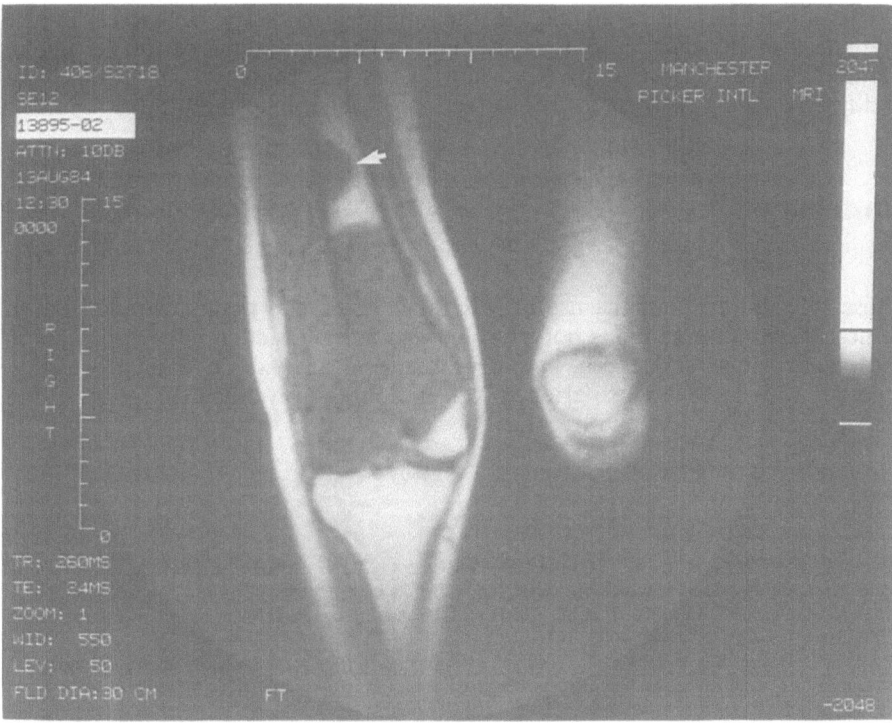

Fig. 7.17. An osteosarcoma of the distal right femur shown in a coronal T_1-weighted (SE 260/24) image. The tumour has extended to the knee joint and laterally into the soft tissues. The delineation between tumour and muscle is better seen on a T_2-weighted image (see Fig. 7.15b). A "skip lesion" is also seen (*arrow*).

7.16) or fatty infiltration produce characteristic changes in signal intensity. In addition areas of necrosis and cystic change are characteristic within tumours.

In primary bone tumours MRI is superior to CT, not only in demonstrating the extent of tumour within the cancellous bone (Fig. 7.17) but also in assessing involvement of the growth plate, joint space and adjacent soft tissues. MRI also has advantages compared with CT in the assessment of tumour recurrence in post-operative patients with non-ferromagnetic metallic prostheses and metallic surgical clips *in situ*, which can produce significant degradation of the CT image. CT is, however, superior to MRI in demonstrating pathological fractures and in the assessment of pulmonary metastases.

Work is in progress to obtain characterisation of musculoskeletal tumours by MRI, and early results are encouraging (Pettersson et al. 1985b). To date it has been shown that measured *relaxation times* of different groups of musculoskeletal tumours differ significantly but with some overlap, making the use of these parameters difficult for tumour differentiation in individual cases. An exception has been in lipomas, since fat gives specific T_1 and T_2 values. Significant changes have also been observed in the measured *relaxation times* following chemotherapy and radiotherapy.

Therefore MRI, if available, is the imaging modality of choice in the evaluation of bone and soft tissue tumours. The limitations of the technique should however be borne in mind and in osseous tumours CT remains the preferred imaging method for the detection of pulmonary metastases.

Conclusion

These selected areas of the use of MR for imaging and tissue characterisation demonstrate its tremendous potential in oncological practice. Developments in equipment, pulse sequences, contrast-enhancing agents and data processing, together with increased experience, will undoubtedly validate its place in the management of patients with cancer.

References

Beynon J, Foy DMA, Roe AM, Temple LN, Mortensen NJMcC (1986) Endoluminal ultrasound in the assessment of local invasion in rectal cancer. B J Surg (in press)

Bryan PJ, Butler HE, Lipuma JP et al. (1983) NMR scanning of the pelvis: initial experience with a 0.3 Tesla system. AJR 141: 1111–1118

Bryant DJ, Payne JA, Bailes DR, Young I (1984) Effect of slice distortion in MR imaging on accuracy of measurement. In: Proceedings of the Third Annual Meeting of the Society of Magnetic Resonance in Medicine, New York. Society of Magnetic Resonance in Medicine, Berkeley, CA, pp 109–110

Butch RJ, Stark DD, Wittenberg J, Brady TJ, Ferrucci JT (1985) Magnetic resonance and computed tomography in evaluation of rectal cancer. In: Proceedings of the Fourth Annual Meeting of the Society of Magnetic Resonance in Medicine, London. Society of Magnetic Resonance in Medicine, Berkeley, CA, pp 216–217

Choyke PL, Thickman D, Kressel HY et al. (1985) Controversies in the radiological diagnosis of pelvic malignancies. In: Symposium on new imaging technology: pitfalls and controversies. Radiol Clin North Am 23: 531–549

Clarke LR, Jaffe MH, Choyke PL, Grant EG, Zeman RK (1985) Pancreatic imaging. In: Symposium on new imaging technology: pitfalls and controversies. Radiol Clin North Am 23: 489–501

Dixon AK, Kelsey Fry I, Morson BC, Nicholls RJ, York Mason A (1981) Preoperative computed tomography of carcinoma of the rectum. B J Radiol 54: 655–659

Fisher MR, Hricak H, Tanagho EA (1985) Urinary bladder MR imaging. Radiology 157: 471–477

Frodin L, Hemmingsson A, Johansson A, Wickland H (1980) Computed tomography in the staging of bladder carcinoma. Acta Radiol [Diagn] (Stockh) 21: 763–767

Haaga JR (1984) Magnetic resonance imaging of the pancreas. Radiol Clin North Am 22: 869–877

Hickey DS, Checkley DR, Aspden RM, Naughton A, Jenkins JPR, Isherwood I (1986) A method for the clinical measurement of relaxation times in magnetic resonance imaging. B J Radiol 59: 565–576)

Hodson NJ, Husband JE, McDonald JS (1979) The role of computed tomography in the staging of bladder cancer. Clin Radiol 30: 389–395

Hricak H, Williams RD, Spring DB et al. (1983a) Anatomy and pathology of the male pelvis by magnetic resonance imaging. AJR 141: 1101–1110

Hricak H, Alpers C, Crooks LE, Sheldon PE (1983b) Magnetic resonance imaging of the female pelvis: initial experience. AJR 141: 1119–1128

Husband JE, Hodson NJ, Parsons GA (1980) The use of computed tomography in recurrent rectal tumours. Radiology 134: 677–682

Isherwood I, Hickey DS, Jenkins JPR (1986) Magnetic resonance imaging: an approach to tissue characterisation using measured relaxation times. In: J Valk (ed) Neuroradiology 1985/1986. Elsevier, Amsterdam, pp 27–35 (Excerpta Medica International Congress Series 698)

Jeffrey RB, Palubinskas AJ, Federle MP (1981) CT evaluation of invasive lesions of the bladder. J Comput Assist Tomogr 5: 22–26

Jenkins JPR, Hickey DS, Zhu XP, Machin M, Isherwood I (1985a) MR imaging of the intervertebral disc: a quantitative study. B J Radiol 58: 705–709

Jenkins JPR, Isherwood I, Hickey DS, Machin M, Grant J, Blacklock NJ (1985b) Quantitative magnetic resonance imaging in prostatic disease. In: Proceedings of the Fourth Annual Scientific Meeting of the Society of Magnetic Resonance in Medicine, London. Society of Magnetic Resonance in Medicine, Berkeley, CA, pp 227–228

Jenkins JPR, Braganza JM, Isherwood I, Hickey DS, Machin M (1987) Quantitative magnetic resonance imaging in pancreatic disease. B J Radiol 60 (in press)

Johnson RJ, Jenkins JPR, Isherwood I, James RD, Schofield PF (1987) Quantitative magnetic resonance imaging in rectal carcinoma. B J Radiol (in press)

Koss JC, Arger PH, Coleman BG, Mulhern CB, Pollack HM, Wein AJ (1981) CT staging of bladder carcinoma. AJR 137: 359–362

Lee JKT, Stanley RJ, Sagel SS, Levitt RG, McClennan BL (1981) CT appearance of the pelvis after abdomino-perineal resection for rectal carcinoma. Radiology 141: 737–741

LiPuma JP, Bryan PJ (1985) Magnetic resonance imaging of the genito-urinary tract. In: Kressel HY (ed) Magnetic resonance annual 1985. Raven Press, New York, pp 149–196

Pettersson H, Hamlin DJ, Mancuso A, Scott KN (1985a) Magnetic resonance imaging of the musculo-skeletal system. Acta Radiol [Diagn] (Stockh) 26: 225–234

Pettersson H, Spanier S, Sloane R, Fitzsimmons JR, Scott KN (1985b) MRI relaxation characteristics of musculo-skeletal tumours and surrounding tissue. In: Proceedings of the Fourth Annual Meeting of the Society of Magnetic Resonance in Medicine, London. Society of Magnetic Resonance in Medicine, Berkeley, CA, pp 96–97

Poon PY, Macullum RW, Henkelman MM et al. (1985) Magnetic resonance imaging of the prostate. Radiology 154: 143–149

Saini S, Sullivan J, Ferrucci JT, Stark DD, Wittenberg J (1986) Particulate iron oxide (magnetite) as a potential bowel contrast agent for MRI. Magn Reson Imag 4: 179–180

Seidelmann FE, Cohen WN, Bryan PJ, Temes SP, Krauss D, Schoenrock G (1978) Accuracy of CT staging of bladder neoplasms using the gas filled method: report of 21 patients with surgical confirmation. AJR 130: 735–739

Stark DD, Moss AA, Goldberg HI, Davis PL, Federle MP (1984) Magnetic resonance and CT of the normal and diseased pancreas: a comparative study. Radiology 150: 153–162

van Waes PFGM, Ruben Koehler P, Feldberg M (1983) Management of rectal carcinoma: impact of computed tomography. AJR 140: 1137–1142

Waterton JC, Checkley DR, Jenkins JPR et al. (1984) Use of the total saturation recovery sequence in magnetic resonance imaging: an improved approach to measurement of T_1. In: Proceedings of the Third Annual Meeting of the Society of Magnetic Resonance in Medicine, New York. Society of Magnetic Resonance in Medicine, Berkeley, CA, pp 736–737

Zheng G, Johnson RJ, Eddleston B, James RD, Schofield PF (1984) Computed tomographic scanning in rectal carcinoma. J R Soc Med 77: 915–920

Zhu XP, Checkley DR, Hickey DS, Isherwood I (1986) Accuracy of area measurements made from MR images compared with computed tomography. J Comput Assist Tomogr 10: 96–102

Zimmer WD, Berquist TH, McCloud RA et al. (1985) Bone tumours: magnetic resonance imaging versus computed tomography. Radiology 155: 709–718

8   Ultrasound Techniques in Oncology

Keith Dewbury

Historical Aspects

The history of ultrasound goes back many decades. It is impossible to give a precise date for the discovery of diagnostic ultrasound, since its foundations lie in the basic research into the physics of sound, which took place over a century ago. By the early nineteenth century the existence of inaudible high-frequency sound waves had been well established, and different methods of generating ultrasound had been developed. The basic principles of pulse echo techniques for the measurement of distance and detection of under-water bodies was given impetus by the First World War, and in 1916 Chilowsky and Langevin produced the first working version of a marine sonar system. Within a relatively short time, high-frequency pulse echo techniques were being applied to the detection of flaws in metallic structures.

It is extremely difficult to determine who first decided that ultrasound had potential medical diagnostic use. It is most likely that several different groups working independently in different countries, including Germany, America and England, came to this conclusion. Today, almost all diagnostic ultrasound equipment relies upon reflection of ultrasound and the production of images by a pulse echo technique, rather than by transmission. A number of groups were investigating such techniques, notably Howry and Bliss in Denver, Colorado. They produced a water immersion B-scanner during the late 1940s and published their first clinical images in 1952. Such immersion scanners could not easily be applied to routine clinical examination, and the world's first contact compound

B-scanner was developed by Brown in the late 1950s. Surprisingly good compound images were produced by this machine, which was used on a wide variety of patients by Donald during the early 1960s. The large majority of early commercial B-scanners continued to use a bistable oscilloscope display until the mid 1970s, when the development of the television scan converter tube stimulated the ultrasound equipment manufacturers to introduce grey-scale imaging. The same result is usually achieved today with a digital memory. The other major technical development to occur during the 1970s was the real-time scanner. Undoubtedly the most commonly used ultrasound equipment today is a high-resolution real-time machine, either with a linear array or a sector transducer.

Principles of Ultrasound

Diagnostic procedures using ultrasound are painless, harmless, relatively inexpensive and have no contraindications at the intensities used with commercial equipment. Scanners utilise very short pulses (about one millionth of a second) of sound of high frequency, usually two to five million cycles per second. At this very high frequency, sound can be focused into a fine beam a few millimetres in diameter, and when the beam impinges on the junction between two substances of different density and elasticity (acoustic impedance) a proportion of it is reflected, as in marine echo sounding. Diagnostic scanners employ a transducer which acts as both a transmitter and receiver of the sound. The sound transmitted from the transducer takes the form of a fine beam which is then scanned through the patient to interrogate the structures within a thin slice of the patient.

The scanning action may be performed either manually or automatically. In the traditional, manually operated static scanner the transducer is held in contact with the patient, and moved by hand in a linear fashion or an arc over the area of interest. The returning echoes are compiled into a static image of the structures beneath the transducer's path. These static scanners currently produce the highest resolution but require considerable operator expertise, and cannot be used to observe moving structures. An ever-increasing proportion of modern diagnostic ultrasound makes use of the more recently introduced real-time scanners. These devices vary widely in design but consist of either mechanical or electronic mechanisms that steer the ultrasound beam through the plane of interest. The majority of these scanners perform the scanning so rapidly that a continuously changing or real-time image is displayed. This permits observation of tissue movements and also permits a rapid survey of the anatomy. Although these devices make a greater demand upon the operator's knowledge of anatomy, they have generally resulted in an increase in the speed with which an examination can be performed and their image quality now equals that of static B-scanners.

To ensure good acoustic contact between transducer and skin, the skin is coated with oil or a suitable jelly as coupling medium. The echoes received are displayed as dots on the screen, the position of each dot corresponding to the locus of the interface which gave rise to that echo. In general, there are more echoes from heterogeneous tissues than from homogeneous tissues. As the transducer is moved over the patient an image is built up of all the interfaces contained within the thin slice of the patient over which the transducer has been moved. Ultrasound is an anatomical imaging technique, and a detailed knowledge of anatomy is a prerequisite to the understanding and proper use of ultrasound in diagnosis. Because of the variability of the projections used, particularly with modern real-time scanners, the operator needs to have a truly three-dimensional appreciation of the anatomy being studied, and of the normal variations. In addition, it is necessary for the user to understand at least some of the factors involved in producing the echo pattern which provides the basis of ultrasound imaging. An understanding of these factors aids the interpretation of anatomy and the recognition of artefacts which are frequently seen in ultrasound images (Fig. 8.1).

The structures that produce echoes are not clearly understood. Fundamentally, they are discontinuities, where there is a change in acoustic properties. A simple analogy is the stiffness or rigidity of the tissue, similar to that which may be felt on palpation. This is most marked between tissue and gas or bone interfaces, and so extremely strong echoes (bright) are produced at these interfaces. Fluid-containing structures stand out clearly from surrounding soft tissues, as they generate no echoes and so appear black. Most soft tissue organs return mid-grey level echoes which probably arise from the collagen microskeleton of each organ.

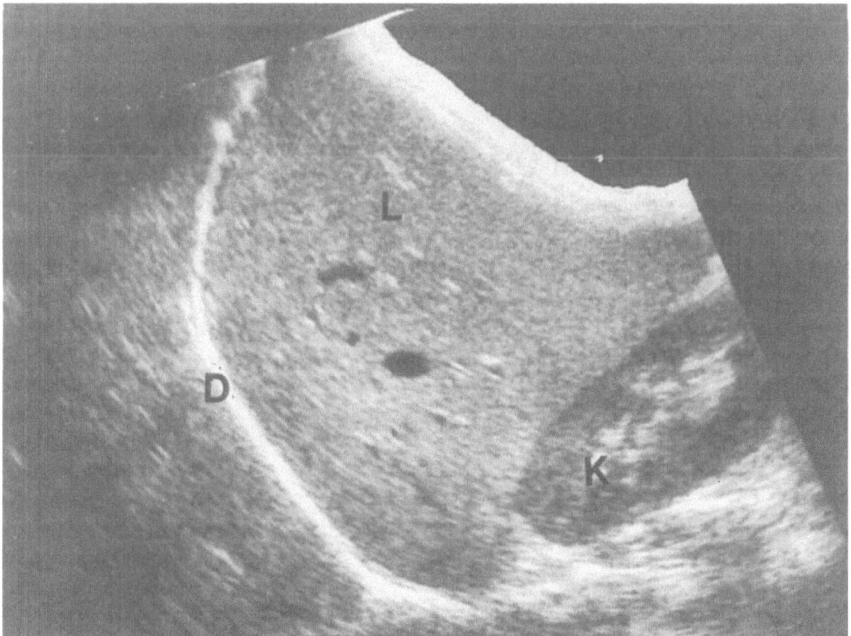

Fig. 8.1. Normal longitudinal scan taken through the right lobe of the liver (L). This shows the bright curve of the diaphragm (D), the normal liver and the normal right kidney (K).

Uses and Limitations of Ultrasound

Ultrasound is a soft tissue imaging technique which produces detailed anatomical tomograms, or slices of information, of the organ at which the examination is directed. The areas of application of ultrasound have increased steadily over recent years and the organs regularly examined with ultrasound today include the following: brain, eyes, thyroid gland, heart, breast, liver, gall bladder, spleen, pancreas, kidneys, abdominal vascular structures, lymph nodes, bladder, prostate, uterus, ovaries, testes, muscles and tendons.

The general advantages of ultrasound as an imaging technique are that it is quick and relatively easy to perform, non-invasive and safe, and relatively inexpensive. The limitations of ultrasound from a physical point of view result from the total reflection of sound at gas/soft tissue interfaces or at bone/soft tissue interfaces. In practice, therefore, ultrasound cannot see through gas or bone, and when the abdominal organs are examined the interposition of ribs or bowel gas between them and the transducer has to be avoided. This is usually possible in the majority of situations by using appropriate acoustic windows, such as, for example, the filled urinary bladder when examining the pelvic structures.

The disadvantages of ultrasound are really only relative disadvantages. The image clarity, reproduction and documentation are such that the inexperienced may have difficulty in interpreting the images. By the same token, a significant degree of operator expertise is required to achieve satisfactory diagnostic results. Ultrasound remains a highly interactive imaging procedure and is best performed to answer rapidly a specific clinical question.

Areas of Application of Ultrasound

The potential and actual uses of ultrasound in oncology are extremely wide and far-ranging. The relative importance of this particular imaging technique in relation to other available techniques will depend on the particular tumour and the clinical problem in question. It is convenient to consider the use of ultrasound under the following five main headings: primary diagnosis, staging, follow-up, complications, and intervention and therapy.

Primary Diagnosis

The primary diagnosis of many different types of tumour remains an important application of ultrasound. Five different organs have been selected, somewhat arbitrarily, to demonstrate here the differing role and value of ultrasound in different areas.

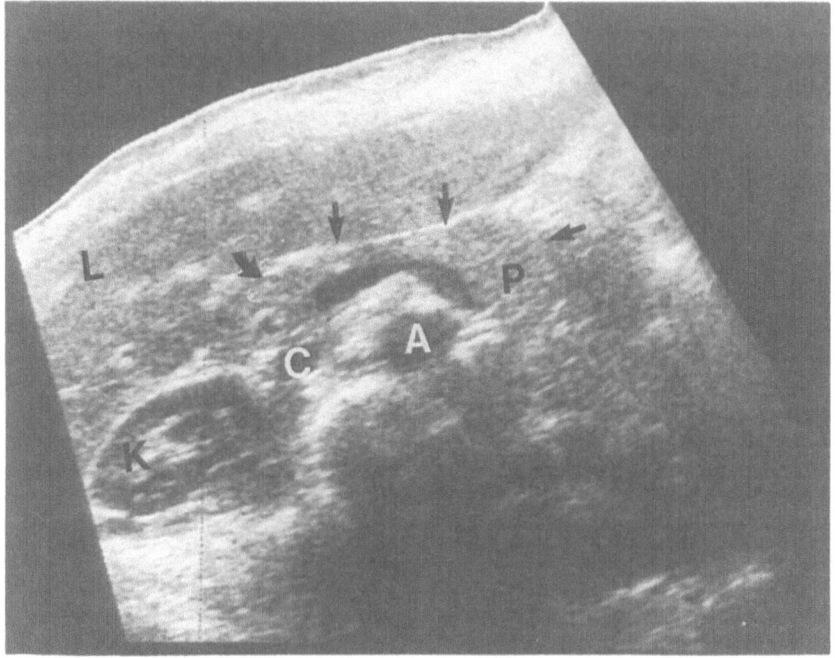

Fig. 8.2. Normal transverse scan taken at the level of the pancreas showing detail of the head and body (*arrows*, P). L, liver; K, kidney; C, vena cava; A, aorta.

Pancreas

At least a portion of the normal pancreas can be demonstrated in the vast majority of patients. The head and body in particular can be seen in 80%–90% of patients (Fig. 8.2). Clear visualisation of the tail of the pancreas may represent something of a problem, since this lies behind the stomach, which will often contain small, if not large, amounts of gas. Whilst various manoeuvres are available to improve visualisation of this region of the pancreas, it may remain non-visualised.

The incidence of pancreatic adenocarcinoma has increased substantially in the Western world over the past 20 years, although the prognosis remains extremely poor with the 5-year survival being in the order of a few per cent. The pancreatic adenocarcinoma is by far the most common variety of pancreatic carcinoma, accounting for over 90% of cases. Two-thirds of these tumours arise in the pancreatic head, frequently causing obstructive jaundice, which may be the main reason for their diagnosis (Fig. 8.3). Ultrasound provides a safe, non-invasive means of evaluating the pancreas for the presence of tumour, and information regarding unresectability may be obtained.

The ultrasonic texture of adenocarcinoma is less echogenic than that of normal pancreas, allowing a clear differentiation of tumour from adjacent pancreatic tissue in the majority of cases. This textural difference allows tumour detection within a gland that is entirely normal in size. Unfortunately, the abnormal texture of adenocarcinoma is non-specific and other tumours, as well

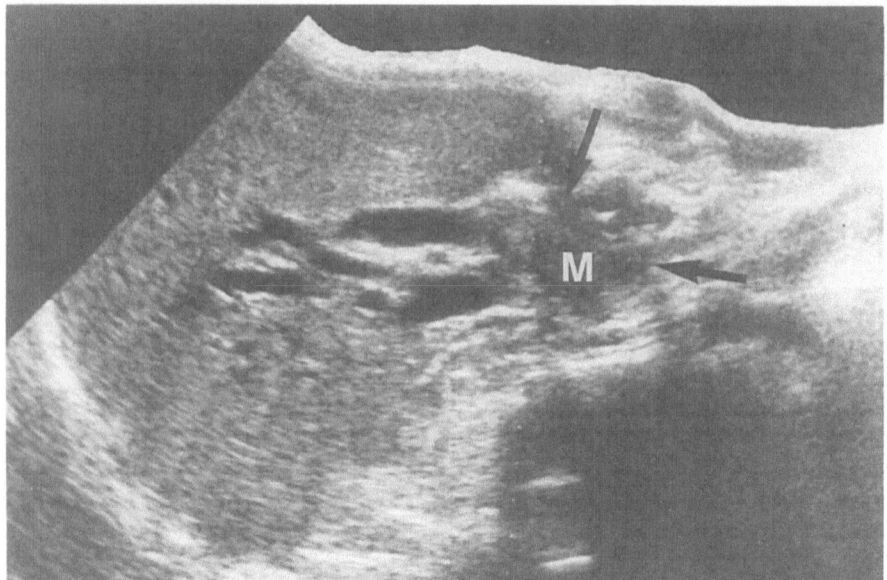

a

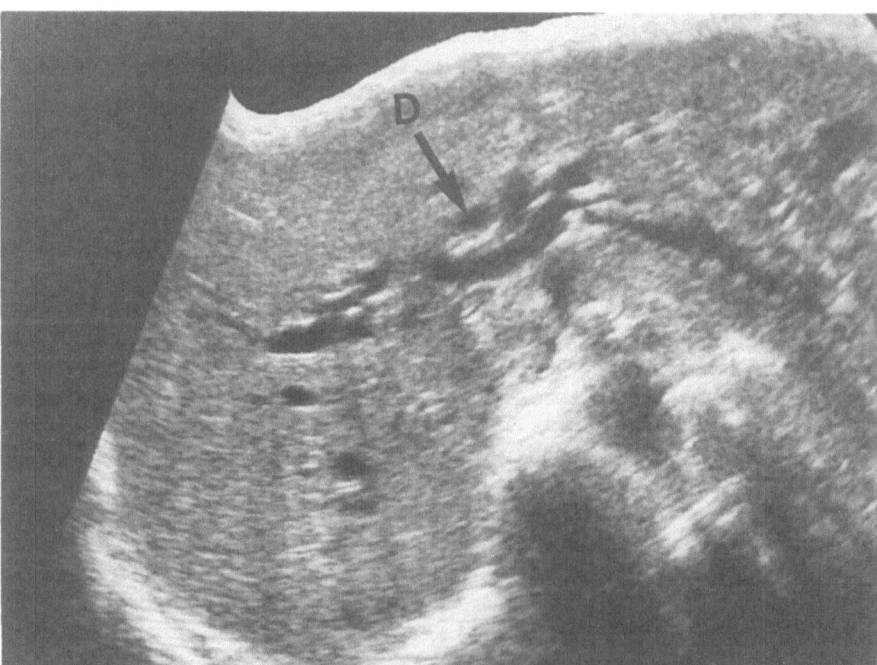

b

Fig. 8.3.a,b. Longitudinal and transverse scans respectively in a patient with a lobular pancreatic carcinoma in the head of the gland (M, *arrowed*) producing marked biliary duct dilatation within the liver (D, *arrowed*).

as focal areas of chronic pancreatitis, may produce a very similar echo pattern. Most pancreatic tumours are focal, lobulated enlargements of the gland. Due to biological variations in gland morphology, size alone is a poor diagnostic criterion for the detection of a pancreatic carcinoma. The shape of the entire gland must be considered in evaluating the region of the pancreas for enlargement. When tumours do occur in the pancreatic head there will commonly be dilatation of the biliary tree, producing a very characteristic and readily recognised pattern on ultrasound. There may even be associated dilatation of the pancreatic duct which can also be demonstrated. Pancreatic adenocarcinomas tend to metastasise early and, typically, liver metastases are small and multiple and show as poorly reflective areas on ultrasound. When the detailed visualisation of a pancreatic tumour is made with ultrasound it will usually not be necessary to proceed to other more complex imaging procedures. However, when visualisation is inadequate or incomplete it would be appropriate to supplement this information with a further imaging procedure, such as a computerised tomographic scan. This technique undoubtedly provides the most detailed visualisation of the pancreas, and so ultrasound should be regarded as the first line of investigation, or the filter.

Kidney

Renal masses are extremely common, especially in elderly people. Fortunately, most of them (95%) are benign renal cysts. Although most renal cysts are innocuous, rarely producing any symptoms, they frequently resemble renal neoplasms on routine intravenous urography (IVU). Ultrasound has been shown over many years to be particularly accurate in differentiating a simple renal cyst from a solid renal lesion, such as a neoplasm, and undoubtedly should be the first follow-up investigation following the suggestion of a mass lesion on the IVU.

The typical characteristics of a cyst on ultrasound are that it has a smooth, clearly defined, uniform wall and contains no echoes within. There is enhancement of the sound beyond the cyst, arising because of the ease with which sound passes through the fluid (Fig. 8.4). Renal tumours show up as solid renal masses containing a variety of echoes of differing intensities (Fig. 8.5). The smallest neoplasms that can be detected with any reliability with ultrasound are in the order of 1 cm in size. Cysts are easier than neoplasms to discriminate from adjacent renal parenchyma since there is such a marked difference in their acoustic properties, and cysts as small as 2–3 mm in size can be seen if they lie in a well-visualised area. Since ultrasound is a tomographic technique, it does not represent a good screening method for the detection of hypernephroma. Neoplasms in locations that are relatively inaccessible to ultrasound, such as the left upper pole, can be missed, and ultrasound should be used as a follow-up to an IVU. Ultrasound is able to outline the size and extent of a tumour and make some assessment of invasion beyond the renal capsule. In addition, it is able to image the renal veins and the inferior vena cava, and so assess the presence of tumour thrombus which may be an important part of the pre-operative evaluation of a patient with a renal tumour (Fig. 8.6). The liver and node-bearing areas in the upper abdomen may also be easily visualised at the same time as examination of the kidneys to assess the presence of metastases in lymph nodes or in the liver.

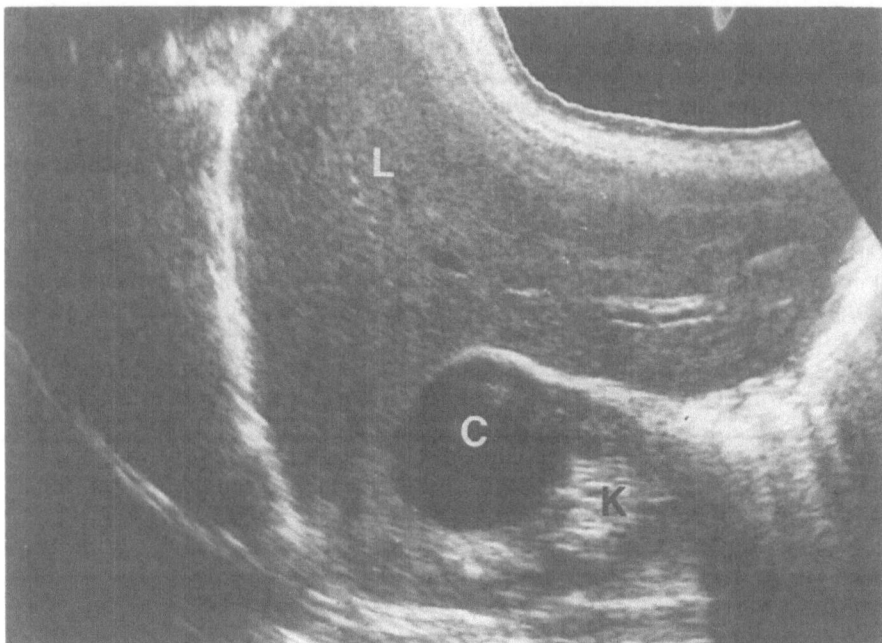

Fig. 8.4. Longitudinal scan through the right lobe of the liver (L) and the right kidney (K) showing a typical 5 cm cyst (C) lying anteriorly in the mid portion of the right kidney.

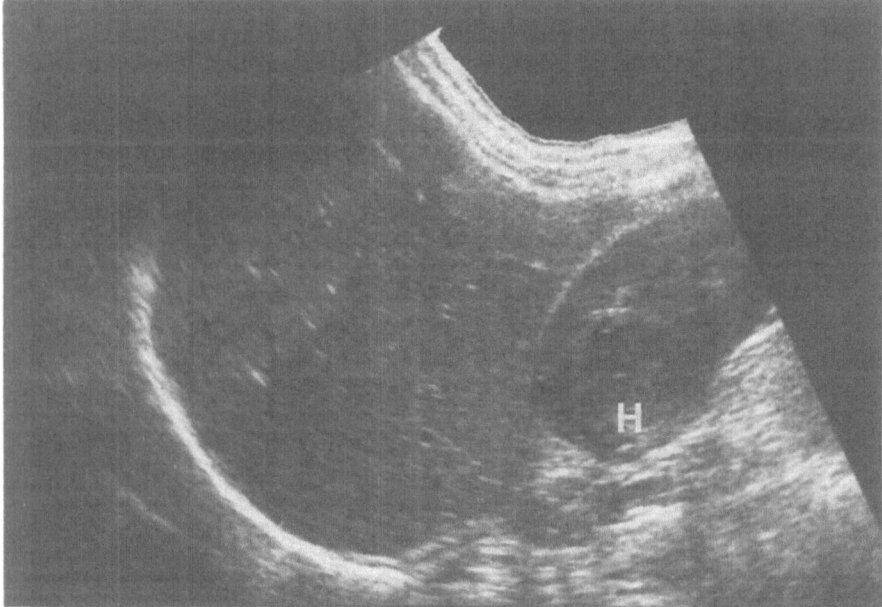

Fig. 8.5. A similar section to Fig. 8.4 showing a solid renal carcinoma in the upper pole (H).

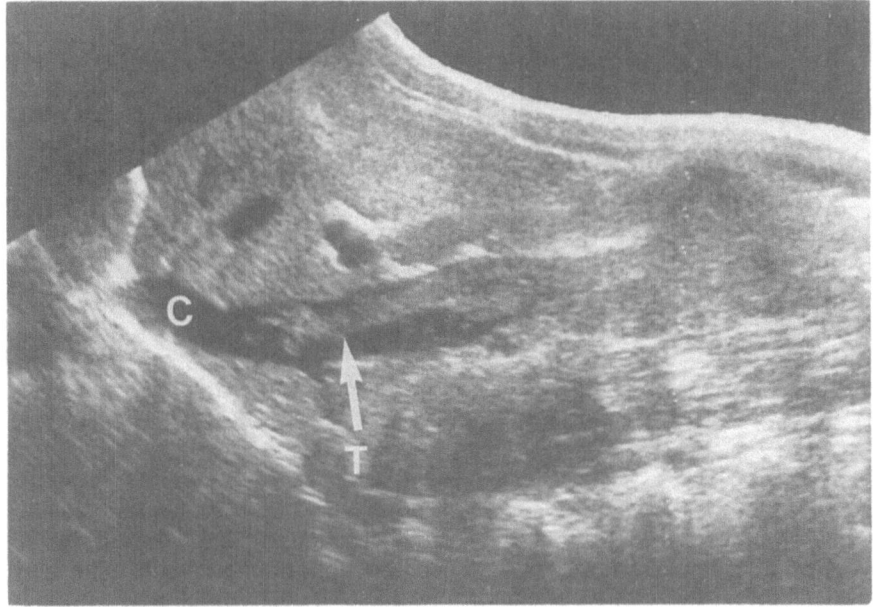

Fig. 8.6. Longitudinal scan through the inferior vena cava (C) in a patient with a right-sided hypernephroma. Tumour thrombus extends into the renal vein and the inferior vena cava and is clearly shown within the lumen (T).

In summary, ultrasound is a reliable and accurate technique for demonstrating the presence of a renal tumour and distinguishing it from benign cysts of the kidney. Accurate staging of renal tumour may also usually be reliably made with ultrasound. It will usually not be necessary subsequently to perform CT scans or arteriography.

Testes

Superficial structures such as the testes lend themselves particularly well to ultrasound scanning. There is no gas or bone to get in the way of the beam and the requirements for penetration by the ultrasound beam are considerably reduced. Consequently, much higher frequency sound beams can be used for imaging, which significantly improves the overall resolution of the images.

One of the major benefits of being able to image the testis is the ability to sort out the anatomy of a scrotal swelling. In many cases it is difficult even for an experienced examiner to determine the origin of such masses. Ultrasound is nearly always able to localise the lesions to epididymis, testicle or a combination of the two. Most masses that involve the epididymis are inflammatory in nature. The epididymis enlarges and takes on a more echo-lucent character. Most testicular tumours present as an area of decreased echogenicity compared with the normal testicular parenchyma. The range of appearances is, however, variable and the ultrasound imaging characteristics of teratoma and seminoma are not significantly different.

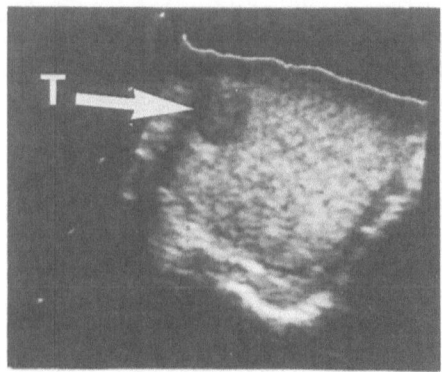
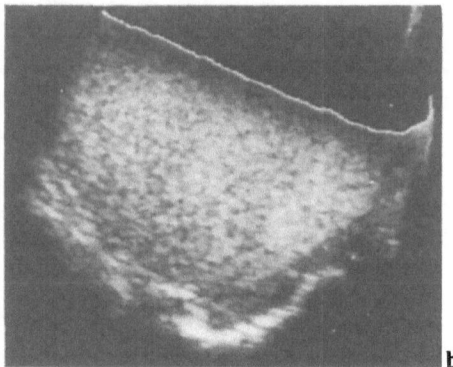

a   b

Fig. 8.7.a Longitudinal scan through the testis demonstrating a small occult teratoma less than 1 cm in diameter (T). **b** Similar section through a normal testis for comparison.

Perhaps the most valuable application of ultrasound in respect of the examination of testes is not in the further elucidation of a palpable mass, but in the confirmation or exclusion of a small occult neoplasm of the testis. This may be in the clinical setting of a patient with florid secondary spread and an occult primary, or in a patient with previous disease when the object is to exclude a second further tumour. An example of a tiny occult testicular teratoma is shown in Fig. 8.7(a).

At present, no other imaging technique is able to demonstrate the testes so well—although both dynamic scintigraphy and Doppler ultrasound will assess the blood flow to the testis, which may be of diagnostic value in differentiating a torsion of the testis from an epididymo-orchitis.

Ovarian Screening

Ovarian cancer comprises about 25% of all gynaecological cancers, causing a little under 4000 deaths per year in the UK. These numbers are higher than the total of those from death due to cancer of the cervix and the body of the uterus. Reducing the mortality from ovarian cancer is one of the more difficult problems facing the gynaecological oncologist today. Despite the introduction of better radiotherapy techniques and new cytotoxic agents, the overall 5-year survival rate has not changed significantly over recent years, and remains at approximately 30%. This poor survival is mainly attributable to late diagnosis. The 5-year survival with stage III or IV disease is 14% and 4% respectively. However, those patients with stage I disease have a 5-year survival of 85%. The failure to detect localised ovarian tumours when surgery could be curative is due to the insidious nature of the disease, to the unreliability of clinical examination and to the lack of an effective early screening technique. Approximately a third of patients with ovarian carcinoma are asymptomatic when the diagnosis is made. Clinical examination is of limited value even when conducted by an experienced gynaecologist.

The routine visualisation of the normal ovaries has long been a part of examining the female pelvis with ultrasound (Fig. 8.8). Accurate measurement of the volume of normal ovaries allows the sensitive detection of departure from normal size. Since 1982, an ovarian scanning clinic has been running at King's College Hospital in London. To date, over 5500 women have been screened, 4% of whom had abnormal results as indicated by an increase in the ovarian volume and/or a change in morphology of the ovary. The vast majority of these tumours were not detected on pelvic examination. Ultrasound does not distinguish benign from malignant tumours, and the definitive diagnosis has to be made by histological examination. In this series there were no false negatives and ultrasound was shown to detect stage I cancers, indicating that ultrasound screening of the ovaries has the potential to be a practical method for early detection of pre-symptomatic ovarian cancer.

One of the very earliest uses of ultrasound was in the definition of larger ovarian tumours; by noting the detailed echo characteristics of ovarian masses, ultrasound will often be able to suggest whether or not they are malignant. The larger tumours are almost always clinically apparent (Fig. 8.9), and perhaps the most useful role ultrasound has is in assessing any associated features, such as the presence of ascites or spread of metastatic disease to lymph nodes or to the liver.

Breast Ultrasound

X-ray mammography of the breast is a well-established diagnostic technique with well-defined diagnostic criteria. It has a high degree of accuracy in the

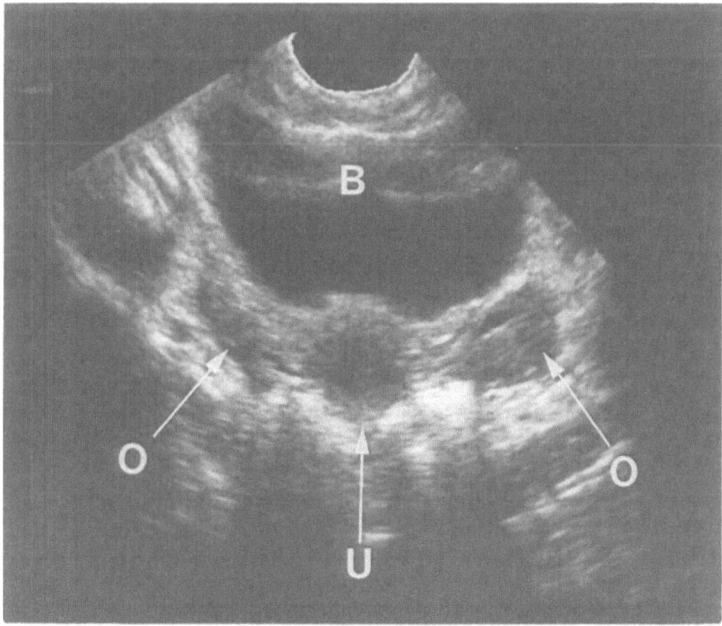

Fig. 8.8. Transverse scan through a female pelvis showing the normal uterus (U) and both normal ovaries (O). B, bladder.

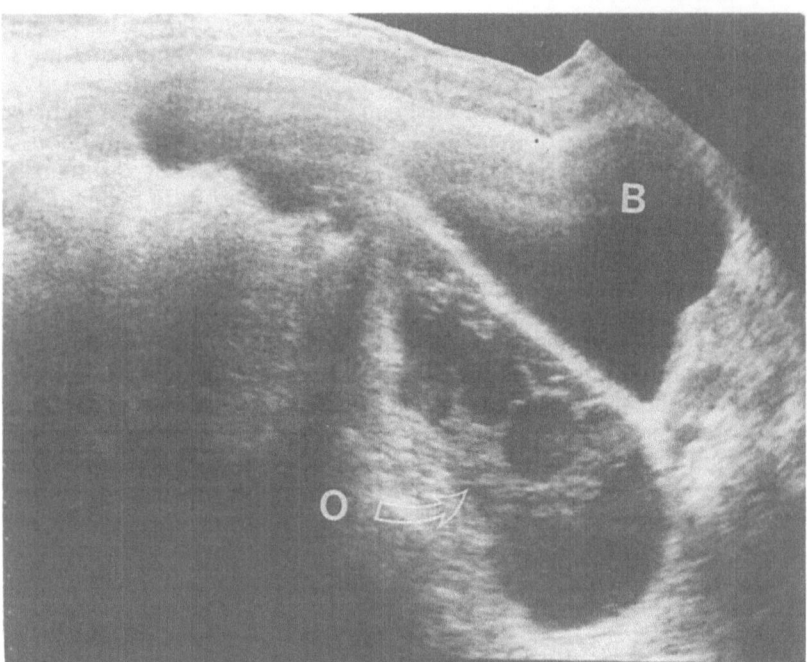

Fig. 8.9. Longitudinal scan through the pelvis showing a large complex mass with solid areas, septae and cystic areas (O). The appearances are typical of a moderately large ovarian cyst adenocarcinoma. B, bladder.

detection of carcinoma; in the numerous series reported in the literature accuracy ranges from 87% to 94%. It may be used for examination of the symptomatic breast or as a screening procedure for the detection of carcinoma, where the pick-up rate is in the order of 3 per 1000 cases. In the latter group the carcinoma is usually detected by the identification of tiny areas of microcalcification. Problems may be encountered, though, in X-ray mammography of some groups of patients: younger patients with dense glandular breasts in whom detailed visualisation of the breast structure cannot be reliably made because of the density of the breast; patients who have had a cosmetic augmentation procedure; and patients with benign diseases of the breast. In these clinical situations ultrasound may be useful as a supplementary procedure to add further diagnostic information to the X-ray mammogram (Fig. 8.10). The accurate preoperative diagnosis of breast lumps is of great assistance in careful patient counselling, the planning of surgery and in the reduction of the number of two-stage procedures.

Cysts in the breast, as elsewhere, have a very characteristic appearance on ultrasound, with a smooth, well-defined wall and posterior enhancement; they can reliably be detected and distinguished from solid lesions. Fibroadenomas are typically rounded and smooth with a homogeneous echo pattern, whereas carcinomas appear as irregular echo-poor masses, often with disruption and disturbance of the surrounding tissue and distortion of the trabecular pattern of the breast. One of the most striking features is the strong distal shadowing seen

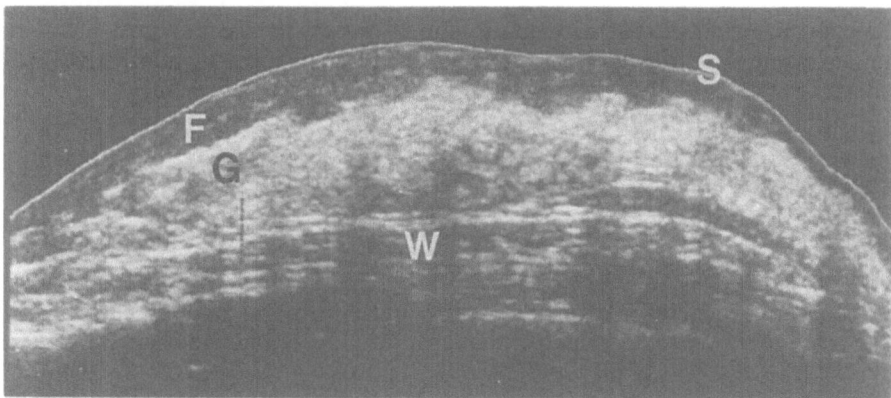

Fig. 8.10. Section through a normal breast showing the pattern of normal glandular tissue (G) and the subcutaneous fat (F). S, skin; W, chest wall.

behind carcinomas (Fig. 8.11). Recent analysis at Southampton General Hospital of a series of 2000 consecutive ultrasound examinations of the breast showed that the sensitivity of ultrasound for the detection of carcinoma was 93%. The use of ultrasound and X-ray mammography together increased the sensitivity of both techniques.

Two other areas in which ultrasound was found to be particularly valuable were firstly as a guide for aspiration cytology, when the pick-up rate was considerably enhanced to nearly 100% for carcinomas, and secondly in the positive identification of benign breast diseases. The diffuse echo pattern changes seen in fibroadenosis and fibrocystic disease of the breast are characteristic on ultrasound, whereas positive identification radiographically can be extremely difficult. Because ultrasound at the present time is not able reliably to detect microcalcification, it is not used as a screening technique for the

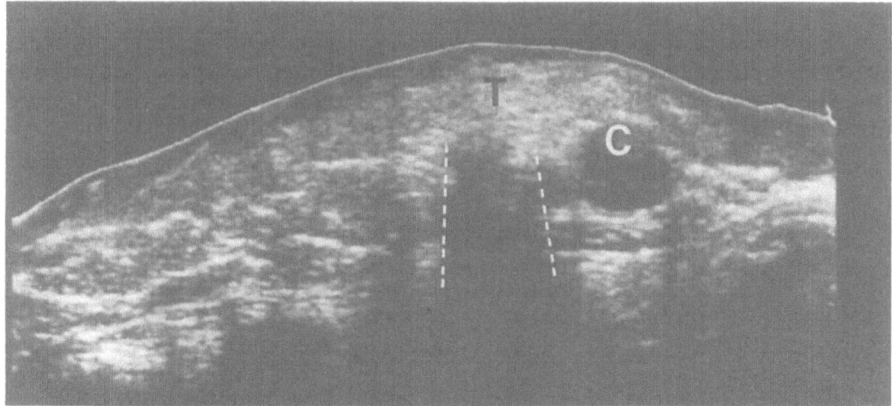

Fig. 8.11. Section through a breast containing a palpable lesion. Ultrasound shows this to be a typical carcinoma ('T') with disruption of the subcutaneous tissues and strong distal acoustic shadowing. Directly adjacent to the carcinoma is a 2 cm cyst (C).

detection of occult breast carcinoma, and this remains the province of X-ray mammography. Ultrasound does, however, remain a useful adjunctive procedure for clarifying the diagnosis in a particular clinical situation.

Staging of Tumours

Liver

Ultrasound is generally regarded as the most sensitive and specific of the available non-invasive imaging techniques for the detection and characterisation of focal liver diseases of all types. Where the histological diagnosis is required, ultrasound-directed biopsy is readily performed and greatly increases the success rate. The accuracy of ultrasound in detecting liver metastases is high, in the order of 80%–90%. However, failures do occur, and if the clinical suspicion remains high in the presence of normal ultrasound scans, further imaging procedures should be performed.

The appearance of liver metastases on ultrasound examination is extremely variable. Hepatomegaly is usual but not invariable and is often associated with a rounding up of the liver that leads to blunting of the normal sharp anterior margin (Fig. 8.12). The enlargement predominates in the affected portion of the liver, and, when superficial, produces localised bumps of the liver contour. These are most easily seen when there is coexistent ascites to outline them. Distortions of the normal hepatic blood vessels can also sometimes be recognised, as can biliary distension of segmental distribution, upstream to areas of obstruction. Whilst these features are non-specific they may provide helpful clues to the presence of metastases. Characteristic alterations in echo pattern usually occur in tumours of the liver. These range from the most commonly seen rounded foci of reduced or increased reflectivity, to normal attenuation when neither shadowing nor distal enhancement is seen. Combinations of increased and reduced reflectivity occur. These are sometimes randomly distributed within one lesion but are often arranged concentrically within a cortex of relatively anechoic tissue arranged around a more reflective central core, giving what is sometimes referred to as the target or bull's eye lesion. Calcification may occur occasionally in metastases, producing extremely intense echoes with strong distal shadowing. Tumours with fluid properties are also encountered and care must be taken in distinguishing these from true cysts.

Nodal Involvement

Lymphangiography has proved particularly accurate in the diagnosis of para-aortic and paracaval lymphadenopathy. It does, however, fail to detect disease of numerous other abdominal sites, including mesenteric, perisplenic and perihepatic lymph nodes. Ultrasound is able to detect retroperitoneal disease and provides additional information not detectable by lymphangiography with respect to the extent of abdominal lymphoma involvement. The characteristic appearance of enlarged lymph nodes on ultrasound is of well-defined, rounded, echo-poor areas in the node-bearing areas (Fig. 8.13). Bowel gas may obscure

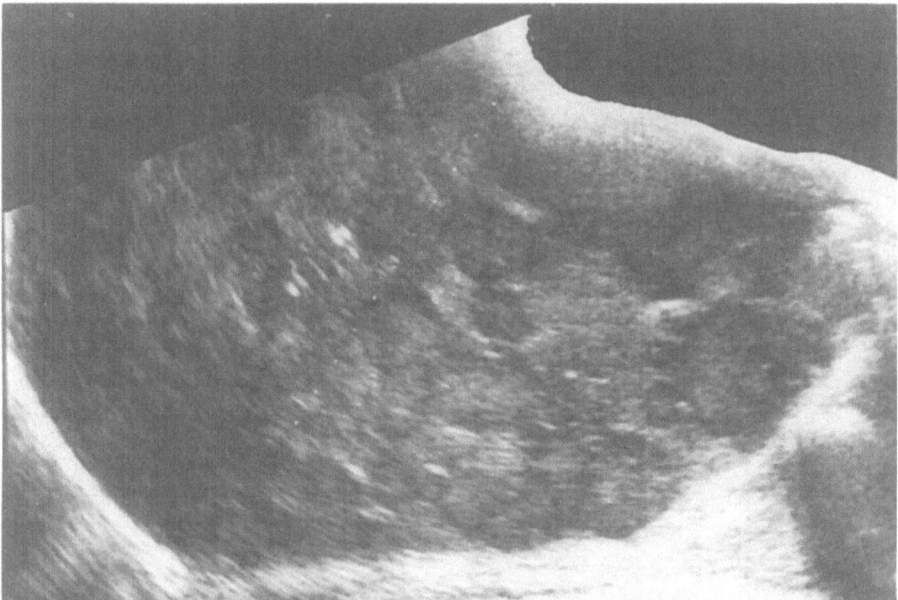

Fig. 8.12. Longitudinal scan through the right lobe of the liver. The liver is enormously enlarged and contains numerous rounded focal lesions. These are producing lobularity and blunting of the inferior margin of the liver. The appearances are absolutely typical of extensive metastatic liver disease (compare with Fig. 8.1).

retroperitoneal structures, and a large amount of retroperitoneal fat degrades sonographic resolution. In larger patients, resolution particularly of the lower para-aortic area may therefore be rather poor. However, ultrasound can usefully be employed as a screen for retroperitoneal disease before proceeding, if necessary, to lymphography or CT scanning.

Follow-up

Clearly, when an abnormality has been satisfactorily demonstrated by ultra-sound, it is appropriate to continue using this simple non-invasive procedure at intervals to show whether any change occurs on therapy. This is an application that is particularly relevant in the follow-up of nodal involvement in lymphoma, either in the para-aortic area or in the mesentery, and in the follow-up of the extent of liver metastases in patients on chemotherapy.

An area of the body where ultrasound is particularly used as a follow-up procedure is in the evaluation of the pelvis following surgery for ovarian tumours. The pelvis is readily visualised with ultrasound, using the acoustic window of the filled bladder, and regular scans may be used sensitively to detect possible recurrences.

Children form a group of patients in whom ultrasound should be carefully considered as a follow-up procedure. With their sparse amounts of body fat they are relatively poor subjects for CT scanning. However their size and lack of fat

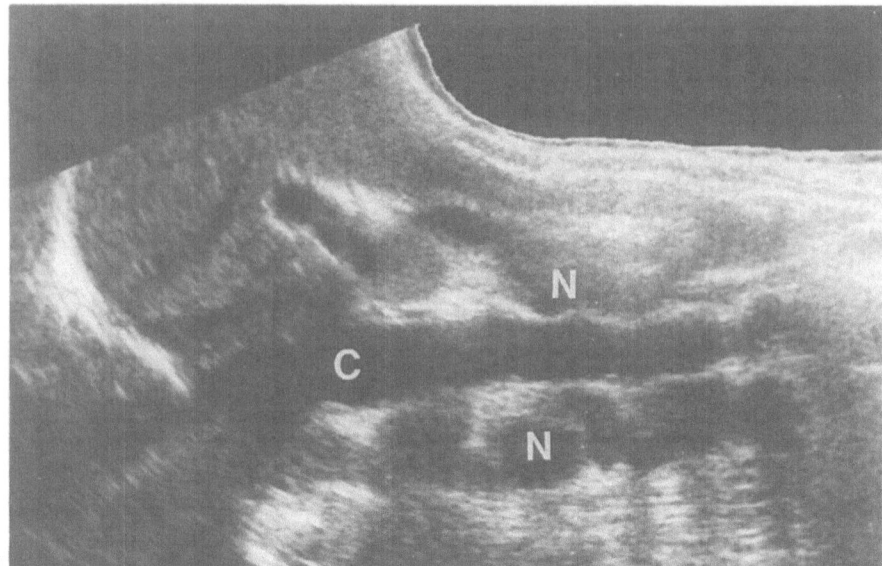

a

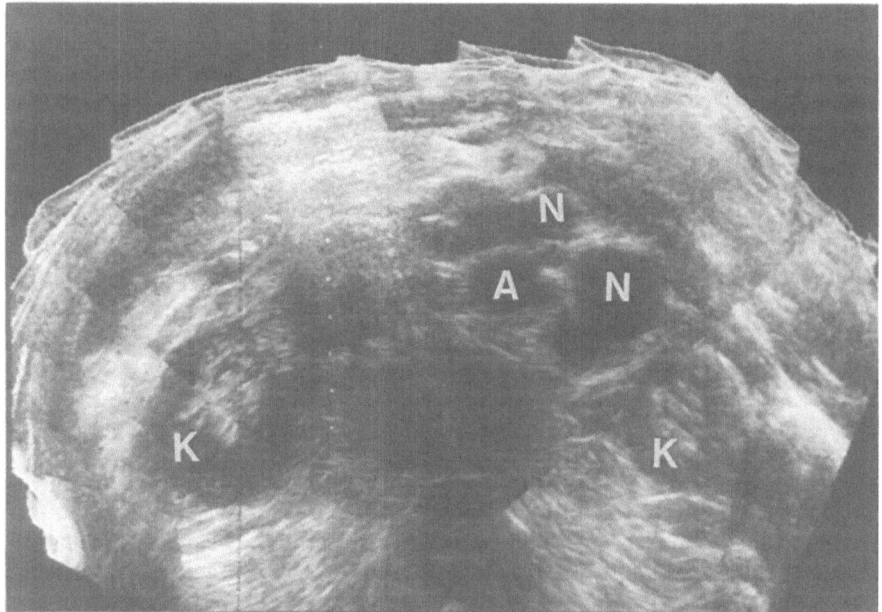

b

Fig. 8.13.a Longitudinal scan of the abdomen over the inferior vena cava (C). **b** Transverse scan at the level of the hilar of the kidneys (K). Typical lobular enlargement of the para-aortic and retro-aortic and retro-caval lymph nodes is shown (N). A, aorta.

make them particularly good subjects for ultrasound examination. This, coupled with the avoidance of ionising radiation, makes ultrasound follow-up of various sorts of paediatric tumours particularly appropriate.

Complications

Clearly there are almost innumerable potential complications in patients with malignant disease. The intention here is to consider only one or two representative areas. One of the great strengths of ultrasound is its ability to answer a specific question, and in certain clinical areas ultrasound remains the best and most appropriate test to undertake.

Jaundice

There are numerous causes for jaundice. It is of considerable importance in the further management of the patient that obstructive jaundice is differentiated from hepatocellular disease. There can be no doubt that where ultrasound is available this should be performed early in the further evaluation of the jaundiced patient. Ultrasound has this central role in the investigation of jaundice because of its great reliability in detecting dilatation of the biliary tree.

The ultrasonic criteria for assessing biliary tree dilatation can be divided into two groups: those concerning the ducts in the liver parenchyma and those concerning the extrahepatic ducts. Normally the intrahepatic biliary vessels are too small to be resolved separately. They run parallel to the portal vein branches and in part contribute to the reflective periportal cuff of echoes. When obstructed, they dilate and can be imaged as duplicate vessels running alongside the portal veins. Cut along their length this produces the parallel channel sign. This distended biliary tree is usually best seen in longitudinal scans where the dilated ducts have rather short straight courses. Multiple branch points may be seen and the directional changes may be sharp and angular. An important diagnostic feature is the acoustic enhancement that may occur beyond dilated biliary ducts—a feature not seen beyond vascular structures. If, as is common, the obstructing lesion is extrahepatic, then the ducts throughout the liver are dilated; but a lobar or segmental pattern of dilatation points to a lesion in the porta hepatis or liver parenchyma. The latter, in a cancer patient, may be a massive lymph node at the porta hepatis, or a critically placed metastasis obstructing the biliary ducts. The normal extrahepatic biliary tree can be routinely identified and measured, and the normal common bile duct should not measure more than 4–5 mm in diameter. This accuracy of measurement allows sensitive detection of even small degrees of biliary duct dilatation. A diagnosis of obstruction is made on the identification of dilated biliary radicals in a jaundiced patient. The next step is to define the level and cause of the obstruction.

Renal Failure

Renal failure is a not uncommon complication in patients with malignant disease, and may be due to many causes. It is important for the further management of the patient in renal failure to decide whether there is an obstructive uropathy present or not. Infiltrative conditions of the kidney, such as, for example, diffuse lymphoma, are readily detectable with ultrasound. In addition, ultrasound is extremely sensitive in positively identifying even minor degrees of hydronephrosis (Fig. 8.14). Having been identified, the obstruction can be relieved by performing percutaneous drainage of the kidneys under ultrasound guidance. This will be discussed further in a later section.

Abcesses

Abscesses remain an important clinical problem, presenting with increasing frequency in patients who are immunocompromised due to steroids or chemotherapy. Proper treatment depends on early and accurate diagnosis, with delay causing increasing morbidity and mortality. Patients with sepsis due to an intra-abdominal abscess, in whom ultrasound is going to be most often used, are usually critically ill and can tolerate only simple diagnostic procedures. The ability of ultrasound to identify, localise and provide guidance for needle aspiration has made it invaluable in this clinical setting. There are certain areas in the abdomen where ultrasound is of particular value. These are in the two subphrenic spaces and in the pelvis. Ultrasound is relatively poor at demonstrating abscesses in the mid portion of the abdomen, unless these are large, because of the interposition of loops of bowel. In this part of the abdomen CT scanning is likely to be more productive.

Most abscesses appear on ultrasound examination as homogeneous, fluid-filled masses with a relatively uniform echo pattern throughout. However, the appearance can vary markedly depending on the precise contents of the abscess.

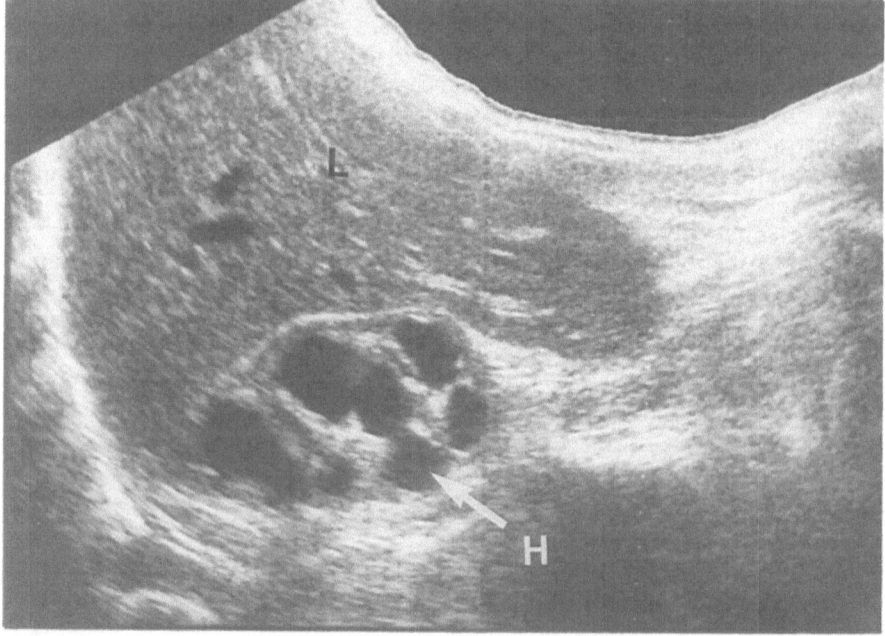

Fig. 8.14. Longitudinal scan through the right lobe of the liver (L) and right kidney showing moderately severe hydronephrosis (H). This scan was carried out immediately prior to proceeding with percutaneous nephrostomy.

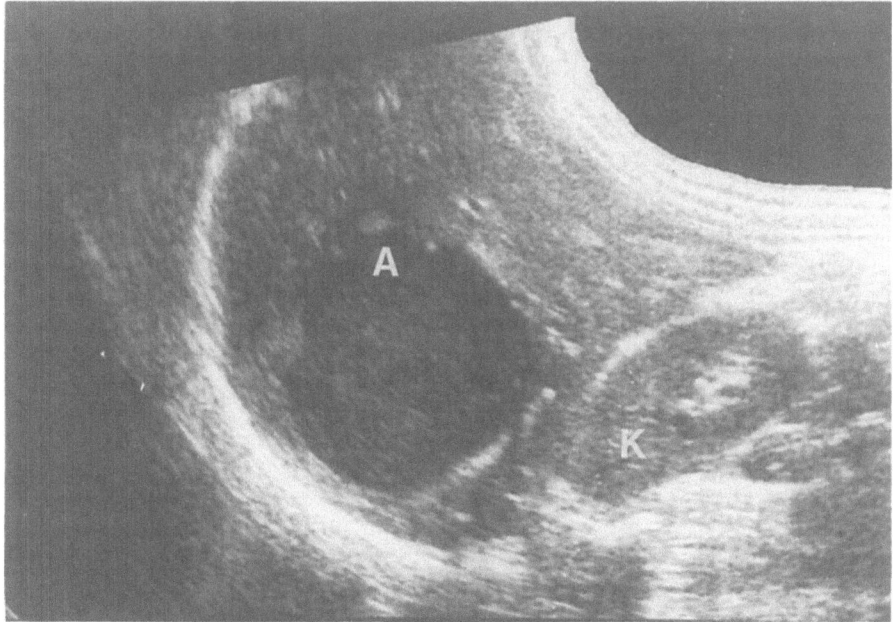

Fig. 8.15. Longitudinal scan through the right lobe of the liver showing a large irregular abscess cavity (A) within the posterior part of the right lobe. Following demonstration of this abcess with ultrasound it was drained under ultrasound guidance. K, kidney.

The walls of abscesses are usually convex outwards and well defined but a little irregular (Fig. 8.15). This lack of wall sharpness is useful in distinguishing abscesses from cysts, ascitic collections and lymphoceles, all of which have very sharp, smooth margins. There are several types of post-operative fluid collections which must be considered in the diagnosis of abscess: biloma, urinoma, seroma, haematoma and lymphocele. It may not always be possible simply on the basis of ultrasound to distinguish these one from another without aspirating some of the fluid.

Intervention and Therapy

This aspect will only be discussed extremely briefly as it has been considered in more detail in Chapter 5 by McIvor.

Fine Needle Aspiration

Aspiration biopsy of abdominal organs and masses under ultrasound guidance was introduced in the early 1970s. Since then, the procedure has become a useful tool in the diagnostic armamentarium. Increasingly widespread use of this technique can in many cases greatly speed up the diagnostic evaluation of the

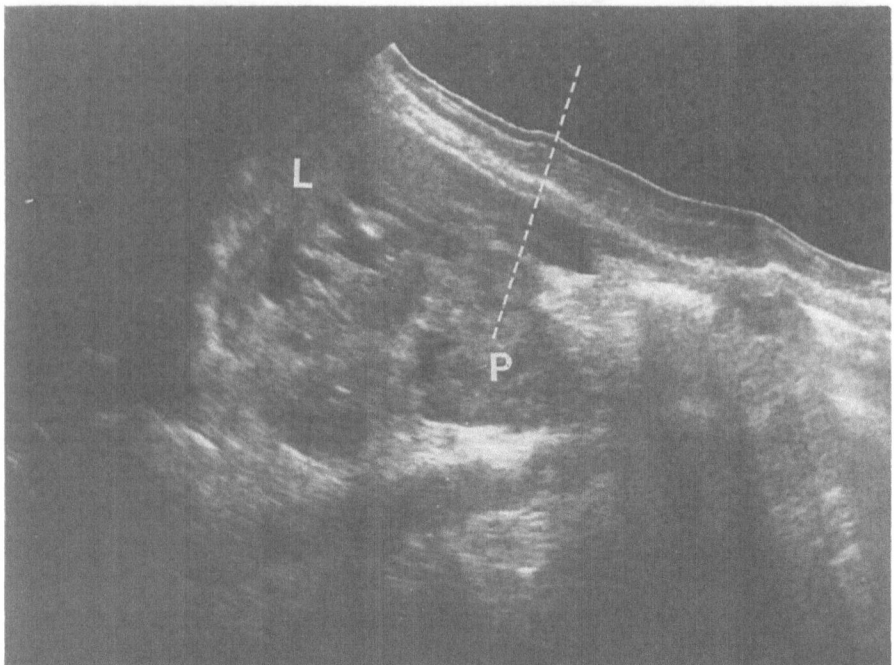

Fig. 8.16. Longitudinal scan through the pancreas (P), which shows lobular irregular enlargement. The line of small marker dots shows the path of the aspiration needle. Fine needle aspiration in this case confirmed the presence of a pancreatic carcinoma. L. liver.

patient, and short circuit more expensive and less informative procedures. Percutaneous aspiration biopsy can be applied to any organ or mass which can be identified on the ultrasound scan (Fig. 8.16). In the evaluation of masses, the fine needle aspiration technique using a 21 or 23 gauge needle is most appropriate. Many thousands of patients have now been examined in this way, and the complication rate is almost negligible. With larger lesions it is satisfactory simply to mark the site of the lesion on the skin and biopsy in the known position. With smaller lesions modern equipment can be used to guide the tip of the needle into the lesion. The needle is not shown with the same clarity as it would be on X-ray examination; however, the tip can usually be sufficiently well identified for accurate localisation. Clearly, ultrasound may be used to guide not only the fine needle, but, where appropriate, a wider-bore needle also.

Abscess Drainage

Comments have already been made above about abscess drainage under ultrasound guidance, and the same comments apply as were made there. If an abscess can be identified with ultrasound, usually it can be drained using ultrasound to guide the needle into the appropriate place. Percutaneous drainage of abscesses is being increasingly frequently used and in many instances this is saving more extensive surgical intervention.

Nephrostomy

Following the identification of a dilated collecting system, ultrasound is the ideal initial guidance method for the puncture of this dilated collecting system. After initial localisation of the system, the remainder of the procedure is performed under X-ray fluoroscopic control.

Conclusion

Clearly the range of applications of ultrasound techniques in oncology is extremely diverse. Ultrasound will rarely be the only technique that is available, although occasionally this may be the case. However, because of its speed, simplicity and safety, ultrasound will often be the first diagnostic procedure to be undertaken in the evaluation of very many problems in the cancer patient.

9   Nuclear Medicine Techniques in Oncology

M. V. Merrick

Nuclear medicine encompasses a number of powerful techniques for assessing function. The quality of anatomical information obtained is in general much weaker. A realisation of this, and the development of techniques for visualising organs which were not accessible to earlier methods of imaging, has resulted in a fundamental shift in the role of nuclear medicine. The scintigraphic search for mass lesions in the liver and brain, although by no means obsolete, has been relegated to a subsidiary role beside ultrasound, computerised tomography and magnetic resonance imaging. Of the older isotope investigations, bone scintigraphy, much the most sensitive technique available for displaying regional differences in bone turnover rate, remains the commonest single scintigraphic examination. It is likely to retain this distinction for the foreseeable future, in large measure because it is widely accepted as an integral part of the staging of a number of common tumours.

A number of new techniques are under development or evaluation. None of these has yet fully established its clinical role. It is clear that it is no longer useful to talk in generalisations and each disease must be considered as a separate entity. There is, moreover, an increasing body of evidence which requires the role of bone scintigraphy to be re-evaluated.

Technical Developments

Gamma cameras are effectively the only instruments still used for scintigraphy. The general tendency in design is towards improved intrinsic resolution, better uniformity and a higher peak count rate capability. It is doubtful whether any of these factors are of practical clinical relevance when imaging bone. Achievable count rates are limited by considerations of radiation dosimetry and the inherent limitations of collimator design. Any camera manufactured within the last 15 years should be able to accept adequate count rates for a clinical examination of the skeleton. Although improvements in intrinsic uniformity and in linearity are of importance in certain fields, the performance of existing cameras, when correctly tuned, is entirely adequate for skeletal scintigraphy. To achieve better resolution most manufacturers now fit 9.5 mm thick crystals rather than the 12.5 mm ones used in older instruments. This has only a minimal effect on sensitivity at the energy of ^{99m}Tc, but causes a substantial loss of sensitivity for ^{131}I. If labelled antibodies achieve clinical importance this will become a significant consideration.

There is no evidence that the higher resolution of the more recent generation of cameras has any effect on lesion detection rate (Hoffer et al. 1984). Improved resolution, by reducing the partial volume effect, increases contrast. This is inevitably offset by poorer count statistics and hence greater noise. In practice, if there is an advantage from higher resolution, it must be too small to have been detected. The study was such that only a large inequality could have been demonstrated. It would take a very large series to confirm a real difference of a magnitude which is credible, taking into account the accuracy of established scintigraphic techniques. Proof that more accurate localisation of abnormalities is of clinical benefit would be even more difficult to adduce.

The major technical innovation attracting attention at the present time is single photon emission tomography. The majority of available systems utilise one or more gamma cameras which rotate around the patient. There are in addition a few specialised systems which employ either a battery of rectilinear scanners with specially designed focused collimators (Kirsch et al. 1981), or a scanning Anger camera with a focused collimator (Freedman 1973). Both have better resolution and greater sensitivity than the rotating gamma camera in its tomographic mode, but are inflexible and lack versatility. They are therefore at present little used.

The clinical role of single photon emission tomography in the examination of the skeleton is not yet established. This is partly for technical reasons. The majority of instruments available hitherto have employed a gamma camera describing a circular orbit. Most had a system resolution of about 20 mm full width at half maximum (FWHM) or worse, compared with 10 mm or better at a depth of 10 cm for static cameras. The combination of poor resolution and limited count statistics in the tomographic studies at least balanced the greater contrast obtained by tomography. Studies claiming an advantage for tomography have compared it with mediocre planar images.

Non-uniformity in the detector is likely to result in circular artefacts, which may give rise to diagnostic confusion. With many of the earlier instruments it was not appreciated that uniformity is affected by the earth's magnetic field and therefore alters as the instrument changes its angle in the course of rotation (Jahangir et al. 1983). Further artefacts in some instruments were due to mechanical instability resulting in the orbit not being a true circle, and no correction was made for this in the reconstruction. Many of these objections have been overcome in newer instruments by the incorporation of magnetic shielding, improved uniformity correction and the introduction of non-circular orbits (Gottschalk et al. 1983) which substantially reduce the geometrical blurring due to the distance of the collimator from the patient whilst at the same time reducing ring artefacts.

At the present time the major applications of single photon emission tomography are the more accurate localisation of skeletal abnormalities for subsequent radiographic evaluation with plain radiographs, and one or other form of transmission tomography, for biopsy localisation, and for improving lesion detection rate with certain radiopharmaceuticals. The major oncological attraction of tomography arises from the increase in contrast which it is capable of giving. There is now some evidence that this may be of real advantage when imaging low-contrast agents such as gallium and the labelled antibodies which have been used experimentally for tumour localisation (Berche et al. 1982, Waxman et al. 1984).

Radiopharmaceuticals

^{99m}Tc-labelled diphosphonates remain the only commonly used pharmaceuticals for bone scintigraphy. The polyphosphates have been entirely superseded as there can now be no reasonable doubt that the active compound was pyrophosphate formed by spontaneous decomposition. Pyrophosphate itself has largely gone out of favour for imaging the skeleton because of the relatively rapid excretion and poor contrast between the skeleton and soft tissue, although it is still widely used for infarct scintigraphy of the myocardium. Methylene diphosphonate (MDP) is probably the most widely used agent, although some centres continue to use ethane hydroxydiphosphonate (EHDP). More recently, methane hydroxydiphosphonate (MHDP) has been advocated. This has a higher uptake in the normal skeleton than MDP (Fogelman et al. 1981) and allows the normal skeleton to be visualised slightly earlier.

There is, however, no evidence that any of these compounds has any significant diagnostic advantage over any of the others. Perhaps the most interesting compound to have been described recently is dimethyl amino-diphosphonate (DMAD) (Subramanian et al. 1983). This was first described some years ago but at the time rejected because of the low contrast between the skeleton and soft tissues which was no better than that achieved with pyrophosphate. However, it has been shown that the contrast between normal and abnormal areas of the skeleton is higher with this compound than with MDP, despite the lower contrast between normal bone and soft tissues (Rosenthall et al. 1982, Smith et al. 1984a,b). Urinary excretion is more rapid.

It is not clear why this better contrast should be, but it has been confirmed in two comparatively small series from different centres. Both also found more lesions in patients in whom some had been demonstrated with MDP, but neither was able to demonstrate a case which was positive with one agent but negative with the other. It is therefore as yet unproven that DMAD has any clinically important advantage, although *a priori* it is to be expected that a compound with a higher contrast would have fewer false negatives. In view of the relatively low false negative rate in well controlled series (see below) a very large study would be required to establish this beyond question. Because of the relatively low uptake of DMAD in normal bone—less than one half that of MDP—the images are less aesthetically attractive. There is in consequence ill-conceived consumer resistance to the introduction of this agent. There must, however, be a useful reduction in absorbed dose to normal subjects and to normal bone in affected subjects.

These observations call into question the criteria conventionally used for selecting agents for skeletal scintigraphy, namely high bone uptake and a high bone to soft tissue ratio at early times after injection. It may well be that agents which are incorporated rapidly and to a large extent into the skeleton reduce the contrast between normal and abnormal areas and hence lead to a lower detection rate of abnormalities. It is unlikely that any radiopharmaceutical will affect the specificity of the examination.

The most important new agent for imaging soft tissue tumours to have become available in recent years is undoubtedly metaiodo-benzylguanidine (MIBG). This compound is most commonly labelled with ^{131}I but has also been labelled with [123]I (McEwan et al. 1985). It localises on the alpha-2 receptors present in tumours of chromaffin origin, especially phaeochromocytoma and neuroblastoma. It is in some cases possible to obtain a high enough contrast between tumour and normal tissues to deliver a therapeutic dose of radiation to the tumour.

A great deal of effort has been devoted to the production of antibodies to "tumour-specific" antigens (Goldenberg 1983), labelled either with ^{131}I, ^{123}I or, with the aid of a bifunctional chelate, [111]In (Rainsbury et al. 1983). A limited amount of success has been obtained. It is not established whether monoclonal (Epenetos et al. 1986) or polyclonal (DeLand and Goldenberg 1985) antibodies, F(ab) fragments or other derivatives are to be preferred. The general applicability of these compounds is not established. Much of the published work has involved tumours of ovarian or testicular origin and dual isotope subtraction, with non-specific blood pool and extravascular markers to increase contrast. The approaches used have in general been unsophisticated. Moreover, like all initial trials, studies have been restricted to subjects with a high *a priori* probability of a detectable tumour. The accuracy achieved under these conditions does not reflect what may realistically be anticipated in clinical use (Goris 1985). False positives due to inflammatory disease have already been reported. As most tumour antigens are in fact dedifferentiation markers, specificity is unlikely to be high.

Although not used for imaging, the synthetic bile acid [75]SeHCAT has an important role in the management of chronic diarrhoea following therapeutic irradiation. It has now been established that there is not a single cause for this distressing iatrogenic complication of treatment (Ludgate and Merrick 1985). [75]SeHCAT is the only simple clinical test able to detect malabsorption of bile acids, which are the immediate cause of the symptoms in about half of the affected patients. As effective specific treatment is available, but selection of the optimum dosage regime requires patience and persistence, it is valuable to have a firm diagnosis before starting treatment. By combining the SeHCAT test with a test for the presence of bacterial colonisation in the small intestine, it is possible to distinguish between the major treatable causes of diarrhoea in this group.

Diagnostic Criteria

The criteria for defining abnormality were inadequate in many of the earlier studies of skeletal scintigraphy. The dichotomy between scintigraphy and radiology is obsolete. They must be considered as integral components of the same examination, neither part of which can be interpreted adequately without the other. Careful examination of radiographs obtained after bone scintigraphy, choosing accurately centred and coned projections of suspected abnormalities, reveals that the "scan positive X-ray negative" patient is a rarity with most tumours, although radiological confirmation is not necessary in every site. If no radiological evidence of metastases can be identified at any site despite the presence of a definite scintigraphic abnormality, transmission tomography, either conventional or computerised depending on the site and the availability of facilities, should be performed. In many cases a definite explanation, either benign or malignant, will thus be revealed. In the few cases which remain, in which there are no proven metastases, it is reasonable to proceed to biopsy. A diagnosis based on scintigraphy alone is undesirable, unreliable and rarely indicated.

Carcinoma of the Breast

Since the early papers by Galasko et al. (1968) and others it has been widely proposed that bone scintigraphy should be part of the routine staging of all new patients with carcinoma of the breast. Galasko (1975) found occult skeletal metastases in 24% of patients with otherwise "early" disease. However not all subsequent reports have been in agreement. The Guy's Hospital group (Chaudary et al. 1983) found no metastases in 241 patients, while the British Breast Group (Adam et al. 1978) reported a multicentre study in which the incidence varied between 1% and 20% for different centres. It is possible to offer explanations for some of these discrepancies. For example, the definition of early used by Galasko included some T3 tumours, which would not have been included in the early category of some later series. Although the patients were unselected by him there is a possibility that there may have been a preselection by referral pattern to his hospital. Some other series included a higher percentage of T0 and T1 tumours.

Whilst Galasko (1975) was subsequently able to confirm the presence of metastases in all of his cases who were available for follow-up, several groups (Sklaroff and Sklaroff 1976, Perez et al. 1983) have found a very high prevalence of false positives. This was in some cases the result of the criteria used to define abnormality, namely the presence of any focal increase in radioactivity in scintigrams viewed in isolation, paying no attention to site or radiological findings. Similarly the range of prevalence reported in the British Breast Group Survey almost certainly reflects the fact that neither the criteria for considering an examination to be abnormal, nor the technical standards, were defined.

Inter-observer variations in interpretation must also play a part. The extent of these may be gauged from two surveys, by Rossing et al. (1982) and by Smith et al. (1985). In the first series, films from other centres were reviewed by different observers, whilst in the second a number of experienced observers were invited to report independently on the same set of studies. The lack of agreement between the observers was both striking and disheartening. Indeed the level of agreement in the second series was little better than would have been expected by random chance. Both series may be criticised because radiographs of the patients were not provided. It is not established whether the addition of radiographs would have as much effect on inter-observer variability as it has on the rate of false positives.

The largest single unit series, and the one with the longest follow-up, was that recently reported from Edinburgh (Kunkler et al. 1985). We reviewed the results of staging scintigraphy in 465 consecutive women with histologically proven carcinoma of the breast followed for a minimum of 2 and a maximum of 9 years or until death. One important difference between this and many previous series was that scintigraphy was interpreted in conjunction with radiographs of any suspicious areas. Studies were classified as normal if there was no scintigraphic abnormality. They were deemed abnormal if there was a definite abnormality with radiographic evidence of metastatic involvement, or alternatively if there were multiple abnormalities for which there was no benign explanation on adequate radiographs. Cases were considered benign if there was a lesion such as osteoarthritis or Paget's disease, and equivocal when there was a non-specific radiographic abnormality such as a collapsed vertebra with intact pedicles, or if the area was not adequately seen on available radiographs.

Using these criteria, as few as 1.5% of patients with T0 or T1 N0 disease had abnormal staging scintigraphy. This rose to 7% for patients with T1N1, T2N0, T2N1 or T3N0 disease. Only in patients with T3N1 or T4 disease was the incidence high, being approximately 17.5%. Taking T1 to T3 N0 and N1 together, the prevalence in the British Breast Group series ranged between 1.9% and 20% carcinoma of the breast. The comparable group in the Edinburgh series gave an incidence of 7.6%. However in our series twice as many patients, 15.7% of the total group, developed overt evidence of skeletal metastases on follow-up as were detected as having metastases at presentation. A similar false negative rate was found by Strender et al. (1981), Roberts and Hayward (1983) and Galasko (1975). As neither scintigraphy nor radiographic follow-up was routinely performed, our figures, which are substantially lower than those found at post-mortem, represent a minimum estimate of the true prevalence of skeletal metastases. It is clear that staging scintigraphy in patients with early disease has a low pick-up rate and even so detects only approximately half of all patients who develop clinical signs of skeletal metastases (Table 9.1). The mean delay between normal scintigraphy and the appearance of overt metastases was 21.7 months, with a range from 6 to 45 months.

The criteria for considering the results of a study to be abnormal must be properly defined and correctly applied. Groups such as Perez et al. (1983), using the laxest possible criteria, that is merely enumerating areas of increased count rate, found bone scintigraphy to be a poor predictor of subsequent radiographically detectable relapse. In our series, using much stricter criteria, 6 of the 44 patients (13.6%) who were considered to have definitely abnormal results appear on follow-up to have been false positives (1.3% of all cases). However as

Table 9.1. Value of bone scintigraphy in carcinoma of the breast, bronchus and bladder

Primary site (number)	Sensitivity	Nonspecificity	Accuracy	Predictive value of positive test	Predictive value of negative test
	$\left(\dfrac{TP^a}{TP+TN}\right)$	$\left(\dfrac{FP}{TN+FP}\right)$	$\left(\dfrac{TP+TN}{Total}\right)$	$\left(\dfrac{TP}{All\ positive}\right)$	$\left(\dfrac{TN}{All\ negative}\right)$
Breast (465)	0.48	0.02	0.84	0.86	0.89
Bronchus (57 post-mortem)	0.89	0.00	0.78	1.0	0.71
Bladder (221)	0.40	0.02	0.91	0.78	0.92

[a]TN, true negative; TP, true positive; FP, false positive; FN, false negative.

many of the patients received adjuvant chemotherapy during the follow-up period this may overestimate the number. Had we applied the criteria of Perez there would have been 137 abnormal studies at presentation, 86 (62%) of which would have been false positives (18.5% of all cases)—an unacceptable level of inaccuracy.

The importance of regarding radiographs as an integral part of the study cannot be over-emphasised. There is a strong case for suggesting that a scintigraphic abnormality in the absence of any radiographic change should be regarded with caution if not frank scepticism. Had we employed the strictest possible criteria and accepted as positive only those cases in whom there was radiographic (or biopsy) confirmation of at least one deposit there would have been no false positives, whilst the false negative rate would have been only slightly increased above its already high level.

There is agreement that the prognosis is worse for those with abnormal staging scintigraphy than for those with normal examinations, at least up to 9 years of follow-up (Kunkler et al. 1985). Despite this there can be little doubt that routine staging scintigraphy cannot be justified in all newly diagnosed cases of carcinoma of the breast. The low pick-up rate, especially in early disease, an appreciable false positive rate and the poor predictive value for the subsequent appearance of symptomatic metastases indicate that the results of this test should not influence management. The false positive rate could be substantially reduced if stricter criteria for defining abnormality were applied, especially as in the majority of patients careful examination of good-quality radiographs and (where appropriate) tomograms usually reveals some radiological abnormality. It is also helpful to rehearse the clinical history and physical examination in patients with a solitary lesion, especially if this is in a rib, or if there are a small number of adjacent rib lesions. These are commonly due to minor trauma and a history can usually be obtained on direct questioning. If these precautions are observed the incidence of false positives should approach zero.

This, however, would do relatively little to improve the accuracy of the investigation because of the low prevalence of deposits in early disease and the number of false negative and, especially, equivocal examinations. There are three possibilities for these. Either the deposits were not present at the time of the staging investigation, they were too small to be detectable or they were wholly lytic and not provoking any osteoblastic response. If they were too small, it might be possible to improve the accuracy by introducing an agent which gives a higher contrast between normal and abnormal bone than the agents currently in general use. The number of equivocal results could be substantially reduced by pursuing the diagnosis more vigorously in such cases, but this in turn would require a clearer definition of the therapeutic consequences of this information.

In recurrent carcinoma of the breast the picture is very different. I have not been able to trace any published series which define the role of bone scintigraphy in patients with recurrent disease, as distinct from those being staged at presentation. We have, however, recently reviewed our results in 315 patients (Kunkler and Merrick 1986) and find a picture which contrasts with that in the staging examination. Not surprisingly, in the presence of both bone pain or tenderness and radiographic abnormalities, scintigraphic confirmation is very common (over 80%). Indeed a principal question is, perhaps, why it is not 100%. There are a number of possible explanations for this, in particular that many lesions become sclerotic and therefore more visible radiologically in response to endocrine therapy or chemotherapy, although they become scintigraphically less active. The phenomenon of osteolytic deposits which are not producing any osteoblastic response is responsible for some cases. Radiographic diagnosis is complicated by the difficulty of distinguishing between fractures in irradiated bone and metastases. Moreover it would certainly be incorrect to assume 100% accuracy of radiographic interpretation, which in our series was made by a wide variety of radiologists of varying levels of seniority and experience.

The scintigraphic pick-up rate in patients with local pain or tenderness suggestive of bone involvement, but negative initial reading of the X-rays, was also very high, being approximately 38%. However the most interesting and important group were those presenting with loco-regional recurrence. In our series 36% of these patients were found to have occult skeletal metastases. This finding substantially alters their management and is therefore of direct practical importance.

Thus in carcinoma of the breast the role of bone scintigraphy has changed appreciably. It can no longer be recommended as a routine staging examination in new patients at presentation. It is, however, of considerable value in those who return with loco-regional recurrence, and should be performed routinely in all such cases. It should also be performed in any patient at any stage of the disease with local pain or tenderness for which there is no satisfactory explanation on plain radiographs. It may have a further role in patients who are asymptomatic but have radiographic changes, in order to determine whether or not these deposits are active at a particular time.

Direct tumour imaging is not yet a routine clinical examination in carcinoma of the breast. DeLand and Goldenberg (1985), using polyclonal anti-carcinoembryonic antigen (CEA), monoclonal anti-CEA or F(ab')2 fragments, reported a 50%–70% detection rate, but it is not clear whether this applies to the primary or to secondary deposits, nor whether these were readily detectable by other means, such as a chest radiograph. Rainsbury et al. (1983) claimed better success with ^{111}In-labelled monoclonal antibody in a small series. Further comparisons in larger series are required. A number of centres have reported encouraging results in animals with labelled oestrogen antagonists (Jagoda et al. 1984, Kiesewetter et al. 1984). No clinical trials with these compounds have yet been published.

Carcinoma of the Bladder

It is salutary to note that, stage for stage, the prevalence of bone metastases, the false positive rate and the false negative rate are similar in bladder and in breast cancer (Davey et al. 1985) (Table 9.1). It has never been seriously suggested that routine bone scintigraphy should be included in the staging protocols for bladder cancer.

Carcinoma of the Prostate

The prevalence of bone metastases in carcinoma of the prostate is much higher than in carcinoma of the breast. In virtually all published series it rises from approximately 10% in patients with T0 disease to 80% in patients with T4 disease or at post-mortem. These high prevalence rates are associated with high scintigraphic pick-up rates and there is fairly general agreement that this justifies routine staging scintigraphy in all patients with this disease. Indeed many centres do routine follow-up scintigrams as well. We have recently reported the results of an extended follow-up in a group of 220 patients with histologically proven carcinoma of the prostate (Merrick et al. 1985). The results indicate that in this condition also, established practice needs to be reviewed.

Survival was unrelated to age at presentation and only weakly correlated with histological grading, being better in patients with well-differentiated tumours than in those who had moderately or poorly differentiated tumours. Not surprisingly, patients with the lower T stages, 0, 1 or 2, had a better survival than those with stage 3 or 4 tumours. The unexpected finding was the relationship between survival, scintigraphy results and enzyme (acid and alkaline phosphatase) levels. Patients with a raised acid phosphatase had a poorer survival than those with a normal acid phosphatase level. Like Lund et al. (1984) we found that those with scintigraphic evidence of metastases had a shorter survival than those without. However the difference in survival was much greater when plasma alkaline phosphatase was also considered. Multivariate analysis confirmed that all the differences in survival could be attributed to the alkaline phosphatase level. Thus in carcinoma of the prostate the most important prognostic indicator is the plasma alkaline phosphatase level. Neither bone scintigraphy nor the acid phosphatase level give any additional prognostic information beyond that obtained from measurement of this enzyme.

There is, however, still an indication for one initial bone scan in those patients in whom the alkaline phosphatase is elevated at presentation, as this finding is non-specific. Benign conditions associated with a raised level, such as Paget's disease, are not uncommon in patients of the age group who also have carcinoma of the prostate (Merrick and Merrick 1985). The prevalence of the various conditions does of course vary in different areas, but in particular that of Paget's disease is relatively high in most parts of the United Kingdom. There is thus a case for scintigraphy in order to distinguish prostatic metastases from various benign bony conditions.

The appearance of scintigraphic abnormalities in previously unaffected patients preceded a rise in the plasma acid phosphatase level and the development of symptoms by a mean interval of approximately 6 months. It is well established that treatment of the asymptomatic patient with carcinoma of the prostate does not improve either survival or the duration of the symptom-free period (Parker et al. 1985). However there is an obvious, although as yet unproven, case for starting treatment when patients convert from scan negative to scan positive, just prior to them developing symptoms, in the hope that this may prevent the appearance of symptoms. Bishop et al. (1985) found that in some cases a rise in alkaline phosphatase level preceded the scintigraphic appearance of deposits. It is not established whether or not this is a constant finding. Until this has been clarified it is reasonable to perform 6-monthly follow-ups on asymptomatic patients with normal bone scintigrams.

The role of bone scintigraphy in assessing response to treatment is more controversial. A number of groups have reported sequential follow-up as a means of assessing patients on treatment. It is accepted that simple analogue evaluation of the images is too subjective to be of value. Some workers count the number of focal abnormalities, but this itself is not entirely objective. In many areas, for example the cervical and upper thoracic spine, pelvis and skull, it is often difficult to determine the exact number of lesions. Moreover, although in some patients the total number of lesions decreases in response to treatment and increases when escape from treatment occurs, in a substantial minority some lesions become less active or disappear whilst simultaneously others become more active and new ones appear. In an attempt to overcome this problem some groups have tried to relate the observed count rate either to the activity of a standard containing a known percentage of the administered dose, or to the activity in an area of non-involved bone.

These methods are unsatisfactory for a number of reasons. To begin with there is an effect, the flare phenomenon, which is seen in many, although not all, deposits as they start to respond to a new treatment. There is more osteoblastic activity, leading to increased uptake. This is presumably, but not definitely, related to a reduction in tumour activity. The time scale of this phenomenon is fairly short, but rather variable. A more important objection is that the scintigraphic appearance of a skeletal deposit is only indirectly related to the tumour activity at the site, being the result of the osteoblastic response to the osteoclastic activity provoked by the tumour. There is no evidence to suggest that this is directly related to other parameters of tumour growth or activity. Thus on balance it cannot be assumed that bone turnover as assessed by bone scintigraphy is a valid method of determining the mitotic activity of tumour metastases in the skeleton.

Thus the indications for scintigraphy in carcinoma of the prostate have, like those in carcinoma of breast, changed considerably. In patients with a normal alkaline phosphatase level, regular follow-up scintigraphy may be indicated in order to anticipate the development of symptoms. In patients with a raised alkaline phosphatase level, a single examination is indicated in order to confirm that this is due to malignant rather than benign bone disease. There is no evidence that scintigraphy is clinically useful for assessing response to treatment nor for estimating prognosis. For the former purpose sequential measurements of acid and alkaline phosphatase are simpler, cheaper and probably more sensitive (Bishop et al. 1985).

Carcinoma of the Lung

In the United Kingdom as a whole lung cancer is the commonest malignant tumour in men and the second commonest in women. All histological types have a poor prognosis, although recent advances in chemotherapy have substantially improved it. Even so, only around 10% of patients presenting with the most chemosensitive small cell tumours survive for more than 2 years.

In approximately three-quarters of all patients with lung cancer it is obvious at presentation, on the basis of a clinical examination, history and plain radiographs of any painful areas, that the patient has disseminated disease (Matthews et al. 1973). There is clearly no indication for further staging investigations. Because most small cell tumours are advanced when first seen, there is an impression that they carry a poorer prognosis than tumours of other cell types. However Little et al. (1983) have suggested that stage may be a more important prognostic factor than cell type. Unfortunately accurate staging of early lung cancer is more difficult, in those patients who do not come to thoracotomy, than in breast or prostatic tumours because of the inaccessibility of the majority of sites of early spread. The two scintigraphic examinations which are widely used for staging are bone and gallium scintigraphy.

With very few exceptions, the majority of published series of bone scintigraphy in carcinoma of the bronchus fail to distinguish between cell types or refer to only one type. In most studies there was neither post-mortem nor clinical follow-up to determine whether or not the scintigraphic interpretation was correct. The relationship of scintigraphic findings to survival is either not considered or is assessed using inappropriate statistical techniques.

We have recently completed a follow-up of 587 patients referred for skeletal scintigraphy up to 1982 (Merrick and Merrick 1986). The end-point of the series was chosen to coincide with the start of a number of trials of chemotherapy, so that our findings represent the natural history of the disease, not influenced by effective systemic therapy. This series comprises approximately one-quarter of all patients in the area served by our hospital who developed lung cancer during this period, the criteria for selection being that the referring clinician considered there was at least a possibility that disease might have been localised to the chest or that skeletal scintigraphy was indicated on other clinical grounds. It includes all patients being considered for surgery or radical radiotherapy, and a number presenting with bone pain, in some of whom scintigraphy preceded the establishment of the diagnosis.

There were no significant differences in survival between patients with the various histological types. Irrespective of cell type, subjects without any scintigraphic abnormality survived significantly longer than those with evidence of bone metastases. The prevalence of scintigraphic abnormalities was highest (62%) in patients who were symptomatic at the time of the examination. Pain itself was an important prognostic factor, the survival being appreciably and significantly poorer in those with pain than those without it.

In contrast to carcinoma of the prostate, the prognostic significance of the alkaline phosphatase level in carcinoma of the bronchus was very limited. It has previously been shown (Williams et al. 1977) that scarcely 50% of patients with bone metastases from bronchogenic primaries have a raised alkaline phosphatase level. In the majority it was less than 10% above the upper limit of their reference range. Moreover there was a high false positive rate, the alkaline phosphatase being raised in 45% of patients without skeletal metastases. This contrasts with the findings of Hooper et al. (1978) who found the alkaline phosphatase to be elevated in all patients with a scintigraphic abnormality. The difference may be the result of the criteria chosen for selection of patients for entry into these two series. Almost half the patients with a raised alkaline phosphatase level in our series did not have bone metastases. Because of the small number with a raised alkaline phosphatase and uncertainties about the completeness of recording normal values, we were not able to assess the effect of a raised level on prognosis. However the high false positive and false negative rates in both the present and previous series indicate that it is unlikely to be an important determinant.

Wide variations have been reported in the prevalence of occult skeletal metastases in this disease: from 63% (Tofe et al. 1975) to as little as 15% (Turner and Haggith 1981). Technical factors are undoubtedly responsible in some cases, whilst selection of patients for study is the reason in others. However it is not always clear why these discrepancies, which are of a magnitude which is unlikely to be due to statistical fluctuations, should have occurred. The prevalence of scintigraphically detectable metastases in our series was similar in all histological types, being approximately half of all patients with apparently early disease whether the patients were examined within 8 weeks of diagnosis or at a later time. The inference is clearly that, in the majority, skeletal deposits, if they are to develop, are present when the patients are first seen.

For staging to be of practical value the findings must have some prognostic or therapeutic significance. In the case of carcinoma of the bronchus, the survival of asymptomatic patients with occult skeletal metastases is significantly worse than that of those with no scintigraphic abnormality ($P<0.01$). Skeletal metastases were indeed the most important single prognostic determinant in asymptomatic subjects. It is also important to be certain of the prevalence of both false positives and false negatives (Table 9.1). We obtained post-mortems in 57 patients, 32 of whom were considered to have skeletal metastases. Thirty of these were confirmed at post-mortem to have metastases. In the other 2 the area of the scintigraphic abnormality was not examined at post-mortem. These must be considered false negative post-mortem examinations, as in both there was unequivocal radiological evidence of metastases at the sites implicated. There were no false positives. Ten of the cases were true negatives and a further 7 false negatives. It is worthy of note that in 3 of these the examination was negative because of technical inadequacies.

The significance of this latter observation must be stressed. There were only 3 technically unsatisfactory examinations in the 57 patients who came to post-mortem. All of these were false negatives. There were 4 false negatives in the 54 technically satisfactory examinations. The false negatives which were technically adequate were small deposits provoking little or no osteoblastic response. One or at most 2 of these might have been detected using an agent giving a higher contrast between normal and abnormal bone. Others, which provoked no osteoblastic response at all, could not have been detected unless they had been large enough for a photon-deficient area to be detectable. This would not have been the case in any of these patients. It is thus evident that false negatives cannot be entirely eliminated.

The remaining examinations were considered equivocal. In many of these cases better radiographs, tomograms or in a few cases biopsy would have been required to eliminate this uncertainty. It is clear from this series that the accuracy which can be achieved by skeletal scintigraphy can never reach 100%. It could be appreciably improved if more strenuous efforts were made to obtain adequate radiographs or tomograms of any equivocal areas, but even so there is a residue which will not be detectable by scintigraphy with existing skeletal imaging agents. It is, however, possible to eliminate false positives by adhering to strict criteria of diagnosis, with only a minimal increase in the false negative rate.

Although it has been known for many years that gallium concentrates in many primary lung tumours, the clinical utility of this information is much less clear. The predictive value of positive gallium scintigraphy for primary lung carcinoma has been put as high as 91% (deMeester et al. 1979) while the predictive value of a negative examination in establishing that a lesion is not a primary lung carcinoma, has been put at 76%. Von Muhe (1971) found gallium scintigraphy to be more accurate than sputum cytology or bronchoscopy in patients with peripheral lung tumours. Indeed some series have found no false negatives. When they do occur they are in general associated with small tumours, less than 1.5 cm in diameter, tumour degeneration or necrosis, other associated lung pathology, recent administration of cytostatic drugs or hepatic activity obscuring tumours in the right lower lobe (Bekerman et al. 1985). However gallium is also taken up by pneumonias and tuberculosis, so that scintigraphy is not useful in differentiating a tumour in the presence of distal infection.

Increasing the administered gallium activity from 100 to 400 MBq (3 to 10 mCi), the use of multiple window pulse height analysers and the introduction of tomography have been associated with a substantial improvement in the detection rate for small peripheral lung tumours. Nevertheless the method is still inferior to radiography, while being considerably more expensive. As ultimately biopsy is always required for final diagnosis, the information provided by gallium in patients with solitary peripheral lesions is of little or no clinical value.

Its role in the detection of hilar and mediastinal metastases is still a matter of controversy. Alazraki et al. (1978, Alazraki 1980) concluded that when there was gallium concentration in the primary tumour but not in the mediastinum, the probability of mediastinal involvement was so low that mediastinoscopy was not indicated and thoracotomy could be considered. However if there was uptake in both sites, the primary failed to concentrate gallium or there was radiographic evidence of mediastinal spread, mediastinoscopy was indicated because of the prevalence of false positive gallium scintigraphy. Other workers (deMeester et al. 1979) found that uptake in the mediastinum in patients with peripheral lesions had a predictive value of 90% with a specificity of 96%. This, however, almost certainly reflects the relatively low probability of occult mediastinal spread in patients with such tumours. The overall accuracy is probably the most useful index. This is 84% for peripheral lesions, falling to

61% for paramediastinal tumours, with a 33% false negative rate for mediastinal nodes.

The differences in interpretation of the significance of their results and in recommendations emanating from different units reflect the difficulty and danger of generalising from small and highly selected series to a more general case. Before advocating any staging procedure it is first necessary to have a clear concept of what effect various possible findings might have on management. At the present time there is no agreement as to how any of these findings should influence treatment. The prognosis is poorer in patients whose disease has extended beyond one hemithorax than in those with limited disease (Ihde et al. 1981) and that of asymptomatic patients with occult bone deposits is worse than that of those without (Merrick and Merrick 1986). The number or site of metastases is not significant. In view of its simplicity, availability, low cost and high true positive rate, bone scintigraphy should be the first investigation for the presence of extrathoracic spread in those patients with lung cancer in whom this information is required. Gallium should be reserved for those with normal bone scintigraphy results.

Conclusion

Scintigraphic procedures thus continue to play an important and varied role in the investigation and management of many common malignant diseases, as part of initial staging, assessment of fitness for therapy, during follow-up, in the detection of toxic effects of treatment and as one of the measures of response. Each technique has a different place in each disease, and it is unwise to generalise. New techniques are continually being developed, and new uses found for old ones. If present and future methods are to be employed to maximum advantage there remains no substitute for meticulous clinical observation and recording. Modern technology greatly eases management of masses of data, but nothing can compensate for incomplete or missing information. Data pollution is evidence only of lack of forethought.

References

Adam NM, Bligh AS, Griffiths PA et al. (1978) Bone scanning in breast cancer. Preliminary statement by British Breast Group on Bone Scanning. Br Med J ii: 180–181

Alazraki NP (1980) Usefulness of gallium imaging in the evaluation of lung cancer. CRC Crit Rev Diagn Imag 13: 249–269

Alazraki NP. Ransdell JW, Taylor AT (1978) Reliability of gallium scan and chest radiography compared to mediastinoscopy for evaluating mediastinal spread in lung cancer. Am Rev Resp Dis 117: 415–422

Bekerman C, Hoffer PB, Bitran JD (1985) The role of gallium-67 in the clinical evaluation of cancer. Semin Nucl Med 15: 72–103

Berche C, Mach JP, Lumbroso JD et al. (1982) Tomoscintigraphy for detecting gastrointestinal and medullary thyroid cancers: first clinical results using radiolabelled monoclonal antibodies against carcinoembryonic antigen. Br Med J 285: 1447–1451

Bishop MC, Hardy JG, Taylor MC et al. (1985) Bone imaging and serum phosphatases in prostatic carcinoma. Br J Urol 57: 317–324

Chaudary MA, Maisey MM, Shaw PJ, Rubens RD, Hayward JL (1983) Sequential bone scans and chest radiographs in the postoperative management of early breast cancer. Br J Surg 70: 517–518

Davey P, Merrick MV, Duncan W, Redpath AT (1985) Bladder cancer: the value of routine bone scintigraphy. Clin Radiol 36: 77–79

DeLand FH, Goldenberg DM (1985) Diagnosis and treatment of neoplasms with radionuclide-labeled antibodies. Semin Nucl Med 15: 2–11

Epenetos AA, Carr D, Johnson PM et al. (1986) Antibody-guided radiolocalisation of tumours in patients with testicular or ovarian cancer using two radioiodinated monoclonal antibodies to placental alkaline phosphatase. Br J Radiol 59: 117–125

Fogelman I, Pearson DW, Bessent RG et al. (1981) A comparison of skeletal uptakes of three diphosphonates by whole-body retention: concise communication. J Nucl Med 22: 880–883

Freedman GS (1973) Radionuclide tomography. Semin Nucl Med 3: 267–284

Galasko CSB (1975) The significance of occult skeletal metastases, detected by skeletal scintigraphy, in patients with otherwise apparently "early" mammary carcinoma. Br J Surg 62: 694–696

Galasko CSB, Westerman B, Li J, Sellwood RA, Burn JI (1968) Use of the gamma camera for early detection of osseous metastases from mammary cancer. Br J Surg 55: 613–615

Goldenberg DM (1983) Tumour imaging with monoclonal antibodies. J Nucl Med 24: 360–362

Goris ML (1985) Sensitivity and specificity of common scintigraphic procedures. Year Book Medical Publishers, Chicago

Gottschalk SC, Salem D, Lim CB, Wake RH (1983) SPECT resolution and uniformity improvements by noncircular orbit. J Nucl Med 24: 822–828

Hoffer PB, Neumann R, Quartararo L, Lange R, Hernandez T (1984) Improved intrinsic resolution: does it make a difference? (Concise Communication). J Nucl Med 25: 230–236

Hooper RG, Beechler CR, Johnson MC (1978) Radioisotope scanning in the initial screening of bronchogenic carcinoma. Am Rev Resp Dis 118: 279–286

Ihde DC, Makuch RW, Carney DN, Bunn PA et al. (1981) Prognostic implications of stage of disease and sites of metastases in patients with small cell carcinoma of the lung treated with intensive combination chemotherapy. Am Rev Resp Dis 123: 500–507

Jagoda EM, Gibson RE, Goodgold H et al. (1984) (I–125)17α-iodovinyl-11β-methoxyestradiol: in vivo and in vitro properties of a high-affinity estrogen-receptor radiopharmaceutical. J Nucl Med 25: 472–477

Jahangir SM, Brill AB, Bizais JC, Rowe RW (1983) Count-rate variations with orientation of camera detector. J Nucl Med 24: 356–359

Kiesewetter DO, Kilbourn MR, Landvatter SW et al. (1984) Preparation of four fluorine-18-labeled estrogens and their selective uptakes in target tissues of immature rats. J Nucl Med 25: 1212–1221

Kirsch C, Moore SC, Zimmerman RE et al. (1981) Characteristics of a scanning, multidetector, single-photon ECT body imager. J Nucl Med 22: 726–731

Kunkler IH, Merrick MV (1986) The value of non-staging skeletal scintigraphy in breast cancer. Clin Radiol 37 (in press)

Kunkler IH, Merrick MV, Rodger A (1985) Bone scintigraphy in breast cancer: a nine-year follow-up. Clin Radiol 36: 279–282

Little AG, DeMeester TR, MacMahon H (1983) The staging of lung cancer. Semin Oncol 10: 56–70

Ludgate SM, Merrick MV (1985) The pathogenesis of post-irradiation chronic diarrhoea: measurement of SeHCAT and B_{12} absorption for differential diagnosis determines treatment. Clin Radiol 36: 275–278

Lund F, Smith PH, Suciu S (1984) EORTC Urological Group. Do bone scans predict prognosis in prostatic cancer? A report of the EORTC protocol no. 30762. Br J Urol 56: 58–63

McEwan AJ, Shapiro B, Sisson JC, Beierwaltes WH, Ackery DM (1985) Radio-iodobenzylguanidine for the scintigraphic location and therapy of adrenergic tumours. Semin Nucl Med 15: 132–153

Matthews MJ, Kanhouwa S, Pickren J, Robinette D (1973) Frequency of residual and metastatic tumour in patients undergoing curative surgical resection for lung cancer. Cancer Chemother Rep 4: 63–67

deMeester TR, Golomb HM, Kirchner P (1979) The role of gallium-67 scanning in the clinical staging and preoperative evaluation of patients with carcinoma of the lung. Ann Thorac Surg 28: 451–464

Merrick MV, Merrick JM (1985) Observations on the natural history of Paget's disease. Clin Radiol 36: 169–174

Merrick MV, Merrick JM (1986) Bone scintigraphy in lung cancer: a reappraisal. Br J Radiol 59 (in press)

Merrick MV, Ding CL, Chisholm GD, Elton RA (1985) Prognostic significance of alkaline and acid phosphatase and skeletal scintigraphy in carcinoma of the prostate. Br J Urol 57: 715–720

von Muhe E (1971) Der Szintigraphische Nachweis von Bronchialkarzinomen mit 67 Gallium Zitrate. Thoraxchirurgie 19: 440–443

Parker MC, Cook A, Riddle PR, Fryatt I, O'Sullivan JO, Shearer RJ (1985) Is delayed treatment justified in carcinoma of prostate? Br J Urol 57: 724–728

Perez DJ, Powles RJ, Milan J et al. (1983) Detection of breast carcinoma metastases in bone: relative merits of X-rays and skeletal scintigraphy. Lancet II: 613–616

Rainsbury RM, Ott RJ, Westwood JH et al. (1983) Location of metastatic breast carcinoma by a monoclonal antibody chelate labelled with indium-111. Lancet II: 934–938

Roberts MM, Hayward JL (1983) Bone scanning and early breast cancer: five year follow-up. Lancet I: 997–998

Rosenthall L, Stern J, Arzoumanian A (1982) A clinical comparison of MDP and DMAD. Clin Nucl Med 7: 403–406

Rossing N, Munch O, Nielsen SP, Andersen KW (1982) Early bone scans in breast cancer. In: Proceedings of the Third World Congress of Nuclear Medicine and Biology Vol 1. Pergamon Press, Oxford, pp 838–841

Sklaroff RB, Sklaroff DM (1976) Bone metastases from breast cancer at the time of radical mastectomy as detected by bone scan: eight-year follow-up. Cancer 38: 107–111

Smith ML, Martin W, McKillop JH, Fogelman I (1984a) Improved lesion detection with dimethyl-amino-diphosphonate: a report of two cases. Eur J Nucl Med 9: 519–520

Smith ML, Martin W, McKillop JH et al. (1984b) DMAD and MDP: a qualitative and quantitative comparison. Nucl Med Commun 5: 240

Smith ML, Martin W, McKillop JH et al. (1985) Bone scan interpretation: a multicentre analysis. Paper presented at the European Nuclear Medicine Congress

Strender LE, Lagergren C, Wallgren A et al. (1981) Role of bone scans in the initial assessment of operable patients with breast cancer. Acta Radiol Oncol 20: 187–191

Subramanian G, McAfee JG, Thomas FD et al. (1983) New diphosphonate compounds for skeletal imaging: comparison with methylene diphosphonate. Radiology 149: 823–828

Tofe AJ, Francis MD, Harvey WJ (1975) Correlation of neoplasms with incidence and localization of skeletal metastases: an analysis of 1335 diphosphonate bone scans. J Nucl Med 16: 986–989

Turner P, Haggith JW (1981) Preoperative radionuclide scanning in bronchogenic carcinoma. Br J Dis Chest 75: 291–294

Waxman AD, Julien PJ, Brachman MB et al. (1984) Gallium scintigraphy in bronchogenic carcinoma. Chest 86: 178–183

Williams SJ, Green M, Kerr IH (1977) Detection of bone metastases in carcinoma of bronchus. Br Med J i: 1004

10 Positron Emission Tomography in Oncology

Terry Jones

Introduction

Functional differences are sought between the tumour and normal tissue in order to design methods for improving the treatment of cancer. The aim is to exploit these differences in order to achieve a therapeutic advantage. There is a need, therefore, to measure in vivo the regional tissue biochemistry, physiology and pharmacology. These help form a rationale not only for treatment but for objectively assessing therapeutic response and mechanisms of cell killing. This paper discusses one of the most advanced methods for non-invasively measuring regional tissue function in man. The physical aspects of this investigative speciality are described together with some examples of its use.

The use of gamma-ray-emitting radioisotopes as labels for detecting the regional tissue content of a biological compound in vivo provides a non-invasive means for examining functional aspects of focal tissue disease. This is already an established routine diagnostic procedure known as nuclear medicine that is discussed in Chapter 9 of this volume. In order to exploit the technique of positron emission tomography, gamma-ray-emitting radioisotopes of the elements that constitute biological compounds are required. However, radioisotopes in this category have short radioactive half-lives: oxygen-15, nitrogen-13 and carbon-11, with half-lives of 2.1, 10 and 20.1 minutes respectively, are the longest-lived gamma-ray-emitting isotopic forms of these elements. There is no suitable gamma-ray-emitting isotope of hydrogen, but flourine-18, with a half-life of 110 minutes, can be used as a hydrogen substitute for labelling. All of these short-lived isotopes have two common features. First, they can be manufactured by bombarding specific stable elements with high-energy ionic beams of radiation as produced using a particle accelerator such as a cyclotron. Secondly, when they undergo radioactive disintegration these isotopes emit positrons—positively charged electron-like particles. These travel away from the exploding nucleus, but because they are captured by electrons they penetrate no further than a few millimetres in living matter. Fig. 10.1 shows this process and that following capture. Both the electron and the positron involved annihilate. The energy of this loss of matter is expressed as two photons, each 511 KeV in energy, emitted at approximately 180° to each other. Hence, from a subject containing a positron emitter, correlated pairs of photons emerge from the body in opposite directions.

The emitted photons have to be recorded in such a way that computerised tomographic reconstruction can be made of their spatial distribution. To effect this, positron emission tomography (PET) scanning is employed. This provides accurate quantitative values of the tissue's concentration of a positron-emitting isotope. Such measurements, in combination with the use of biologically compatible radiotracers, represent one of the most advanced means for studying in vivo the regional tissue biochemistry, physiology and pharmacology in man. The following describes how these tomograms are achieved and how quantitative values of tissue function can be realised. The performance of the PET scanners themselves continues to be refined. Indications are given as to the ultimate spatial resolution that will be achieved with these machines. Also discussed are the more advanced and specific pathways of regional tissue function that may be followed in the future and how these investigative techniques may be exploited in oncology.

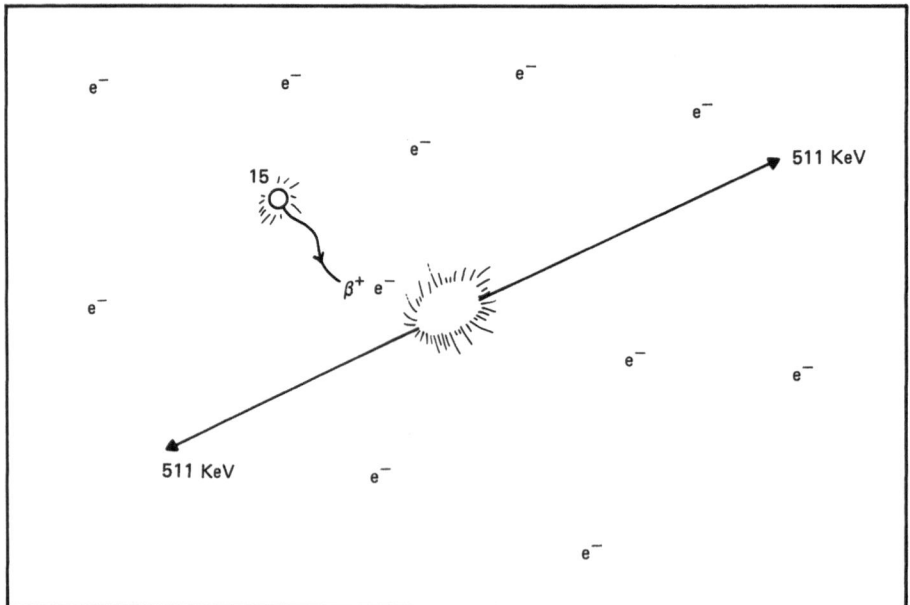

Fig. 10.1. The positively charged, beta-like particle, the positron (β^+) is emitted from the disintegrating oxygen-15 atom. This travels at most a few millimetres in tissue before it is captured by an oppositely charged electron (e^-). Both particles annihilate and the energy of this loss of matter is expressed as two photons, each 511 KeV in energy, emitted at approximately 180° to each other.

PET Scanner Design

The pairs of annihilated photons emitted are registered by placing detectors on opposite sides of the body which operate in coincidence with each other. When one detector registers an event, electronic time windows, of less than 15 nanoseconds, open and shut. If, during this brief period, a detector on the opposite side of the body also registers a photon event, the two detectors concerned record a coincident event. For this to happen a positron–electron capture much have occurred somewhere along the line of sight between the two coincident detectors. In order to achieve tomographic reconstruction, a 360° sampling of such coincident lines around the body is required. This has been achieved in the past with polygon arrays of coincident detectors arranged around a single or series of transaxial planes through the body.

A paper in the previous volume in this series (Beaney 1986) illustrates the whole-body hexagonal array PET scanner that was in use at the Hammersmith Hospital, London, between 1979 and 1985 (Phelps et al. 1978, Williams et al. 1979). Fig. 10.2 shows this system in which the individual banks of detectors translate and rotate to record the angular information needed for computerised reconstruction of the transaxial tomographic distribution of the positron-emitting radioisotope. Octagonal arrays of coincident detectors have also been used for a brain PET scanner (Hoffman et al. 1983a). Present generations of machines have circular detector configurations.

The spatial resolution of a PET scanner relates directly to the individual detector apertures used. Although high spatial resolution is sought, the result of using too small a detector aperture is that sufficient counting events may not be registered and the system becomes too insensitive to record meaningful tomograms. Initial PET tomographs such as that shown in Fig. 10.2 were a compromise design in which statistically adequate tomograms could be recorded in man with spatial resolutions of around 17 mm full width at half maximum (FWHM) of the line spread function. These early scanners were only able to record one plane of transaxial data at a time. Nevertheless, their detection accuracy is representative of the most important quantitative aspects offered by this form of scanning. Later, the physical characteristics of the current generation of PET scanners are discussed as well as their expected future performance.

Accuracy

The geometrical arrangement of the coincident detectors is the key to the accuracy they exhibit for measuring tissue concentrations of positron-emitting tracers. Central to this is the need to ensure that the spatial resolution is uniform throughout the recorded transaxial tomogram. Also the vulnerability of the system to registering false coincident radiation (due either to random events or events in which one of the photons was scattered prior to detection) has to be minimised. In an optimally designed PET scanner these sources of error have been overcome by placing the coincident detectors sufficiently far apart (100 cm in the body scanner shown in Fig. 10.2) and shielding the sensitive elements from

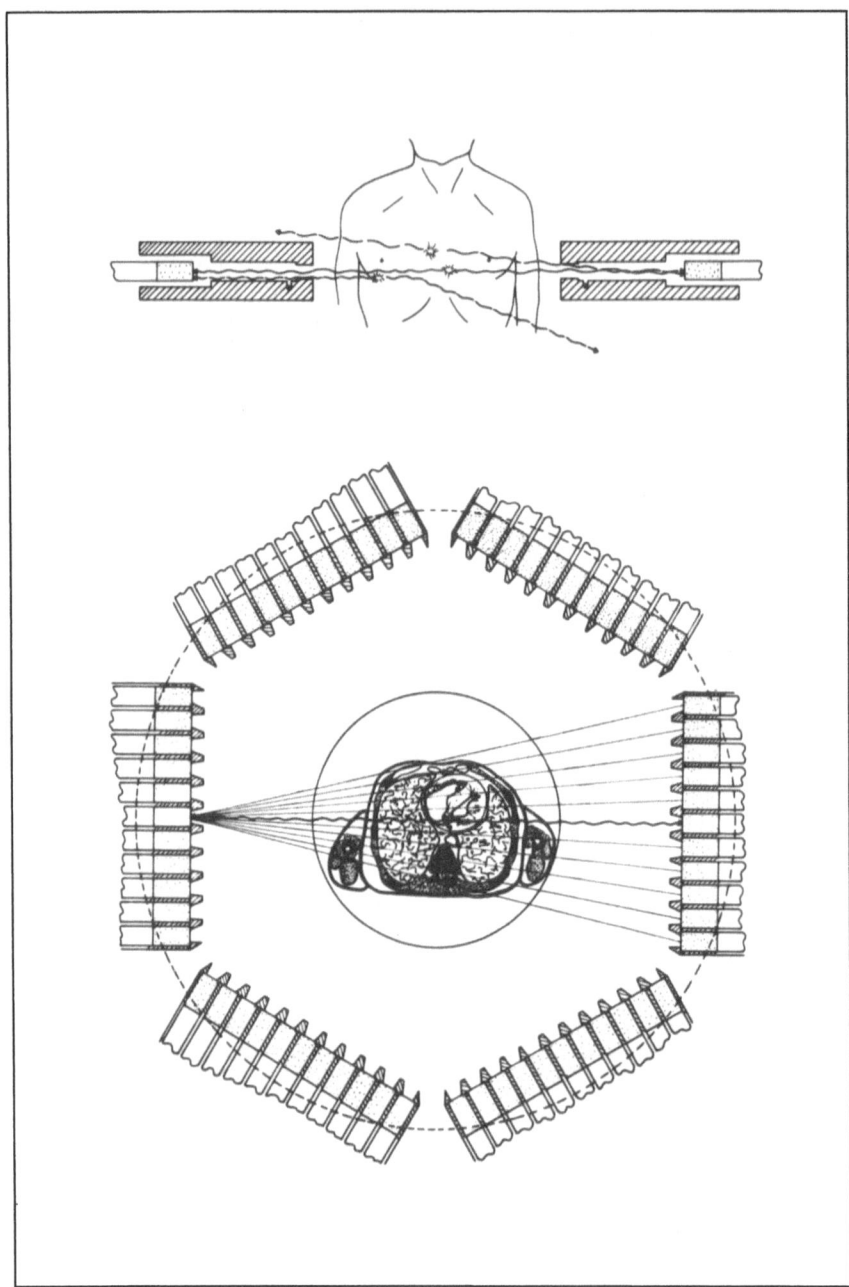

Fig. 10.2. The construction of a first-generation PET scanner. The pairs of emitted annihilation photons are recorded by coincidence radiation detectors placed on opposite sides of the body. A hexagonal array of detectors is shown arranged around a single tomographic plane through the body. Each detector on a hexagonal face can record a coincidence event with eleven detectors on the opposite face. A total of 363 coincident pairs may be registered. Using this arrangement, and with the detectors translating and rotating, sufficient angular information is recorded for the tomographic distribution of a positron-emitting tracer to be reconstructed by computer routines.

their sides. Minimal interference arises from radioactivity outside the coincident plane. Also, the comparatively narrow solid angle for detection ensures that if one of the annihilation photons arising within the plane is scattered, it is unlikely to be registered (Fig. 10.2). The inherent accuracy of such a scanner as determined from physical phantom studies has been reported by Phelps et al. (1978), Soussaline et al. (1979) and T. Jones et al. (1985). In summary, the spatial resolution of a 17 mm FWHM machine is uniform to within 1 mm throughout a tomographic reconstruction of a 20 cm diameter object. False coincidences arising from the registering of scattered and random events is of the order of a few per cent of the levels of activity recorded within the active regions.

A final aspect of accuracy offered by a PET scanner is that absolute corrections can be made for the loss of signal due to attenuation in the body of the emitted photons. The goal is to measure tissue concentration of tracer. Therefore, distortion due to loss of counts has to be accounted for irrespective of the isotope's location and the tissue media surrounding it. For any pair of coincident detectors the effective attenuation length is the thickness of the body that intervenes in the direct line between the two detectors. If a positron is captured near one side of the body, one of the annihilation photons only has to pass through air before meeting a radiation detector. However, the other photon emitted at 180° has to pass through the total thickness of the body before it reaches the coincident detectors on the opposite side. Hence the probability of not registering a coincidence relates to the effective attenuation length, i.e. the total thickness of the body. If on the other hand the positron capture occurs on the other side of the body, then the photon which in the above case had only to pass through air has now to traverse the total thickness of the body before it can be registered. Its partner has only to pass through air. Once again the probability of not registering this event relates to the total thickness of the body. For positron capture occurring in the middle of the body, each photon has to traverse half the body's thickness and here again the probability of the coincidence event not being recorded is the sum of the attenuation lengths, i.e. the total thickness of the body. This attenuation effect is unlike that occurring in conventional nuclear medicine procedures which involve the detection of single photon-emitting radioisotopes. For example, with a gamma camera viewing the body and recording ^{99m}Tc (single 140 KeV photon emitter) the image counts obtained will depend on the relative depths at which the tracer is located. The signal in this case is dependent on both the tissue's concentration of tracer and its depth in the body.

The tissue attenuation effect of positron emitters means that for any two coincident detectors the strength of the recorded signal is independent of the depth in the body where the tracer resides. This unique feature is exploited to realise absolute correction for attenuation. It is achieved by surrounding the subject with a ring source of a positron-emitting isotope (e.g. gallium-68) and recording a transmission scan prior to administering the tracer (Beaney 1986). For any line pair of coincident detectors, the ratio of the signals recorded from the ring source in air (in the absence of a patient) to that when the patient is in the scanner gives the attenuation factors for that line pair. These are the same as those imposed on the pairs of photons emitted from within the patient. The accuracy of this means of attenuation correction was tested using phantoms of the brain and chest. For a point source placed within the chest phantom, after effecting attenuation corrections with the ring source method, the picture element counts from a region of interest around the point source were the same as when the source was scanned in air with no surrounding attenuation medium. Also a common solution of a positron-emitting isotope was placed in a heart compartment within the chest phantom and in a brain phantom. When both phantoms were scanned and corrected for attenuation with the ring source transmission scan, the same picture element counts were found for the heart as the brain. These simple examples represent a range of attenuating conditions and indicate that tomographic distributions of a positron-emitting tracer can be registered and corrected such that the picture element counts become independent of whereabouts in the body the isotope is located.

In effect one is able, with such an attenuation correction, to record tomographic distributions of isotope that would have been registered if the tissues were fully transparent to the emitted photons. This in turn means that the picture element response, within the attenuation-corrected tomogram, can be calibrated against a laboratory well counter. Fig. 10.3 illustrates this, where a phantom, uniformly filled with a solution of a positron emitter, is scanned and at the same time an aliquot of the solution measured in a well counter. From this, the scanner's picture element response as counts per picture element per second can be expressed as counts per second per millilitre in the well counter. By calibrating the well counter against a universal standard, the counts in the PET images can be converted into microcuries per millilitre of tissue. As demonstrated above, the calibration is universal to any part of the body. Hence during a tracer study in a subject, well counter measurements of the dose of isotope administered or in withdrawn blood samples and the resulting image counts can

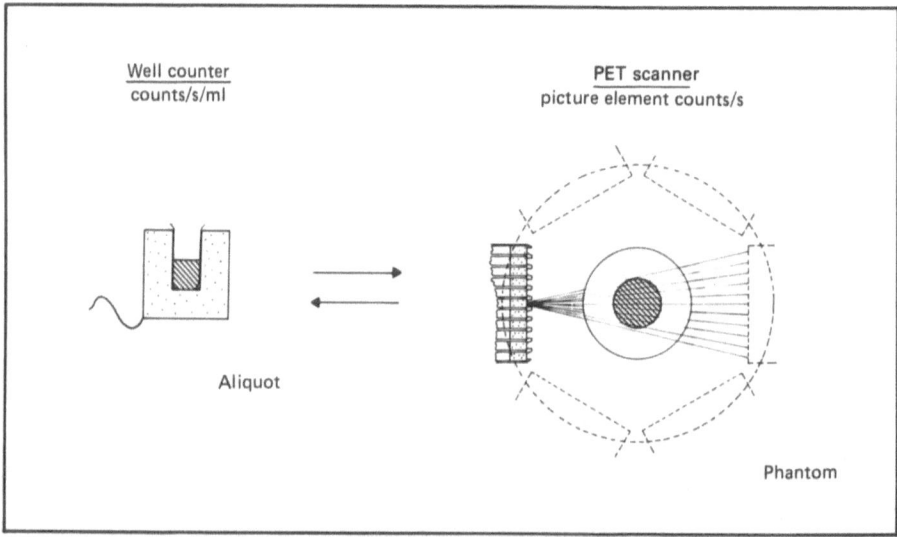

Fig. 10.3. The picture element response of the PET scanner may be calibrated against the laboratory well counter response. Hence a picture element count per second recorded for a regional tissue in man, can be converted into what would have been recorded per second if a millilitre of that tissue were measured in a well counter. Blood samples, injected dose and tissue activities can all be measured in the same units. This enables specific tracer model equations to be solved directly to obtain absolute values of the functional parameters being measured.

be expressed in the same units. This provides an in vivo assay of tracer and allows specific tracer models to be solved to provide absolute values for the functional entities being traced.

In summary, the physical accuracy of a correctly designed PET scanner provides uniform spatial resolution within the body, low noise due to false recordings and an ability to measure absolute tissue concentrations of positron-emitting isotope. The principal limitation for quantitation is the actual spatial resolution itself. The partial volume effect states that the concentration of tracer within an object cannot be correctly measured if the object's physical size is less than twice the scanner's spatial resolution (FWHM) (Hoffman et al. 1979). Hence for a first-generation machine as shown in Fig. 10.2, true quantitative (μCi/ml of tissue) could not be achieved if the tissue were smaller than a 34 mm diameter sphere. Although it was possible to detect and visualise structures of smaller dimensions, full recovery of counts could not be realised. However, if the object's size is known and the tracer is uniformly distributed within it, then corrections can be made for the under-sampling from corresponding phantom data. For further information on the performance of PET scanners the review by Hoffman and Phelps (1986) is recommended.

Applications of PET in Oncology

The use of PET in oncology practice to date has centred mainly on brain tumours, not least because the major applications of PET in medicine have been in neurology and psychiatry. Beaney (1986), in the previous volume in this series, devoted to tumours of the brain, reviewed the use of PET in cerebral neoplasms. Further review chapters, including PET studies of non-cerebral tumours, have been written (Beaney 1984, Beaney and Lammertsma 1985). Here some examples are given of the use of PET in studying tumour biochemistry, physiology and pharmacology. The nature of future studies is also discussed, together with applications.

Biochemistry

Recent studies of lung carcinoma using the glucose analogue [^{18}F]fluorodeoxy-glucose have shown 10 times the uptake of tracer by tumour compared with surrounding lung (Nolop et al. 1985, 1986). This high tumour uptake has also been seen in brain neoplasms (Rhodes et al. 1983, Di Chiro et al. 1984) and liver metastases (Yonekura et al. 1982). Fig. 10.4 shows quantitative values of blood flow and of utilisation of glucose and oxygen in human brain tumours and the surrounding cerebral tissues. This demonstration in vivo of the high preferential aerobic glycolytic activity of human tumours adds support to therapeutic regimes aimed at inhibiting mitochondrial function and biogenesis (Gear 1974, Bernal et al. 1983). A recent report of the high use in brain tumours of ^{11}C-labelled Putrescine (Hiesiger et al. 1986), a polyamine, offers an additional lead for selective inhibition of a neoplasm's metabolism.

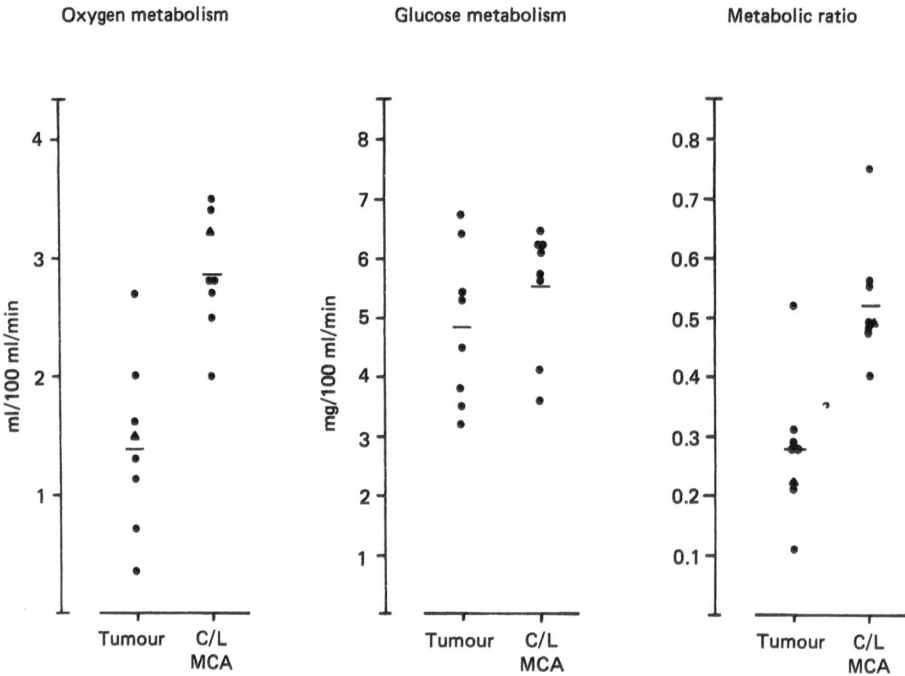

Fig. 10.4. Quantitative values of oxygen (^{15}O) and glucose (^{18}FDG) utilisation for gliomas and contralateral cerebral cortex tissue (C/L MCA, contralateral middle cerebral artery) for a series of patients. (▲, one of 16 patients who did not have a correction made for the presence of intravascular tracer. ●, the other 15 patients whose values were corrected.) Note the relatively low use of oxygen by the tumours and their decreased metabolic ratio (oxygen utilised per unit of glucose utilised). This indicates the tumour's preferential aerobic glycolytic metabolism (Rhodes et al. 1983).

Physiology

An example of physiological studies of non-cerebral tumours comes from work on breast carcinoma. Beaney et al. (1984) measured in both the tumour and normal breast tissue, blood flow, fractional blood volume, oxygen utilisation and the fractional extraction of oxygen within the capillary bed. Fig. 10.5 shows that the blood flow of the tumours studied was in all cases higher than that in the normal breast tissue. This is relevant to drug delivery and the application of hyperthermia, where means for the differential heating of tumours is sought. The values for the fractional blood volume of the tumours were similar to those measured in the normal breast tissue. This indicates that the tumour vascularity (tissue blood volume) does not develop in parallel to its perfusion, unlike the situation in normal tissue. The fraction of oxygen extracted by the tumour from the arterial blood was significantly lower than the value for normal tissue. This indicates that carcinomas are, at least macroscopically, not ischaemic in that the blood draining into the veins is comparatively well oxygenated (low fractional extraction of oxygen). Similar results have been found in brain tumours (Ito et al. 1982, Lammertsma et al. 1985).

Pharmacology

The sensitivity of a PET scanner for detecting compounds within the body is in the picomolar range. Hence tracer kinetic studies can be carried out in vivo without the danger of the tracer doses interfering with the functional state of the tissues. This is an important consideration, particularly in the study of receptor ligands where very low levels of compounds produce functional effects.

A good example of the use of PET for pharmacological studies in tumours comes from the work of the Montreal group. They have labelled BCNU (bis(2-chloroethyl)-1-nitrosourea) with carbon-11 and studied the tissue kinetics of this chemotherapeutic agent in gliomas. It was found that tumours varied considerably with respect to the uptake and retention of the tracer. Following assessment of tissue pharmacokinetics of [^{11}C]BCNU, they prescribed therapeutic doses of unlabelled drug (often by selective arterial cannulation) (Diksic et al. 1984).

The use of PET and labelled ligands to delineate receptor activity in vivo is currently attracting much attention. From the outset, there have been doubts as to whether or not receptor uptake could be delineated in the presence of non-specifically bound tracer within the tissue. However, by the appropriate selection of markers, the dopaminergic (Garnett et al. 1983, Wagner et al. 1983, Leenders et al. 1984, Farde et al. 1986) and opiate receptors (Frost et al. 1985,

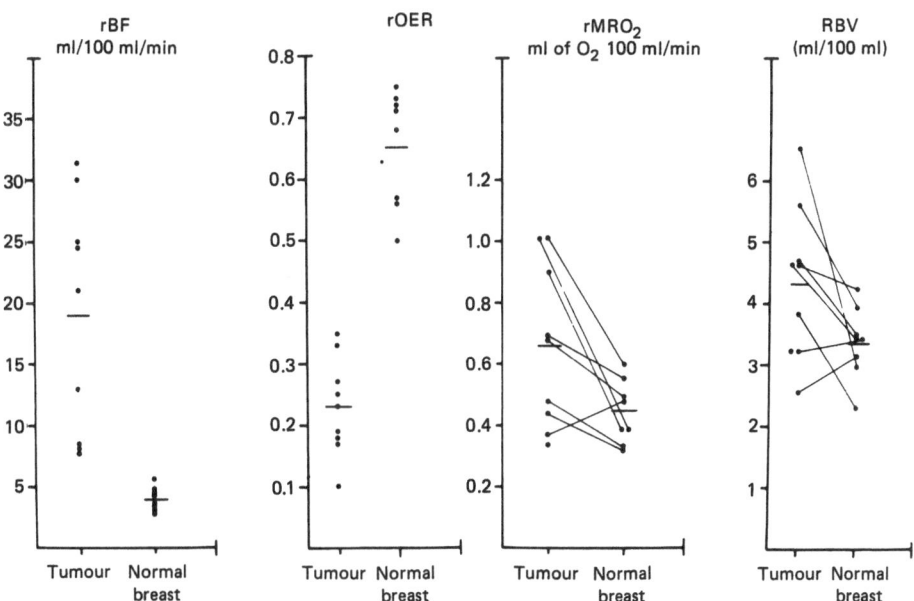

Fig. 10.5. Data from human breast carcinoma and normal breast tissue on values of regional blood flow (rBF), regional blood volume (rBV), regional oxygen utilisation (rMRO$_2$) and the regional fractional extraction of oxygen per single pass through the tissue (rOER). Tumour blood flow is higher than that for normal tissue. Tumour blood volume (vascularity) does not relate to tumour blood flow (perfusion). The tumour's oxygen extraction is low compared with that of normal tissue suggesting that macroscopically the tumour is not ischaemic (Beaney et al. 1984).

A. K. P. Jones et al. 1985) have been delineated in the brain and the muscarinic receptors in the myocardium (Syrota et al. 1984). The levels of material involved are extremely low and the high sensitivity of PET is unrivalled for such in vivo measurements.

Improvements in PET Scanners

It is clear that for visualisation and measurement, the spatial resolution should be as high as possible. Considerable interest has and is being focused on seeking ways to improve resolution together with overall detector sensitivity. The direct approach is to make the individual detector elements as small as possible and to assemble multidetector planes. The original PET scanners used sodium iodide scintillation crystals. These have now been superseded by crystals of bismuth germanate (BGO) which is a much denser compound (Cho et al. 1976). They can be made smaller than those of sodium iodide before cross-talk between detector elements becomes a problem (photons entering one detector and then penetrating into an adjacent element). It has been estimated that BGO crystals as small as 2–3 mm in diameter could be used. As the individual detectors become smaller, the problem arises of how to record their light output. In the earlier machines, each crystal was coupled to a photomultiplier (PM). The smallest practical PM tubes are around 10 mm in diameter. These have been used to construct the present PET scanners (Hoffman et al. 1983b, 1985). One to one coupling of a crystal to PM is not only costly but does not address the problem of readout from the desired smaller detectors.

The new generation of PET scanners will circumvent this problem by sharing the light output from arrays of crystals between comparatively few PM tubes which are physically larger than the individual BGO crystals. A ratio of detector to PM tubes of 8:1 is planned which provides a more cost-effective design (Carroll et al. 1985). Fig. 10.6 shows a comparison between the matrix of small BGO detectors being viewed with comparatively few PM tubes and the detector/PM configuration used in the first-generation PET scanner (Fig. 10.2). This schematic diagram shows round-section PM tubes being used to view the BGO matrix, but in practice these will be of a square section.

The spatial resolution of current PET scanners using BGO crystals is around 5 mm FWHM, which compares with the 17 mm FWHM of early scanners. This means that the volume of tissue within which the tracer concentration can be measured is now 20 times smaller than was possible with the first machines. Also, the multiple crystal planes allow many more transaxial tomograph recordings to be registered simultaneously, and the detectors being arranged in a circle rather than scanning polygons allows the recording of faster time frames of data.

The question remains as to what the limit of spatial resolution is that will be achieved in a PET scanner. This is defined by two physical restraints. The first concerns the distance that the positron travels in tissue, away from the disintegrating nucleus. This depends on the energy of the positron itself. Fig. 10.7 depicts the spectrum of distances which 1.74 MeV positrons emitted by oxygen-15 could travel in tissue. The uncertainty imposed by variable

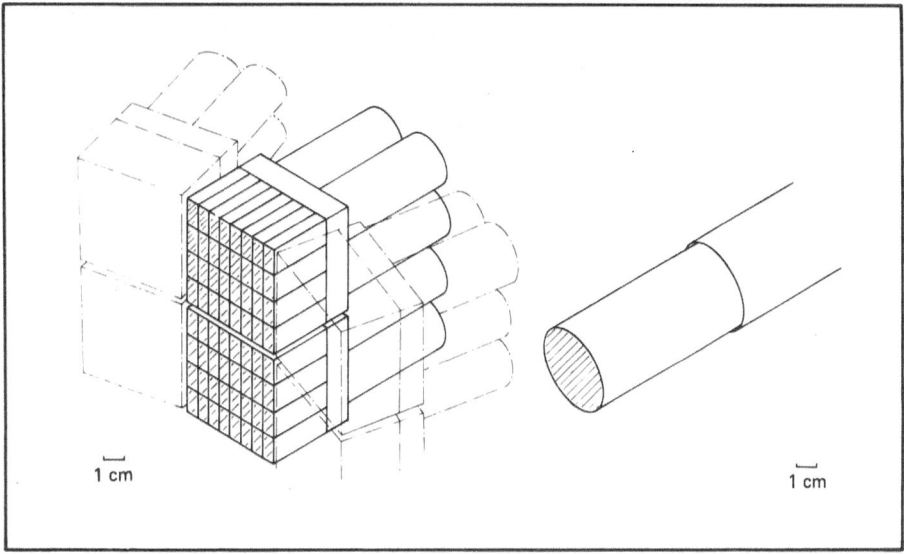

Fig. 10.6. Radiation detector configuration of a new-generation design of PET scanner. Smaller detector elements of bismuth germanate (BGO) are used and viewed by an array of photomultipliers. Compare this arrangement with the single larger detector element (shown on the right) as used in the first-generation scanner illustrated in Fig. 10.2.

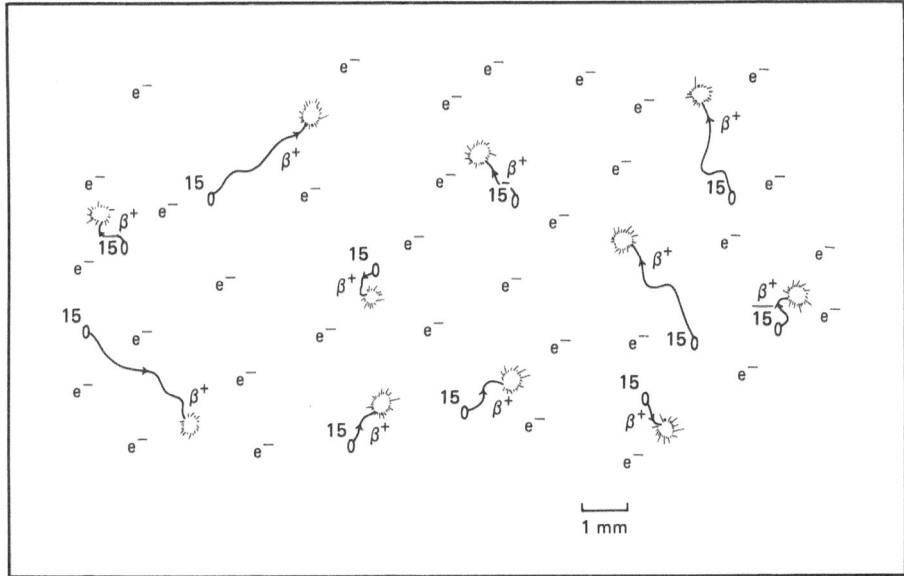

Fig. 10.7. The positrons (β^+) emitted from a radionuclide such as oxygen-15 have a variable path length in tissue before being captured by an electron (e^-). This introduces an uncertainty as to the actual location of the disintegrating radionuclides.

penetration defines the spatial accuracy with which the positron of the radioisotope can be located. For an isotope like oxygen-15, this introduces a spread of around 1.5 mm FWHM (Cho et al. 1976). An additional distortion is the fact that when the positron is captured by an electron, both particles will have some residual kinetic energy. The annihilation photons express this energy, which is in excess of the mass of the two particles, by being emitted at not exactly 180° to each other (De Benedetti et al. 1950). Fig. 10.8 shows the ± 1.25° spread from the 180° emission. This again imposes a distortion on the spatial resolution that can be realised with a PET scanner. The effect becomes more important for the larger 100 cm diameter body machines, where a spread of approximately 1 mm FWHM results. The physical limit in spatial resolution with PET is predicted to be 2–3 mm FWHM.

The remaining potential for further design improvement is in increasing detector sensitivity—by using either more dense detector materials, greater solid angles, or time of flight techniques (Allemand et al. 1980). The increase in solid angles is an attractive approach (Anger and Rosenthal 1959, Burnham and Brownell 1972, Meuhllehner et al. 1976, Jeavons et al. 1983, Bateman et al. 1984). However, care is required since the percentage of false coincidences increases appreciably with increasing solid angle due to the registering of scattered and random coincidences (Derenzo et al. 1975).

PET scanners offer, for in vivo tracer studies, unrivalled spatial resolution and quantitation of tissue tracer concentrations. In a correctly designed system the registering of noise due to false readings is low. The sensitivity for detecting tissue concentration of molecules is in the picomolar range, which is unrivalled by any other non-invasive methodology.

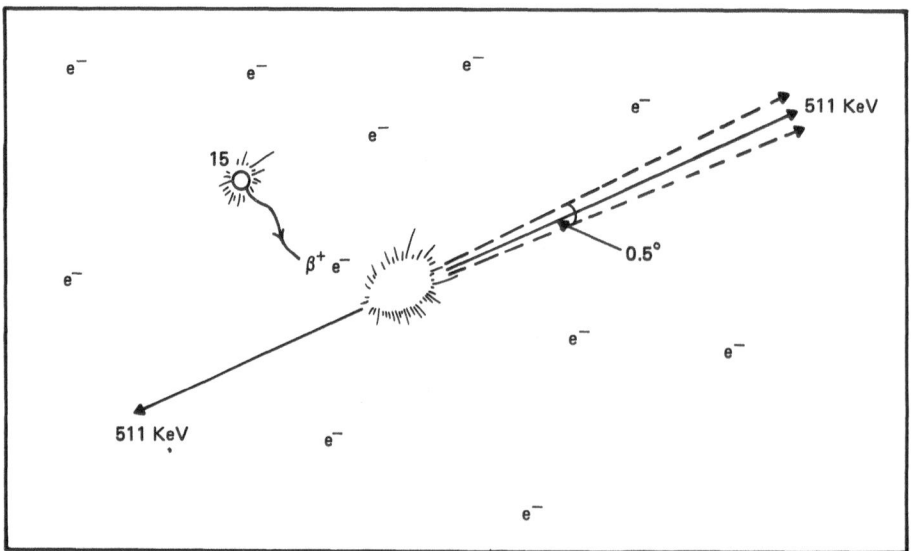

Fig. 10.8. The positron (β^+) at the point at which it is captured will have some remaining kinetic energy and so will the electron (e^-). This additional sum of energy is expressed by a spread (± 0.25°) of the emitted annihilation photons around the 180° emission which introduces some uncertainty as to the actual location of the radionuclide.

Table 10.1. The advantages of positron emission tomography

1.	A wide range of tracer studies for in vivo biochemistry, physiology and pharmacology are possible using ^{15}O, ^{13}N, ^{11}C and ^{18}F
2.	Quantitative measurements (μCi/ml) are possible at low tissue concentrations (picomoles) of labelled molecule
3.	High spatial resolution (< 5 FWHM) is possible uniformly throughout the body

Conclusions

Table 10.1 summarises the principal advantages offered by PET. From the outset, the future role of PET in oncology is as a clinical research tool where the aim is to obtain new information on human cancer and its treatment. The use of PET in oncology outside of brain tumours has to date been under-exploited. The reasons for this are not wholly clear but may lie with the fact that PET images of function have not been so visually eye-catching as images of morphology provided so well with X-ray CT and nuclear magnetic resonance imaging. Maybe the new generation of high-resolution multiplane PET scanners will attract more attention from would-be investigators. The scope for using PET for studying regional tissue function is immense. For example radiochemical synthetic routes have already been identified whereby up to 80% of the drugs in the pharmacopoeia could be labelled with carbon-11 within 40 minutes. For cancer, receptor studies could be of direct interest in breast cancer. Plans are being made to use carbon-11 to label DNA precursors such as thymidine and hence study cellular proliferation in human tumours. Attempts are also being made to label misonidazole to study hypoxic cell fractions. A search continues for a suitable long-lived positron-emitting isotope for monoclonal antibody studies.

The implementation of PET is expensive and involves a range of specific expertise. It will therefore remain for some time within the domain of clinical research. By studying the biochemistry, physiology and pharmacology of human tumours, a means is offered for defining how neoplasms differ from normal tissue. The rationale for therapy may be developed and examined in functional terms and therapeutic responses assessed objectively.

References

Allemand R, Gresset C, Vacher J (1980) Potential advantages of a caesium fluoride scintillator for a time-of-flight positron camera. J Nucl Med 21: 153–155

Anger HO, Rosenthal DJ (1959) Scintillation camera and positron camera in medical radioisotope scanning. International Atomic Energy Agency, Vienna, p 59

Bateman JE, Connolly JF, Stephenson R, Flesher AC (1984) The Rutherford Laboratory Mark I MWPC Positron Camera. Nucl Inst Meth 225: 209–231

Beaney RP (1984) Positron emission tomography in the study of human tumors. Semin Nucl Med 14: 324–341

Beaney RP (1986) Functional aspects of human brain tumours as studied by positron emission tomography. In: NM Bleehen (ed) Tumours of the brain. Springer-Verlag, Berlin Heidelberg New York Tokyo, pp 63–82

Beaney RP, Lammertsma AA (1985) The use of PET in oncology. In: M Reivich (ed) Positron emission tomography. Alan R Liss Inc, New York, pp 425–450

Beaney RP, Lammertsma AA, Jones T, McKenzie CG, Halnan KE (1984) In vivo measurements of regional blood flow, oxygen utilisation and blood volume in patients with carcinoma of the breast using positron emission tomography. Lancet I: 131–134

Bernal SD, Lampidis TJ, McIsaac RM, Chen LB (1983) Anticarcinoma activity in vivo of rhodamine- 1,2,3, a mitochondrial-specific dye. Science 222: 169–172

Burnham CA, Brownell GL (1972) A multi-crystal positron camera. IEEE Trans Nucl Sci NS–19: 201–205

Carroll LR, Nutt R, Casey M (1985) Modelling a multi-crystal detector block for PET. J Nucl Med 26: p 98 (abstr)

Cho ZH, Farukhi MR (1976) Bismuth germanate as a potential scintillation detector in positron cameras. J Nucl Med 18: 840–844

Cho ZH, Chan JK, Ericksson L et al. (1976) Positron ranges obtained from biomedically important positron emitting radionuclides. J Nucl Med 16: 1174–1176

De Benedetti S, Cowan CE, Konneker WR, Primakoff H (1950) On the angular distribution of two-photon annihilation radiation. Phys Rev 77: 205–212

Derenzo SE, Zakland H, Budinger TF (1975) Analytical study of a high resolution positron ring detector system for transaxial reconstruction tomography. J Nucl Med 16: 1166–1173

Di Chiro G, Brooks RA, Patronas NJ et al. (1984) Issues in the in vivo measurement of glucose metabolism of human central nervous system tumors. Ann Neurol 15 [Suppl] S138–S146

Diksic M, Sako K, Feindel W et al. (1984) Pharmacokinetics of positron-labelled BCNU in human brain tumors using positron emission tomography. Cancer Res 44: 3120–3124

Farde L, Hall H, Ehrin E, Sedvall G (1986) Quantitative analysis of D2 dopamine receptor binding in the living human brain by PET. Science 231: 258–261

Frost JT, Wagner HM, Dannals RF et al. (1985) Imaging opiate receptors in the human brain by positron emission tomography. J Comput Assist Tomogr 9: 231–236

Garnett ES, Firnau G, Nahmias C (1983) Dopamine visualized in the basal ganglia of living man. Nature (Lond) 305: 137–138

Gear ARL (1974) Rhodamine-6G: a potent inhibitor of mitochondrial oxidative phosphorylation. J Biol Chem 249: 3628–3637

Hiesiger EM, Fowler J, Brodie JD et al. (1986) Imaging of human brain tumors by positron emission tomography (PET) using [1–11C] Putrescine (11C–PU) and [1–11C]-2-deoxy-D-glucose (11C–2DG). Proc Ann Meet Am Assoc Cancer Res 27:155 (abstr)

Hoffman EJ, Phelps ME (1986) Positron emission tomography: principles and quantitation. In: Phelps ME, Mazziotta JC, Schelbert HR (eds) Positron emission tomography and autoradiography. Raven Press, New York, pp 237–286

Hoffman EJ, Huang SC, Phelps ME (1979) Quantitation in positron emission computed tomography, I. Effect of object size. J Comput Assist Tomogr 3: 299–308

Hoffman EJ, Phelps ME, Huang SC (1983a) Performance characteristics of a multiplane positron tomograph designed for brain studies. J Nucl Med 24: 245–257

Hoffman EJ, Ricci AR, van der Stee LMAM, Phelps ME (1983b) ECAT III: basic design considerations. IEEE Trans Nucl Sci NS–30: 729–733

Hoffman EJ, Phelps ME, Huang SC et al. (1985) ECAT III: A new PET system for heart and whole body dynamic imaging. J Nucl Med 26: p 28 (abstr)

Ito M, Lammertsma AA, Bernardi S et al. (1982) Measurement of regional cerebral blood flow and oxygen utilisation in patients with cerebral tumours using ^{15}O and positron emission tomography: analytical techniques and preliminary results. Neuroradioliogy 23: 63–74

Jeavons A, Hood K, Herlin G et al. (1983) The high density avalanche chamber for positron emission tomography. IEEE Trans Nucl Sci NS–30: 1, 640–645

Jones AKP, Luthra SK, Pike VW, Herold S, Brady F (1985) New labelled for in-vivo studies of opioid physiology. Lancet III: 665–666

Jones T, Forse GR, Heather JD, Rhodes CG (1985) Positron techniques. In: ED Williams (ed) An introduction to emission computed tomography. Institute of Physical Science in Medicine Report No. 44, pp 39–45

Lammertsma AA, Wise RJS, Cox TCS, Thomas DGT, Jones T (1985) Measurement of blood flow, oxygen utilisation, oxygen extraction ratio and fractional blood volume in human brain tumours and surrounding oedematous tissue. Br J Radiol 58: 725–734

Leenders KL, Herold S, Brooks DJ et al. (1984) Pre-synaptic and post-synaptic dopaminergic system in human brain. Lancet III: 110–111

Muehllehner G, Buchin MP, Dukek JH (1976) Performance parameters of a positron imaging camera. IEE Trans Nucl Sci NS–23: 528–537

Nolop KB, Brudin L, Rhodes CG, Beaney RP, Hughes JMB (1985) Glucose utilisation by

pulmonary squamous cell carcinomas in man. Clin Sci [Suppl 12] 69: 46p (abstr)
Nolop KB, Brudin L, Rhodes CG et al. (1986) Glucose utilization in vivo by human pulmonary neoplasms. Ann Int Med (submitted)
Phelps ME, Hoffman EJ, Huang SC, Kuhl DE (1978) ECAT: a new computerized tomographic imaging system from positron-omitting radiopharmaceuticals. J Nucl Med 19: 635–647
Rhodes CG, Wise RJS, Gibbs JM et al. (1983) In vivo disturbance of the oxidative metabolism of glucose in human cerebral gliomas. Ann Neurol 14: 614–626
Soussaline F, Todd-Pokropek AE, Plummer D et al. (1979) The physical performances of a single slice positron tomographic system and preliminary results in a clinical environment. Eur J Nucl Med 4: 237–249
Syrota A, Paillotin G, Davy JM et al. (1984) Kinetics of in vivo binding of antagonist to muscarinic cholinergic receptor in the human heart studied by positron emission tomography. Life Sci 35: 837–845
Wagner HN Jr, Burns HD, Dannals RF et al. (1983) Imaging dopamine receptors in the human brain by positron tomography. Science 221: 1264
Williams CW, Crabtree MC, Burgiss SG (1979) Design and performance characteristics of a positron emission axial tomograph: ECAT II. IEEE Trans Nucl Sci NS–26: 619–627
Yonekura Y, Benua RS, Brill AB, et al. (1982) Increased accumulation of 2-deoxy-2-[^{18}F]fluoro-D-glucose in liver metastases from colon carcinoma. J Nucl Med 23: 1133–1137

11 Recent Advances in Radiotherapy and Oncology and Expectations for the Future

Jerzy Einhorn

Introduction

This volume has detailed some of the major techniques available in the practice of oncology. I shall attempt to put these in the perspective of cancer incidence, prevention, diagnosis and treatment.

First some figures. It is believed that every third person living in Europe in the year 2000 will develop a cancer during his or her lifetime. A recent initiative of the European Communities on a joint European Action Programme Against Cancer (EEC 1985) has indicated that by that year 100 000–150 000 lives in Europe could be saved annually from death from cancer by applying knowledge already available today. This statement of the EEC agrees well with calculations made by groups of experts appointed by the World Health Organisation Regional Office for Europe (WHO 1985). These predict that by the year 2000 mortality from cancer in people under 65 in Europe could be reduced by at least 15% by applying knowledge which is already available. Of all the assumptions in these documents this one is the most difficult to confirm and accept.

Sweden has a population of 8.1 million people. If nothing unexpected happens to cause a dramatic change in the age distribution of the population or the incidence of cancer in the different age groups, 31% of all persons living in Sweden in 1982 will develop a cancer during their lives. This represents 30% of the men and 32% of the women, and a total of 2.5 million people (Eklund and Carstensen 1986). This confirms the first assumption made by the EEC. I do not have similar data for the United Kingdom, but the corresponding number would be 17 million out of the population of 56 million if it is assumed that the age-specific incidence and life span will be the same as in Sweden.

Theoretically, the effects of cancer can be counteracted by prevention; early diagnosis; treatment; rehabilitation; and, perhaps most important of all, by research which increases our knowledge in all these fields. These topics will be considered in turn below.

Prevention

The first major discovery in cancer epidemiology was made in England in 1775, when Sir Percival Pott pointed out that boy chimney-sweeps had a high incidence of what was otherwise a very uncommon type of tumour: skin cancer of the scrotum. This gave the signal for clinical and later also experimental research based on this observation. Almost all subsequent major discoveries in cancer epidemiology concerned the reasons for such signal tumours. These are tumours of a generally very uncommon type that suddenly increase in a small limited population, often as a result of an occupational exposure. The only exception concerning rarity was the discovery, also in England, of the relationship between the use of tobacco and the very frequent incidence of lung cancer.

The advent of modern computer technology in the last decade has made possible developments in cancer epidemiology by allowing large quantities of information on numbers of people to be handled in a way that was previously quite inconceivable. As a result it has been observed that there are major differences in the incidence of tumour diseases between different countries and geographical regions. There are also large differences between different countries and regions with regard to the availability of medical care, diagnostic criteria and the reliability of cancer registration. However, these cannot explain the magnitude of the differences that were observed. The possibility cannot be excluded that the explanation as to why cancer of the prostate is 40 times more common in the USA than in Japan, or primary cancer of the liver 100 times more common in Mozambique than in England, or cancer of nasopharynx 40 times more common in Singapore than in England, could provide us with a basis for rational and possibly realistic preventive measures. However, of more importance is the fact that in countries in which there is reliable cancer registration, it has been found that the incidence of some types of tumours may increase or decrease dramatically over a relatively short period of time (Fig. 11.1). This could indicate that the cause is not genetic but related to other factors which are of major importance for the incidence of these tumours, and that these factors are responsible for the observed rapid and very considerable short-term changes in incidence. For example, if it was known why in Stockholm the age-adjusted incidence of malignant melanoma has increased by about 350% over 23 years and the incidence of cancer of the stomach has decreased to half over the same period of time in both women and men (Fig. 11.1) then this could provide us with a useful basis for realistic preventive measures.

A summary presenting the best estimates of the relative importance of different factors in the incidence of cancer was published recently in the USA (NRC 1982). Table 11.1 shows a corresponding summary prepared by experts on

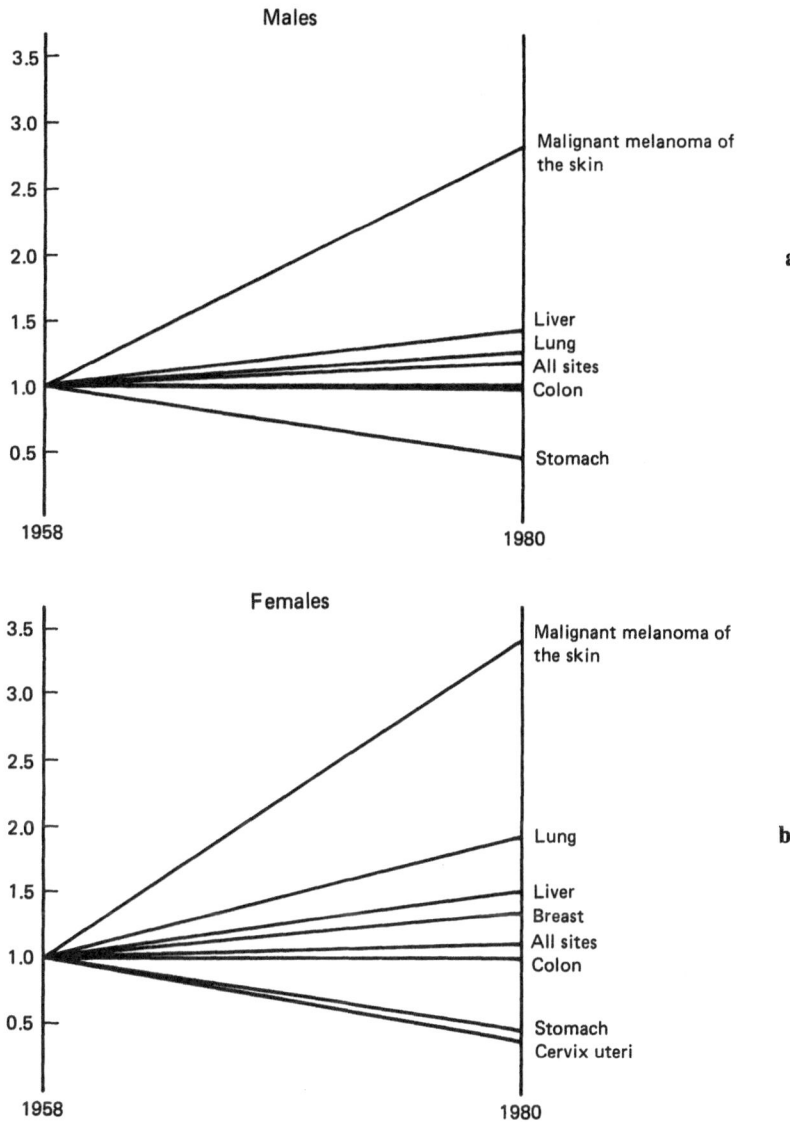

Fig. 11.1. Relative changes in the age-adjusted incidence of some tumours in males (**a**) and females (**b**) in Stockholm between 1958 and 1980. (Based on figures from the Cancer Registry for the Stockholm-Gotland region (Regional Cancer Registry 1985).)

a Cancer Committee appointed by the Swedish government (Swedish Cancer Committee 1984). This too must be regarded as the best possible guess based on incomplete information. Both reports, however, claim that dietary habits are an important factor in the incidence of cancer in these countries.

The development of cancer epidemiology will also in the future provide a rapidly increasing number of observations on statistical relationships between several of our most common forms of tumour and our living habits. These

Table 11.1. Best estimates of the relative importance of different factors in the incidence of cancer in Sweden (based on the report of the Swedish Cancer Committee (1984))

Factor	Percentage of all cancer incidence
Diet	30
Tobacco	15 (12–20)
Sex and reproduction	10
Sun and ultraviolet light	5
Ionising radiation (incl. radon)	3
Infections	2
Occupation	2
Air pollution	1

statistical relationships are not sufficient to demonstrate causal relationships. But when supported by the results of several independent studies using exposure of animals under controlled conditions, then it must be accepted that there are indications for the existence of a causal relationship. This will create a new and often difficult situation for society to deal with.

It is relatively simple to adopt an attitude to the use of tobacco, as it is possible to live without tobacco provided one does not start the habit. However, there is growing evidence that, for example, the high consumption of fat in western Europe might be related to the high incidence of some of our most common tumours: cancer of the breast, prostate, colon–rectum and uterine corpus. For most of us there are no serious disadvantages in reducing our fat consumption from its present average level of 40%–45% of total calorie consumption. However, for many persons and for the economy of large groups in our society a strong recommendation to reduce fat consumption produces problems.

If and when the data linking cancer and living habits become more certain, the problem will be how to use the information. The explanation for the dramatic 300% increase in the incidence of malignant melanoma in women in Sweden over the last 23 years is better travel communications and a higher standard of living. This has made it possible for almost everyone in Sweden to travel to southern Spain, northern Africa or the Canary Islands right in the middle of the long Nordic winter, when we have the lowest values for pigment in the skin and are unprotected from the sun. Then, on the first day after our arrival, we often expose ourselves for several hours to a sudden sun-shock and turn on the proliferation of melanin-producing cells in a way which is presumably completely unphysiological and to which our skin is not adapted. However, for many people in Sweden, being able to travel to a warm and sunny country in the middle of the long dark winter is one of the most significant advantages of a uniformly high standard of living. Should public information campaigns be initiated that will destroy this pleasure? My opinion is that they should not.

For many people good food is a great source of pleasure which the medical profession must also be careful not to destroy. Fat is not a poison. Fat is a cheap and useful source of energy. The problem is that in the West we use too much of it and therefore have an unbalanced diet. And doctors must certainly not involve themselves in people's sexual habits using cancer as a threat (Table 11.1) to prevent an early start to a sex life and to having several sexual partners.

Society must be very careful when using the ever greater flow of scientifically more or less proven information on prevention of cancer as a basis for changing attitudes, standards and habits. At the same time, the most important method available for reducing the total cancer incidence seems to be information on health, and it is very probable that quite soon the knowledge we now possess must be used. The question which then arises is who should have the responsibility for formulating and spreading this public health information? My opinion is that the practising oncologists who have daily contact with human cancer should be involved. This will, however, necessitate that oncologists make themselves familiar with the scientific, ethical and human aspects of the problems involved in disseminating this new knowledge to the public. In formulating the strategy for this health information it should be borne in mind that the fear of cancer is already a heavy burden for cancer patients. This also is true for the two out of every three people in Europe who have not and who never will have a malignant disease.

In two of the three largest towns in Sweden, during the last 5 years the age-adjusted incidence of cancer has in fact significantly decreased for men. The same decrease has not been found among the rural population or among women in large towns. The explanation is a significant reduction in the number of lung cancers among men in large towns, which has resulted from a decrease in the number of male cigarette-smokers. The total consumption of tobacco in Sweden has not diminished, since the number of women who smoke has increased and smokers of both sexes have not reduced their consumption—in fact some have probably increased it to compensate for lower nicotine contents of cigarettes.

Early Diagnosis

The second major approach available for diminishing the effects of malignant tumours is early diagnosis. This is usually taken to mean detecting the tumour before it is clinically manifest, i.e. before it gives rise to any symptoms. This implies mass screening of apparently healthy persons. In Europe there are currently major projects for mass screening for carcinoma of the uterine cervix, breast cancer and colorectal cancer. This is an area which is clearly most relevant to the subject of this symposium on imaging techniques in oncology.

The most extensive experience available is in the mass screening for early diagnosis of cancer of the uterine cervix. These projects were started on the optimistic assumption that the results would be so convincing that controlled trials to prove the usefulness of mass screening would not be necessary. Now, after these methods have been in use for more than 30 years, it is still not possible to give a definite assessment of their usefulness in relation to the unfavourable effects which always accompany the mass screening of apparently healthy persons.

In Great Britain the mortality from cervical cancer has diminished over a 10-year period from 2430 in 1968 to about 2150 in 1978 (Pettersson et al. 1985). One cannot of course be sure whether this can be accredited to mass screening. During the last few years, however, the results of very sophisticated statistical analyses, not least in the Scandinavian countries, have begun to be seen. These give quite strong indications that mortality from cervical cancer really has diminished as a result of mass screening for early diagnosis (for example the results recently published from Stockholm by Pettersson et al. (1985)). Such retrospective analyses cannot, though, take the place of the information which would have been provided by controlled trials on large randomised samples. Lack of such trials is regrettable, since the effects of mass screening on the women examined and the expenditure made by society are very considerable.

In 1959 in Sweden there were 882 new registered cases of invasive carcinoma of the uterine cervix; in 1982 the number had fallen to 580 (Swedish Cancer Registry 1959, 1982). This means that there was a reduction of 300 cases per year of invasive cervical cancer. We cannot be sure that this reduction is wholly the result of mass screening. At the same time to achieve the reduction, one million smears were taken annually in Sweden and about 6000 surgical interventions were performed as a result of the screening. The cost to society was about 25 million pounds sterling per year for the screening alone.

The lessons that have been learnt are being applied in the evaluation of mass screening for early diagnosis of breast cancer by mammography. Results of three major prospective trials on randomised samples in the USA (Shapiro et al. 1982), the Netherlands (Verbeek et al. 1984) and Sweden (Tabar et al. 1985) have been published. In the first of these, the Health Insurance Plan study in New York (Shapiro et al. 1982), the women included in the study group were offered clinical examination every year and training in self-palpation; they were advised to contact the doctors as soon as they felt anything unusual in a breast; and finally they were given mammography. The total sample was 62 000 women randomised to a study group or control group. The compliance was poor. However, after 7 years of follow-up a statistically significant reduction of about 30% has been found in the death rate for the study group compared with the control group (Shapiro et al. 1982).

Breast cancer is the most common type of tumour in Sweden, constituting 24% of malignant tumours in women. If nothing happens to change the present incidence and mortality rates, of the women now living in Sweden more than 7% will develop breast cancer during their lifetime and about 3.5% will die as a result. Recently, the results were published of a Swedish study (Tabar et al. 1985) which at the present time is the largest randomised study to have evaluated the usefulness of mammography in mass screening. About 163 000 women aged 40 years or more in two Swedish counties were randomly allocated at the municipal level into two groups: a study group which was offered screening at 2- or 3-year intervals and a control group. The women were asked to fill in a simple questionnaire, but no clinical examination was included in this study. The examination used was a single medio-lateral oblique-view mammograph. The study was started in October 1977 in one county and in May 1978 in the other. Of particular interest is the group of women aged between 40 and 74 years at entry—altogether about 135 000 women representing 334 000 observation years. In this age group the compliance was very high, being 89% for the first and 83% for the second screening. At present the mortality from breast cancer in the study group has been about 30% lower than in the control group, and the difference in mortality between the two groups is statistically significant ($P = 0.013$: Tabar et al. 1985). During the follow-up of up to 7 years, there has so far been no tendency for the gap in the cumulative mortality rate to narrow between the study group and the control group.

It has therefore now been shown and confirmed by independent groups that mass screening for early diagnosis of breast cancer, and probably also for carcinoma of the uterine cervix, can diminish the mortality. A large number of randomised and non-randomised trials for early diagnosis of different types of tumours are in progress in various countries all over the world. These trials will yield further data which practising oncologists will have to live with. They will also present new problems, such as how small a lesion can be considered to represent a histologically confirmed malignant tumour, and what the natural history of these small preclinical lesions is.

There are indications that it might be possible to develop tests, for example using nuclear DNA analysis as is done in Sweden, for differentiating small lesions that are proliferating rapidly from lesions which will not proliferate or which proliferate slowly (Fallenius et al. 1986). At present, however, such tests are not available, and it cannot be determined with certainty which of these lesions will or will not develop into clinically overt malignant tumours. Treatment must therefore be offered to all patients with these early preclinical lesions. It is thus unavoidable that one result of mass screening will be not only that many will be alarmed and worried, but also that some will be treated unnecessarily. Both society and individuals are involved in considerable expense and sometimes unpleasantness. We practising oncologists cannot avoid our share of the responsibility. We must use our influence to ensure that studies of mass screening are planned in such a way that conclusions as to the advantages and disadvantages can be drawn in the future, and that well-justified questions from patients can be answered. We should not find ourselves once again in the situation which obtains with the mass screening for early diagnosis of cervical cancer, when its usefulness cannot with any certainty be weighed against its disadvantages.

In the background material provided as the basis for review of the European Community (EEC 1985) it was stated that mass screening for early diagnosis will contribute to the reduction in the mortality from malignant tumours by the year 2000. I am not sure that this statement is correct, because I am not wholly sure that when all the facts are known they will favour the continuation of mass screening.

Treatment

Cures for cancer were very uncommon at the turn of this century. In Table 11.2 all figures for the following decades for 5-year survival after treatment for cancer are estimates with considerable degrees of uncertainty, although some of the figures, such as those for 1968 and 1978, are calculations based on the Swedish Cancer Registry and mortality statistics. When malignant tumours are diagnosed earlier during the progress of the disease, survival will be improved without any real improvement in the treatment results. This must always be considered when the types of comparisons given in Table 11.2 are presented. At the same time, it should be borne in mind that calculations indicate that the difference between

Table 11.2. Best estimates of 5-year survival
for all cancer patients 1900–2000

Year	5-year survival(%)
1900	<5
1949	25
1968	33[a]
1978	42[a]
1985	50
2000	60[b]

[a] Swedish Cancer Registry (1959, 1982).
[b] National Cancer Institute estimate.

the 5-year survival and the 5-year cure is at present quite small, if all tumour types and clinical stages are included.

The main explanation for the improvement in the results is earlier diagnosis. This is due to the greater awareness of both the general public and physicians of the early signs of malignant tumours, and also to improved diagnostic facilities. Both factors lead to diagnosis at a stage when a cure is more often possible. In addition, however, there have been real improvements in the results of treatment, although unfortunately not yet for the types of malignant tumours which are most common in Europe. For the most common types and clinical stages of carcinoma of the testis the results have improved dramatically. They have also improved for carcinoma of the urinary bladder (mainly because of advances in radiotherapy); for the most common type of malignant lymphoma in Europe, Hodgkin's lymphoma; for the most common types of malignant tumours in children such as nephroblastoma, Wilm's tumour and acute leukaemia; and for choriocarcinoma, which is one of the most common types of tumour in women in the most densely populated parts of the world in south-east Asia.

During the 1950s there were two principal methods of treatment for malignant tumours: surgery and radiotherapy. During the last 40 years developments have taken place in radiotherapy which have changed it from quite an inaccurate method to one with a degree of exactness unparalleled in other branches of medicine. Nowadays, radiotherapy can be applied to any part of the body with an accuracy that cannot be achieved by any pharmacological method, and with efficient shielding of the surrounding non-invaded tissues. The papers in this volume confirm the fact that these developments will continue and that the main problems for radiotherapists will be to define and limit the tumour region, and to learn how to combine radiotherapy with other available methods of treatment and if possible enhance their biological efficacy.

Furthermore, during the last three decades methods for endocrine manipulation have been developed, and more than 30 clinically useful drugs for chemotherapy have become available. Further possible new methods are under development, including the use of interferons, monoclonal antibodies and interleukines. In addition to using new techniques oncologists are endeavouring to improve the results of old approaches that have been given new names, such as adjuvant therapy and neoadjuvant therapy.

Another development of the last few years is the increasing emphasis on rehabilitation. Cure with organ preservation is usually the most efficient rehabilitation measure. There is at present no other method which has contributed so much to this as radiotherapy. There is the increasing possibility of curing retinoblastoma with preservation of the eye. Radiotherapy is also the best method of preserving good functioning of the larynx in early laryngeal carcinoma and it often makes it possible to cure cancer of the urinary bladder with preservation of the bladder. There is now a growing interest too in preservation of the breast in breast cancer.

Thirty years ago the few practising clinical oncologists were dealing almost entirely with curative treatment. If treatment with curative aim could not be offered, patients were seldom admitted to specialised units. It is my personal opinion that the greatest advance in the clinical practice of oncology since that time is not the improvement in the overall cure rate in cancer but the fact that oncologists have a vastly greater and growing store of experience, practical knowledge and motivation for taking care of the half of their patients whom they cannot cure.

During the last two decades the number of alternative treatments has increased dramatically. When a decision has to be made on the choice of treatment, I often feel that I am entering a labyrinth with a large number of alternative paths and very few signposts. More signposts are needed, but unfortunately in many situations they can only be won by using the very tedious approach of carrying out controlled clinical trials on sufficiently large randomised samples of uniformly treated cancer patients. Another approach which, it is to be hoped, will be increasingly useful in the future is the use of predictive tests, which will make it possible to individualise the treatment more efficiently than can be done today, when decisions are based on statistical evaluations of large or small patient samples.

Analysis of the hormone receptors in tumour cells already makes it possible to select patients for endocrine treatment. Efforts at predicting the effects of different cytostatic drugs and dosages in the individual patient have not yet been very successful. There have been, however, interesting developments in methods which might help to predict the proliferation and growth potential of tumour cells by measuring the thymidine index, using various other types of analysis of the cell and especially the nuclear contents. There are strong indications that in the not too distant future methods based on different types of cell analysis will provide predictive tests that will be increasingly useful in guiding decisions in the present labyrinth of clinical practice in oncology. The first two chapters in this volume have indicated different possibilities for this development.

Summary and Conclusions

If nothing happens to change the present situation two million people in Europe will develop cancer each year by the year 2000 and one million of them will die from it. The Commission of the European Communities has stated (EEC 1985) that by using knowledge which is already available the mortality from cancer in Europe could be reduced by 10%–15%, which would mean 100 000 to 150 000 fewer deaths per year. Groups of experts appointed by the WHO Regional Office for Europe (WHO 1985) estimated that by the year 2000 the mortality from cancer in persons under 65 in Europe could be reduced by at least 15%. Are these estimates and hopes realistic? I believe they are; I even believe that these estimates are quite conservative.

The use of tobacco has already begun to drop in the male populations of large towns in Western Europe. In some groups in countries where the cancer registration is reliable, there has also been a substantial and statistically significant decrease in the incidence of lung cancer over the last few years. Propaganda over a number of years based on solid scientific facts is beginning to have an effect. What has been achieved is a change of attitudes so that it is no longer fashionable to smoke. From information available in the scientific literature, increasing numbers of groups of scientists are claiming that the current indications for a connection between the high fat content of the diet in western Europe and the incidence of some of the most common types of tumours are strong enough to justify action. There are no indications that reducing the fat content of our diet will have any undesirable effects on our health, but strong indications that it will diminish the incidence of carcinoma of the breast, of the prostate, of the colon-rectum and endometrial cancer. I believe that it will be easier to influence dietary habits than it was to reduce the habit of using tobacco.

Increasingly convincing results of an increasing number of studies indicate that the most important method of reducing the total cancer incidence at the present time would appear to be information on health. However, great caution is necessary in formulating information with the aim of changing attitudes, standards and habits where cancer is used as a threat. The medical profession must not indicate a need for sacrifices that would in any way adversely affect the quality of life and must bear in mind that "the purpose of human life is not to prevent cancer". Significant improvement is, however, probably most possible by measures such as reducing the fat content in the diet that would not be connected with any major sacrifice for most of the people in western Europe.

Although there are promising results from studies on mass screening for breast cancer—mortality decreased by 30% for women in certain age groups examined in mammography—I am not equally optimistic about the future possibilities of mass screening for the early diagnosis of cancer. By the year 2000 mass screening will probably be performed for several types of tumours, but there will be major accompanying cost-benefit, psychological and ethical problems, and one of the main difficulties facing practising oncologists will be that no adequate answers can be provided to justified questions from those selected by the mass screening procedures and from those responsible for the political decisions on the future use of these methods.

There will be enormous developments in diagnostic radiology in the future. It will probably be increasingly unjustifiable for a surgeon to operate just "to see what it looks like", since radiological techniques will make it possible to see better without cutting and increasingly often make it possible to take a biopsy or even to perform a surgical intervention guided by radiological devices. Developments in computerised and positron emission tomography, ultrasound, magnetic resonance imaging, digital and interventional radiology have been presented and discussed in papers in this volume. The growing problem will be the integration, if possible into one picture, of the information that will be available from examinations using different methods. The discovery of methods for the production of monoclonal antibodies will probably revolutionise diagnostic work, not least in the area of histopathological diagnostics and prognostics, and will, it is to be hoped, provide the predictive tests that are vital to the provision of individualised treatment.

I am very optimistic about the future developments in therapy, perhaps because I am a practising radiotherapist who has seen within a period of a few decades such enormous developments in radiotherapy and the advent of the whole science of cytostatic chemotherapy. Even if there are no dramatic breakthroughs or completely new methods, many improvements will be made by learning how to make better use of the methods which are already available. Growing numbers of increasingly reliable predictive tests will make treatment less toxic with results which are as good or better than at present. The National Cancer Institute is probably correct in its estimate that it will be possible to cure more cancer patients—maybe 60% by the year 2000. What is more important, though, is that we shall be able to offer better treatment and better care to those patients whom we shall not be able to cure even in the future. I believe that cancer will become, not for all but for an increasing number, a chronic disease with which one can live longer and in a better manner, so that the patient will be able to carry on his or her life at home and in society in the same way that people do with chronic heart, kidney and lung diseases.

References

EEC (1985) Commission of the European Communities. European action programme against cancer. Document UKCCCR 86/8 COM (85), final, annex 1,5, and 6, Brussels, November and December, and document 495312/85 EN, 1985

Eklund G, Carstensen J (1986) Personal communication based on: Cancer incidence in Sweden 1982, Swedish Department of Health and Welfare, and Swedish Mortality Statistics, Life Tables, 1976–1980 (Statistiska Centralbyrån)

Fallenius A, Franzén S, Caspersson T, Auer G (1986) DNA content and prognosis in carcinoma of the breast. To be published

NRC (1982) Diet, nutrition and cancer. Committee on Diet, Nutrition and Cancer. Assembly of Life Sciences, National Research Council, National Academy Press, Washington, DC

Pettersson F, Björkholm E, Näslund I (1985) Evaluation of screening for cervical cancer in Sweden: trends in incidence and mortality 1958–1980. Int J Epidemiol 14: 521–527

Regional Cancer Registry (1985) Stockholm-Gotlands Onkologiska Centrum, Radiumhemmet, Karolinska sjukhuset, Stockholm

Shapiro S, Vennet W, Strax Ph, Vennet L, Roeser R (1982) Ten–fourteen-year effect of screening on breast cancer mortality. J Natl Cancer Inst 69: 349–355

Swedish Cancer Committee (1984) Cancer: Orsaker, förebyggande m.m. betänkande av Cancer-kommittén, (1984) SOU 1984: 67, Socialdepartementet (Cancer Committee, Swedish Department of Health and Welfare, Stockholm, Sweden)

Swedish Cancer Registry (1959, 1982) Cancer incidence in Sweden. National Board of Health and Welfare, Stockholm, Sweden

Tabar L, Fagerberg CJ, Gad A et al. (1985) Reduction in mortality from breast cancer after mass screening with mammography. Lancet I: 829–832

Verbeek AL, Hendriks JH, Holland R, Mrvunac M, Sturmans F, Day NE (1984) Reduction of breast cancer mortality through mass screening with modern mammography: first results of the Nijmegen project 1975–1981. Lancet II: 1222–1224

WHO (1985) Targets for health for all. WHO Regional Office for Europe, Copenhagen

Subject Index